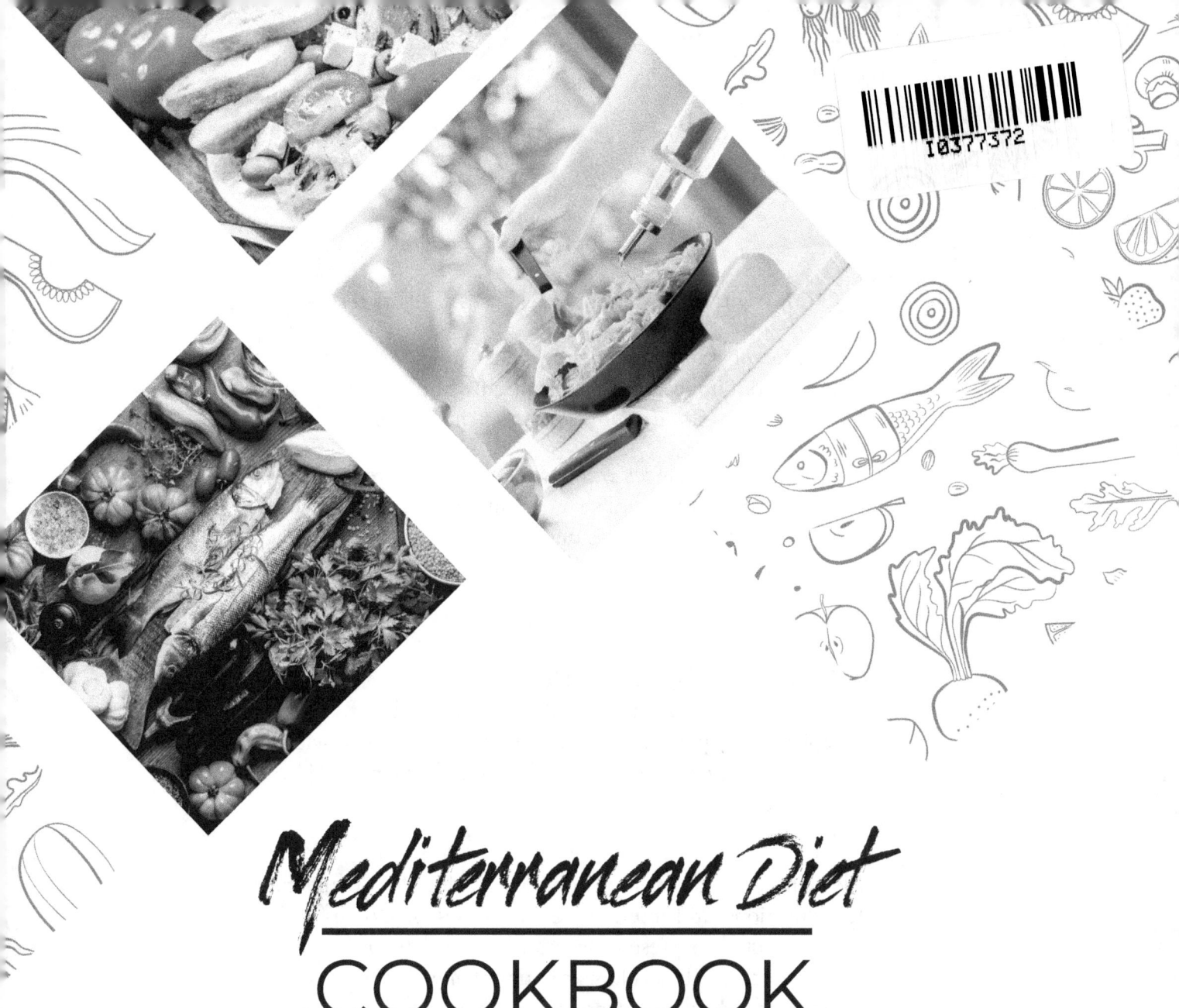

Mediterranean Diet
COOKBOOK

600+ Easy and Flavorful Recipes to Start and Maintain a Healthy Lifestyle. 4-Week Weight Loss Meal Plan to Make your Health Journey Easier

Marlene Buckley

© Copyright 2020 Marlene Buckley - All rights reserved.

The content contained within this book may not be reproduced, duplicated or transmitted without direct written permission from the author or the publisher.

Under no circumstances will any blame or legal responsibility be held against the publisher, or author, for any damages, reparation, or monetary loss due to the information contained within this book. Either directly or indirectly.

Legal Notice:

This book is copyright protected. This book is only for personal use. You cannot amend, distribute, sell, use, quote or paraphrase any part, or the content within this book, without the consent of the author or publisher.

Disclaimer Notice:

Please note the information contained within this document is for educational and entertainment purposes only. All effort has been executed to present accurate, up to date, and reliable, complete information. No warranties of any kind are declared or implied. Readers acknowledge that the author is not engaging in the rendering of legal, financial, medical or professional advice. The content within this book has been derived from various sources. Please consult a licensed professional before attempting any techniques outlined in this book.

By reading this document, the reader agrees that under no circumstances is the author responsible for any losses, direct or indirect, which are incurred as a result of the use of information contained within this document, including, but not limited to, errors, omissions, or inaccuracies.

TABLE OF CONTENTS

CHAPTER 1 • Introduction 5

CHAPTER 2 • The Mediterranean Diet 7

CHAPTER 3 • Eat and Live Healthy 13

CHAPTER 4 • How To Get Started With The Mediterranean Diet 21

CHAPTER 5 • 4-Week Meal Plan 27

BREAKFAST 30

ANTIPASTI, TAPAS, MEZE AND STARTER 50

PASTA AND COUSCOUS 68

RICE AND GRAINS 96

SOUPS AND STEWS 123

SALAD AND SIDE DISHES 143

VEGETARIAN DISHES 167

SNACKS 196

PIZZA 221

POULTRY AND MEAT 240

FISH AND SEAFOOD 279

FRUITS, SWEETS AND DESSERTS 316

RECIPES TABLE OF CONTENTS **342**

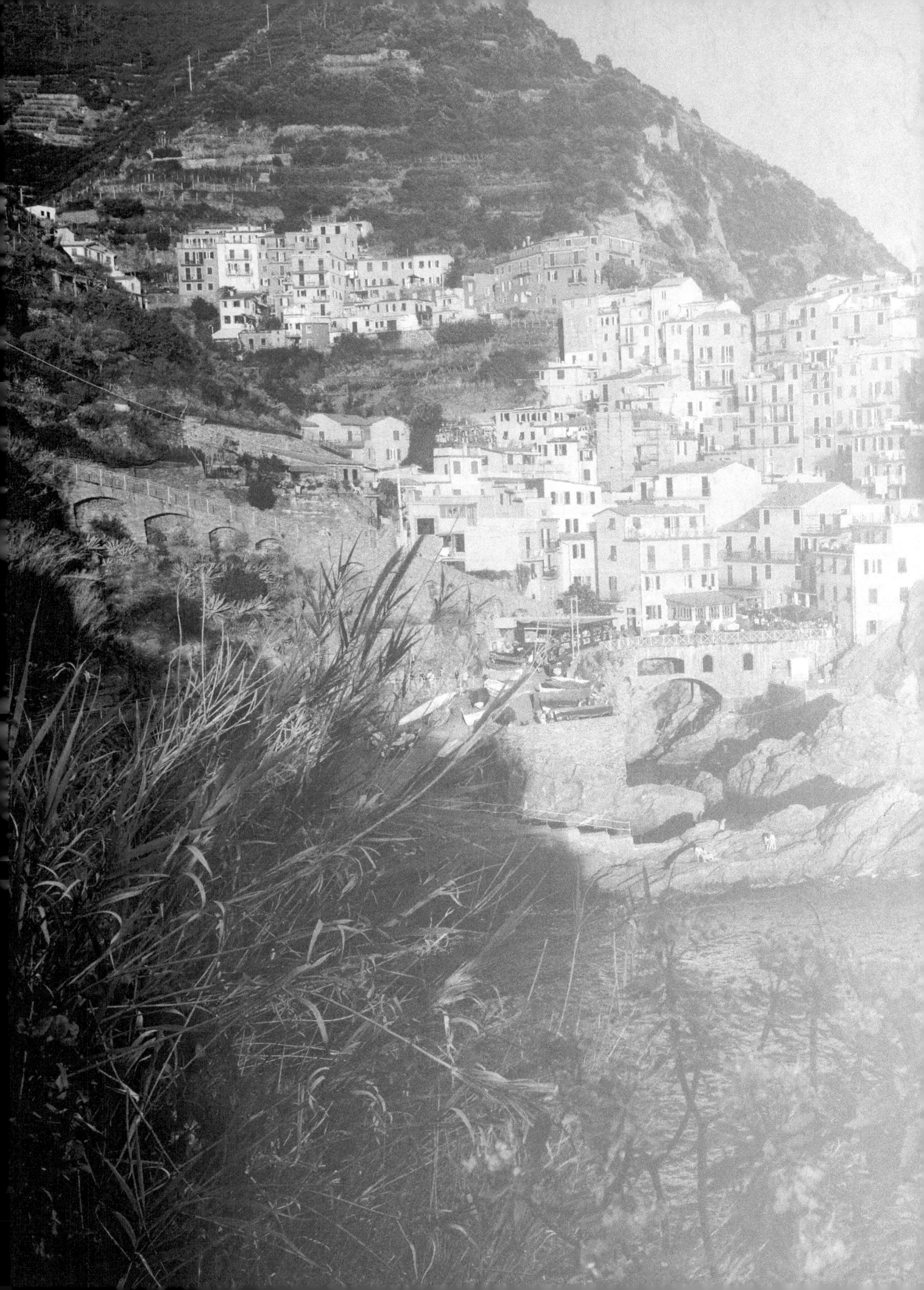

CHAPTER 1

Introduction

Over the decades, the Mediterranean diet saw a slow rise in the Western world. Many countries of the west were slow to pick it up, but once they did, they realized that they had discovered the key to the Elixir of Life.

The Mediterranean diet not only helped people rely on a wholesome and healthy diet, but it helped them lose weight, power up their immune systems, improved their vitality, and even contributed to healthy skin.

In other words, the Mediterranean diet helped people feel good and look good.

The combination of benefits changed people's perception about what they should be having and question their eating habits.

For example, many people often skip breakfast because they feel that having a meal in the morning adds more weight to their body. However, the Mediterranean diet does not skip breakfast. On the contrary, it considers breakfast the most important meal of the day.

The countries that relied on the Mediterranean diet saw its benefits way before any scientific research was conducted. They didn't have any research conducted to guide them toward a particular eating pattern or food content. They relied on habits and suggestions dropped down from one generation to another, dating back to ancient Rome and Greece. Even those ancient civilizations took inspiration from cultures that preceded them. After all, the Roman civilization began around 753 BC, but olive oil was first produced around 2,500 BC., and guess where the oil was first created? You are right. In the Mediterranean region.

Essentially, the diet has been refined over millennia, as newer methods of cooking were introduced. But the adherence to a healthy form of diet remained, no matter how old the diet grew.

Just how did the Mediterranean diet evolve to what it is today while still maintaining its component?

It all comes down to what we eat, when we eat it, and in what quantities.

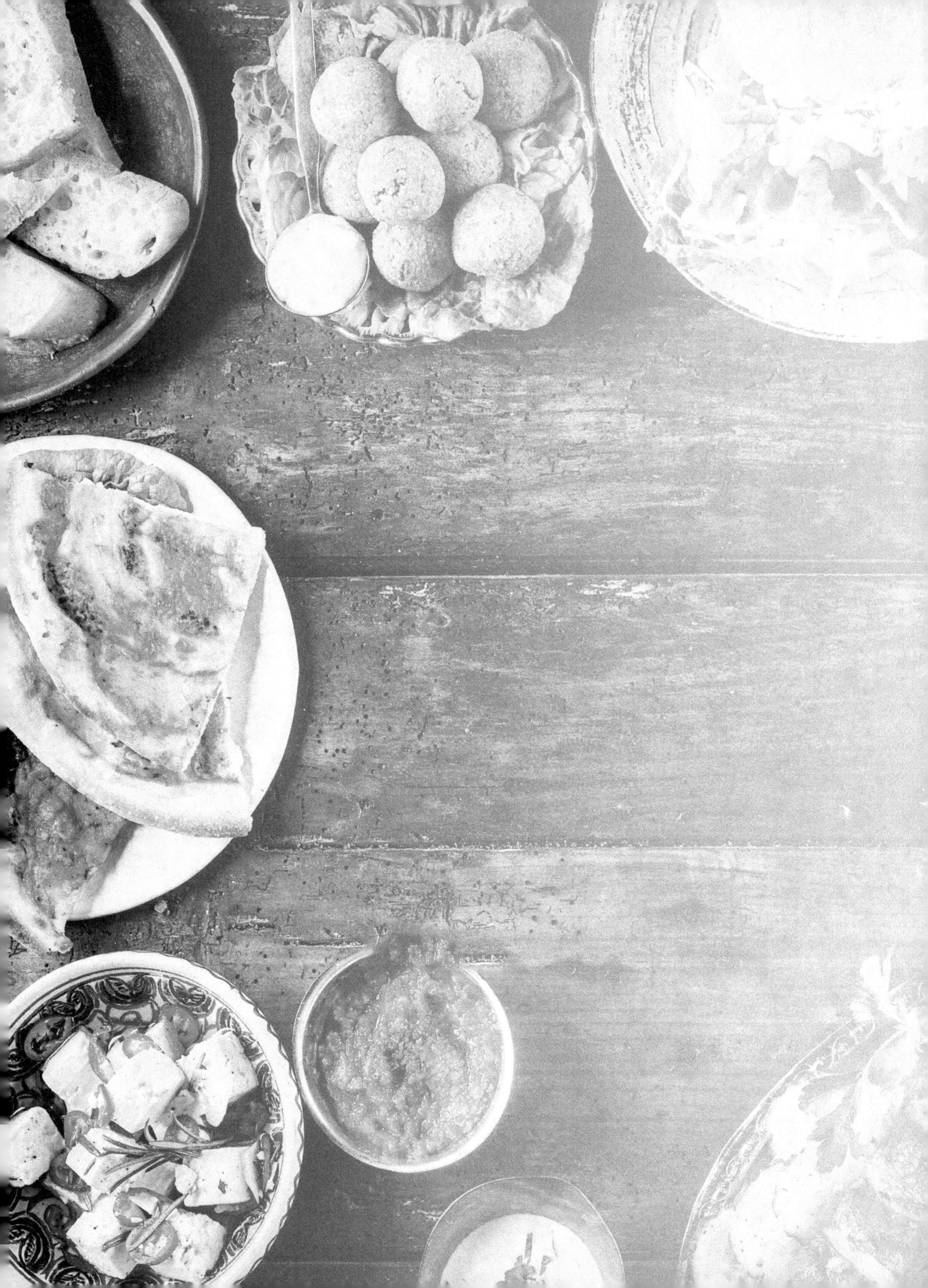

CHAPTER 2

The Mediterranean Diet

The Mediterranean diet is more than just a diet. It is a way of life. It's a method of eating so as to carry on with a full and solid life. When following along these lines of eating you'll get in shape, yet you'll likewise reinforce your heart and give your body all the best possible supplements important to carry on with a long and healthy life. Individuals following the Mediterranean diet have been connected to a lower risk of Alzheimer's disease, better cardiovascular health, and a longer life expectancy.

This eating routine incorporates expending heaps of vegetables and grains, organic products, rice, and pasta while constraining fats, replacing salt with herbs and flavors, and eating fish and poultry rather than red meat. The Mediterranean diet doesn't contain a ton of red meat. Nuts are a solid piece of this eating routine, even though they are high in calories, so they should be consumed in small doses.

The diet also might include a glass of red wine every day, and regular physical exercise to complement the right eating habits. The Mediterranean eating routine reflects different dietary patterns of the nations close to the Mediterranean Sea, for the most part Southern Italy, Greece, Morocco, France, and Spain. Because of their one of a kind territory, the atmosphere bolsters new organic products, vegetables, and a portion of the world's best fish.

This diet isn't centered around constraining your complete utilization of Fat, rather, it centers around settling on more brilliant decisions about the sorts of Fat you devour. It discourages individuals from eating trans-fats and soaked Fats, the two of which have been connected to coronary illness.

Grains utilized in the Mediterranean diet are ideally whole, which contain no undesirable trans-fat. Bread is a significant piece of the Mediterranean way of life; it should be covered with margarine or other types of Fat spreads, but rather sprinkled with olive oil or eaten plain..

Last but not least, the king of the Mediterranean diet: Olive oil. The Mediterranean Diet's main characteristic is the use of olive oil as an essential Fat. In addition to its Fatty acid advantages, the use of olive oil is correlated with a strong food intake due to its use as a seasoning for salads, fruits, and dried legumes. Olive oil is used regularly in stews, fried rice, salads, and even sweets in Mediterranean countries.

Spain's extra virgin olive oil includes vitamin E, which is essential for its antioxidant properties. It is also rich in phenols and makes it such an effective source of antioxidants.

In reality, Spain boasts high-quality olive oils and the longest life expectancy in Europe at 82.2 years, according to the WHO, thanks largely to the Mediterranean Diet and lifestyle.

The value of olive oil is unquestionable and rests on its other qualities, both gastronomic and linked to wellness. We might argue that without olive oil, the Mediterranean Diet wouldn't work because we wouldn't be able to make the bulk of their dishes without it.

The History of the Mediterranean Diet

Just like it sounds, the Mediterranean diet comes from the dietary traditions of the people of the Mediterranean isle region such as the Romans and Greeks. The people of these regions had a rich diet full of fruits, bread, wine, olive oil, nuts, and seafood. Despite the Fatty elements in their diet, the people of this region tended to live longer and overall healthy lives with relatively less cardiovascular heart issues. This phenomenon was noticed by American scientist Ancel Keys in the 1950s.

Keys was an academic researcher at the University of Minnesota in the 1950s who researched healthy eating habits and how to reverse the decline in American cardiovascular health. In his research, he found that poor people in the Mediterranean region of the world were healthier compared to the rich American population, which had seen a recent rise in cardiovascular heart issues and obesity. Compared to wealthy New Yorkers, the lower class in the Mediterranean lived well into their 90s and tended to be physically active in their senior years. Keys and his team of scientists decided to travel the world and study the link between the region's diet and the health of the people who lived there. In 1957, he traveled and studied the lifestyles, nutrition, exercise, and diet of the United States, Italy, Holland, Greece, Japan, Finland, and Yugoslavia.

Keys' research found that the dietary choices of the people from the Mediterranean region allowed them to live a longer lifespan and one that kept them more physically active compared to other world populations. The people of Greece, in particular, ate a diet that consisted of healthy fats like seafood, nuts, olive oil, and fatty fish. Despite the amount of fat in these sources, their cardiovascular health stayed consistent without the risk factors for a heart attack or stroke. His study became a guideline for the United States to set its own nutritional standards, and he became known as the Father of nutritional science.

With Keys' work leading the way, further research and clinical trials have been conducted on the Mediterranean diet which gives evidence for its health-improving properties. Not only will you lose weight, but you could lower your LDL "bad" cholesterol, lower your blood pressure, and decrease and stabilize blood sugar levels. With a decrease in these signs of cardiovascular heart disease, you can greatly reduce your risk of suffering from heart attack, stroke, or premature death.

It's important to point out that the Mediterranean diet cannot alone bring about these changes to someone's health. It will depend on a variety of other factors in their lifestyle such as genetics, physical exercise, smoking, obesity, drug use, etc. Part of the combination of the Mediterranean diet is incorporating physical exercise into your life. That's how it goes from the Mediterranean "diet" to a Mediterranean "lifestyle" that truly mimics the people of that region. The people of Greece tend to live an active lifestyle with some sort of daily physical activity they partake in.

Whether that is walking, sailing, rowing, swimming, or hiking, coupling that physical exercise with a healthy diet can bring about beneficial health results. In our current environment, physical activity could mean a session at the gym or even just a walk around the block. It doesn't have to be highly intensive, but the important part is incorporating some sort of physical activity in your day to truly gain the benefits of following this diet.

Before we begin listing a rudimentary list of what you can and cannot eat, it's important to highlight that the Mediterranean region consists of many countries with their own unique dietary choices. With this diversity come many recipes that you can incorporate into your dishes as long as you are still following the healthy tenets of the Mediterranean diet. This gives a basic outline of which foods you should include on your shopping list and then you can look for recipes from there!

What does the basic Mediterranean diet look like?
- Your diet should consist heavily of whole-grain bread, extra virgin olive oil, fresh fruits and vegetables, herbs and spices, nuts and seeds, fish and seafood
- You should moderately eat: poultry, cheese, egg, and yogurt
- You should try to limit the consumption of: red meat and organ meat
- You should avoid the following: processed snacks, refined oils (canola oil or vegetable oil), refined grains (white bread), sugary drinks (juice, soda), processed meats (hot dogs, sausages, bacon), trans fats
- You should drink: water, wine

Health Benefits of the Mediterranean Way of Eating

Boosts Your Brain Health
Preserve memory and prevent cognitive decline by following the Mediterranean diet that will limit processed foods, refined bread, and red meats. Have a glass of wine versus hard liquor.

The Med Diet Improves Poor Eyesight
Older individuals suffer from poor eyesight, but the Mediterranean diet has provided noted improvement in many cases. An Australian Center for Eye Research discovered that the individuals who consumed a minimum of 100 ml (0.42 cup) of olive oil weekly, were almost 50% less likely to develop macular degeneration versus those who ate less than one ml each week.

It Helps Reduce Risk of Heart Disease
The New England Journal of Medicine provided evidence in 2013 from a randomized clinical trial implemented in Spain, whereas individuals did not have cardiovascular disease at enrollment but were in the 'high risk' category. The incidence of major cardiovascular events was reduced by the Mediterranean diet that was supplemented with extra-virgin olive oil or nuts. In one study, men who consumed fish in this manner reduced the risk by 23% of death from heart disease.

The Risk of Alzheimer's disease is reduced
In 2018, the journal Neurology studied 70 brain scans of individuals who had no signs of dementia at the onset. They followed the eating patterns in a two-year study resulting in individuals who were on the Med diet had a lesser increase of the depots and reduction of energy use - potentially signaling risk for Alzheimer's.

It Helps Reduce the Risk of Some Types of Cancer
According to the results of a group study, the diet is associated with a compelling lessened risk of

stomach cancer (gastric adenocarcinoma).

It Decreases Risks for Type 2 Diabetes
It can help stabilize blood sugar while protecting against type 2 diabetes with its low-carb elements. The Med diet maintains a richness in Fiber, which will digest slowly while preventing your blood sugar variances. It also can help you maintain a healthier weight, which is another trigger for diabetes.

It Suggests Improvement for Those with Parkinson's disease
By consuming foods on the Mediterranean diet, you are adding high levels of antioxidants that can prevent your body from undergoing oxidative stress, which is a damaging process that will attack your cells. The menu plan can reduce your risk factors in half.

The Med Diet Can Fight Inflammation:
The Mediterranean diet uses fatty fish (high in omega-3s), including salmon, mackerel, and tuna. Enjoy them broiled or baked and resist the urge to salt, dry, or fry them.

The Diet Can Help Strengthen Your Skin
Omega 3 Fatty acids, once again, will provide you with nutrients for elastic and healthier skin cells.

Rheumatoid Arthritis Improvements
The diet plan offered using the Mediterranean diet has provided rheumatoid patients with an increase in physical function and improved vitality with the reduction of inflammatory activity.

It Can Help With Depression & Anxiety
By consuming the menu offered by the Mediterranean eating patterns, you are absorbing essential nutrients linked to depression prevention, including fish, legumes, cereals, nuts, fruits, and veggies.

It Promotes Healthy Weight Management
Your body has no choice when you boost your health with the cuisine offered, including whole grains, veggies, healthful Fats, fruits, and much more.

The Med Plan Is Excellent for Your Gut
The diet plan was studied in a study at the University Medical Center in the Netherlands and concluded that healthy Fats and omega-3s were fabulous for boosting good bacteria in your gut; therefore, reducing inflammation.

It May Reduce Risk of Old Age Frailty
Nutrition is considered a vital role in the complex pathogenesis of frailty. Strengthened bones may help to prevent osteoporosis. The studies were mixed and inclusive at this time, but the diet plan provides you with abundant plant foods that are essential for healthier bones.

The Med Diet Is Excellent for Postmenopausal Women

Studies have been provided that women who adhered strictly to the Mediterranean diet, had higher muscle mass and bone density, versus those who didn't. This led to the possibility of how the diet can be useful in the prevention of osteoporosis and fractures in postmenopausal women.

The Mediterranean Diet May Help Ease Pain
Olive oil is a compound composed of oleocanthal, which may have a similar effect to NSAIDs. The oleocanthal has an anti-inflammatory and antioxidant component, which is contained in aspirin and ibuprofen.

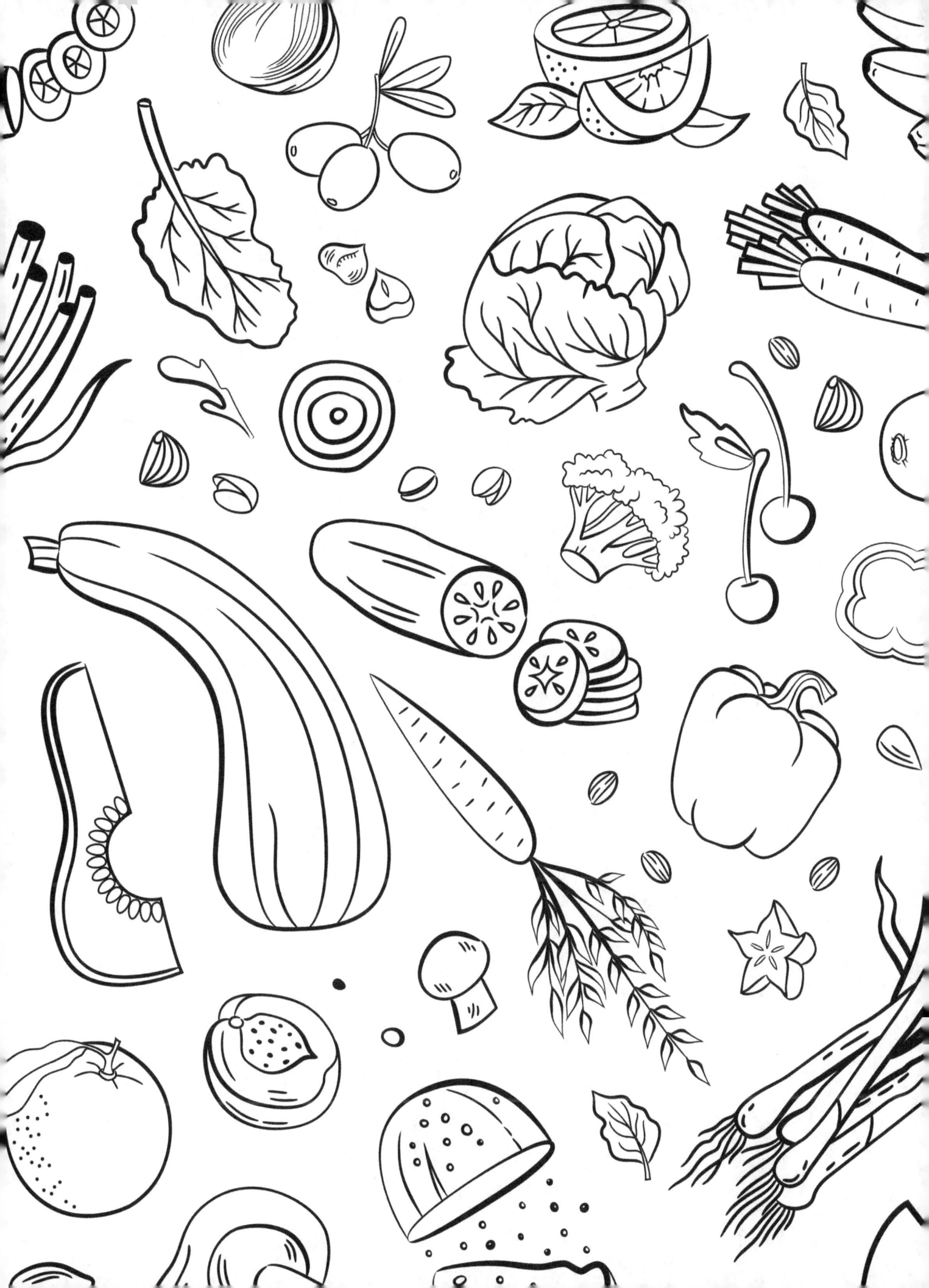

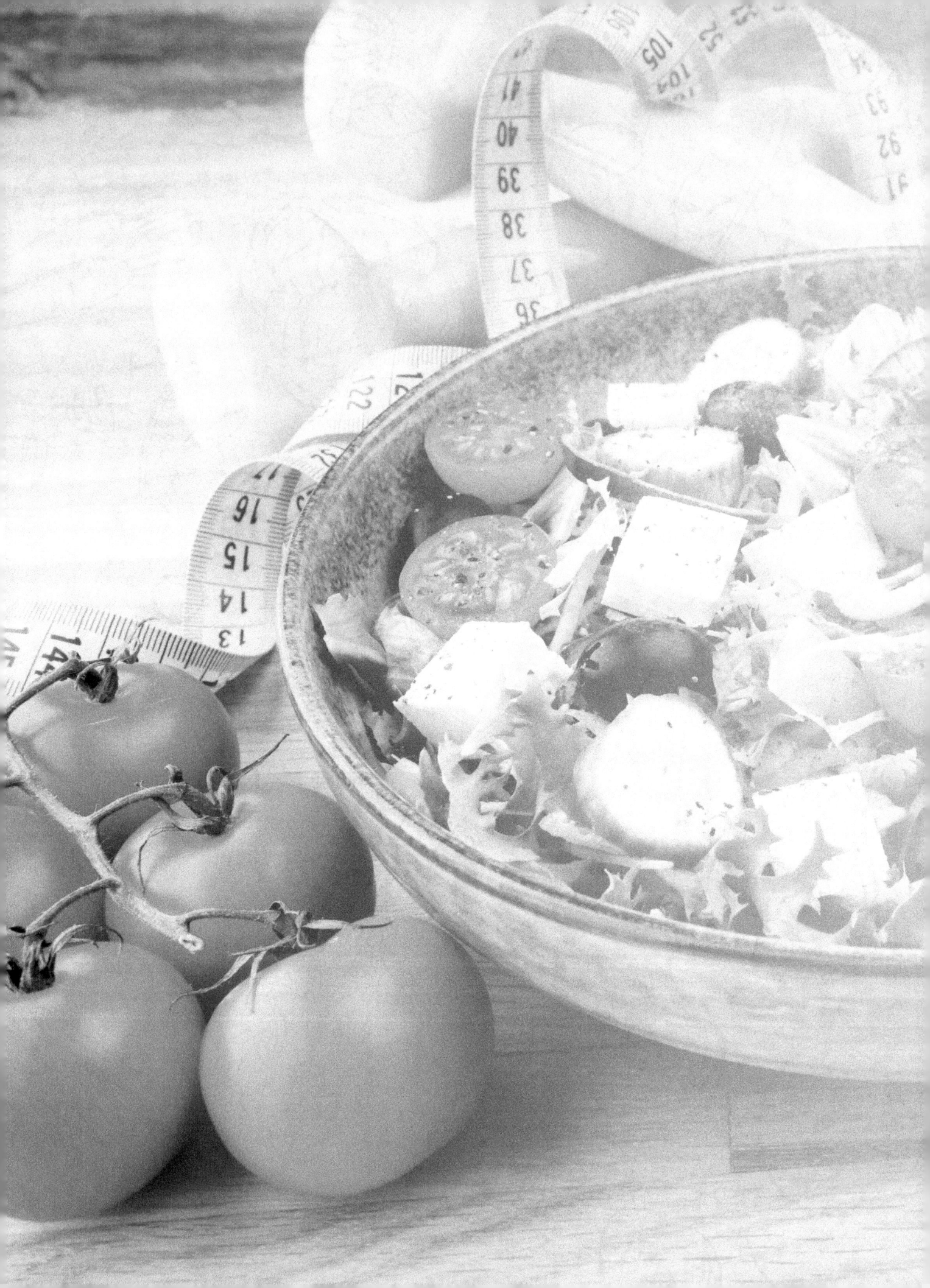

CHAPTER 3

Eat and Live Healthy

What You Can Eat
The foods you can eat while you are on a Mediterranean diet fall into two categories. There are those foods that you can eat regularly, and there are those that you should only eat in moderation. Here is an extensive list of both categories.

Foods to eat regularly
- Healthy fats like avocado oil, avocados, olives and extra virgin olive oil
- Fruits like peaches, figs, melons, dates, bananas, strawberries, grapes, pears, oranges, and apples. Note that you can eat most fruits while on this diet
- Vegetables like cucumbers, Brussels sprouts, artichoke, eggplant, carrots, cauliflower, onions, spinach, kale, broccoli and tomatoes. Those are just popular examples but basically, all vegetables are allowed in the Mediterranean diet
- Whole grains like pasta, whole wheat, whole grain bread, corn, buckwheat, barley, rye, brown rice and whole oats.
- Nuts and seeds like pumpkin seeds, cashews, pistachios, walnuts, almonds and macadamia nuts
- Herbs and spices; the best herbs and spices are mostly fresh and dried like mint, rosemary, cinnamon, basil and pepper.
- Tubers like sweet potatoes, yams, turnips and potatoes.
- Legumes like chickpeas, peanuts, pulses, lentils, peas and beans.
- Fish and seafood, which are actually your primary source of Protein. Good examples include shellfish like crab, mussels and oysters, shrimp, tuna, haddock and salmon.

Foods You Should Eat In Moderation
You should only eat the below foods less frequently when compared to the foods in the list above.

- Red meat like bacon, ground beef and steak
- Dairy products low in fat or fat free. Some of the popular examples include cheese, yogurt and low fat milk
- Eggs, as they are good sources of Proteins and are healthier when poached and boiled
- Poultry like duck, turkey and chicken
- Note that chicken are healthy when their skin is removed. This is because you reduce the cholesterol in the chicken.

Foods to Avoid

The below list contains foods that you need to completely avoid when on a Mediterranean diet. This is because they are unhealthy and when you eat them, you will be unable to experience the benefits of a Mediterranean diet. These foods include;

- Processed meat- you should avoid processed meats like bacon, sausage and hot dogs because they are high in saturated fats, which are unhealthy.
- Refined oils - stay away from unhealthy oils like cottonseed oil, vegetable oil and soybean oil.
- Saturated or Trans-fats - good example of these fats include butter and margarine.
- Highly processed foods – avoid all highly processed foods. By this, I mean all the foods that are packaged. This can be packaged crisp, nuts, wheat etc. Some of these foods are marked and labeled low fat but are actually quite high in sugar.
- Refined grains - avoid refined grains like refined pasta, white bread, cereals, bagels etc
- Added sugar- foods, which contain added sugar like sodas, chocolates, candy and ice cream should be completely avoided. If you have a sweet tooth, you can substitute products with added sugar with natural sweeteners.

Reasons to Love the Mediterranean Diet

Surprise! No Calorie Counting

For that meal plan, you won't need a calculator. You trade bad Fats for heart-healthy ones, instead of adding up amounts. Instead of butter, go for olive oil. Consider seafood or poultry instead of red meat. Love the fresh fruit and miss the trendy, sugar desserts.

Eat your veggies and beans full of flavor. Nuts are good, so stick to a couple of them a day. Bread and wine can be whole-grain but in moderate amounts.

The Food Is Really Fresh

You are not going to have to walk the frozen food lane or visit a fast-food drive-thru. The emphasis is on seasonal food which is processed in clear, mouthwatering ways. Build a savory spinach salad, cucumbers, and tomatoes. Attach traditional Greek ingredients such as black olives, and feta cheese with a recipe for Fast Light Greek Salad. You can also whip up a fun bowl of Grilled Tomato Gazpacho, packed with vegetables.

You Can Have Wine

In many Mediterranean countries, a glass with meals is popular, where eating is often leisurely and social. Several studies suggest that up to one glass a day can be good for your heart for some individuals, for women and two for men. Red wine is actually safer than normal. Check with your doctor to see if you think this is a good idea.

You Can Lose Weight
If you are eating nuts, chocolate, and fats, you would think it would take a miracle to lose any pounds. But those Mediterranean basics (and the slower eating style) help you to feel satisfied and whole. And this helps you stay on with a diet. Regular exercise often forms an important part of a lifestyle.

Your Heart Will Thank You
Quick everything that's good for your heart in this diet. Olive oil and nuts help to bring down "evil" cholesterol. Fruits, vegetables, and beans help to clear arteries. Fish helps lower blood pressure and triglycerides. Even a glass of wine per day can be good for your heart!

You'll Stay Sharper Longer
Always good for your brain is the same goods that protect your skin. You don't eat bad fats and processed foods, which can result in inflammation. Alternatively, foods rich in antioxidants render the eating style a brain-friendly alternative.

A Convenient Course in Health Eating
The Mediterranean diet is essentially quite easy. The diet consists of very simple, quick to prepare food items. Furthermore, the Mediterranean diet includes various relatively inexpensive food items. So you can choose to adopt the Mediterranean diet and not disrupt the routine or break the bank in the process.

Fundamentals
Understanding the Mediterranean diet's fundamentals will empower and encourage you to stick with this healthy way of eating. There has been much controversy surrounding good fats vs. bad fats, red meat, and olive oil. In this chapter, I will bring some more clarity to these areas to help you understand how the Mediterranean diet functions, and how it will also benefit your health in the long-term. This is a mere introduction, but it should be fascinating nonetheless.

Good Fats vs. bad Fats – how do you choose?
When it comes to weight loss and health benefits, the fats you eat play a vital role. The dominant fat in your diet will either aggravate cardiovascular diseases, diabetes, cancer or obesity, or it will assist in regulating your moods, keep you mentally alert and regulate your weight.

How do you choose the Fat that will give you benefits?
Knowing good fat from a bad one is the secret to a healthy life. Saturated and trans fat fall under the "bad fats" category. Saturated fat is usually found in lard, fatty red meats, poultry skin, high fat dairy, and tropical oils such as coconut oil or palm oil. These saturated fats increase LDL (bad cholesterol), which is further aggravated when consumed with refined Carbs. Saturated fats increase the risk of cardiovascular diseases and type 2 diabetes.

Trans fats are even worse than saturated fats. They are found in margarine, fast foods, fried foods, vegetable shortening, processed snack foods, cookies, cakes, and pastries. These fats do not only raise LDL cholesterol, they also suppress HDL (good cholesterol), thereby elevating the risk of cardiovascular diseases three times higher than the risk involved in consuming saturated fats.

So what are the good fats?
So, good fats are monounsaturated fats and polyunsaturated fats. These fats can be found in natural products. Monounsaturated fats are found in nuts, avocados, vegetable oils, and olive oil.

Polyunsaturated fats are found in seafood, seeds and nuts. The best type of polyunsaturated fat is the omega-3 fatty acids found in salmon, sardines, trout, flaxseeds, or walnuts. Fish is the best source for these fatty acids.

Another fantastic polyunsaturated fat is the omega-6 fatty acids found in tofu, walnuts, seeds, eggs, poultry, and so on.

These good fats improve blood cholesterol and reduce the risk of heart disease. Since fat generally has a high calorie content, moderation should still be used even when consuming good fats.

Wine And Benefits

In the Mediterranean diet, wine is an enjoyable addition to a meal. Red wine is preferred over white wine for its heart benefits. Red wine seems to have a higher level of antioxidants than white wine. These antioxidants are a large contributor toward a healthy heart although it has not been concretely established.

Red wine contains flavonoids, which are high in antioxidants. Flavonoids are found in the grape skin. So if you can't have alcohol in your diet for various reasons, that's OK. You can still receive similar benefits by drinking red grape juice. Flavonoids lower LDL while increasing HDL. They also assist in reducing blood clotting. Flavonoids also help the body to resist allergens, viruses and carcinogens.

When it comes to choosing the red wine to go along with your meal, Merlots and red zinfandels may have more flavonoids than white wine, however, your dryer red wines are rich in flavonoid. Stock up on a few different dry red wines brands to ensure that you get as many flavonoids and antioxidants as possible while enjoying your meal.

Other benefits that red wine seems to bring to its consumers include, assisting with weight loss, maintaining good memory, and controlling blood sugar. All thanks to resveratrol – a natural compound in grapes, peanuts, and mulberries, which is both antioxidant and anti-inflammatory.

Wine yes...but with cautions...

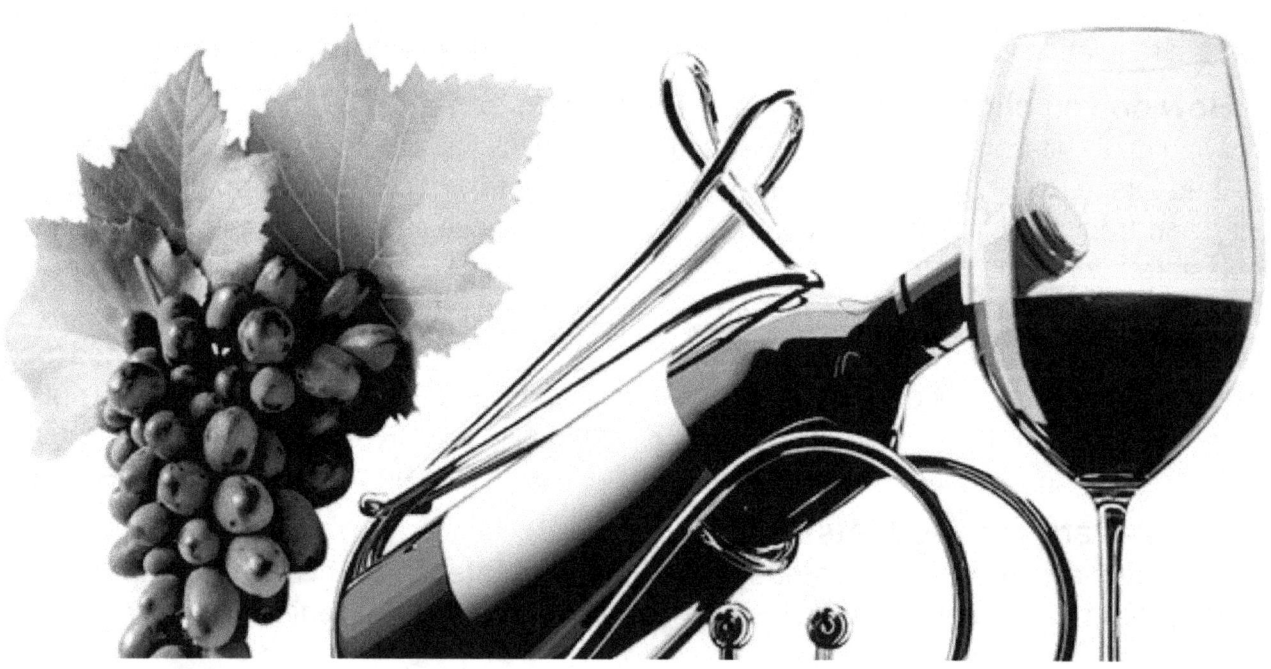

For red wine consumption to be healthy, you must stick to the recommended daily intake. Avoid alcohol if you have pancreatitis, high blood pressure, liver disease, gongestive heart failure.

When you have that delicious wine with your meal, savour your glass of wine, the food and your loved ones. Allow wine to enhance your meal and social experience. Remember, moderation is key for healthy living.

A Word On Red Meat

Currently, there is a conflict that has led to the debate of red meat and its effect on the heart's health. The Mediterranean diet traditionally tends to restrict red meat consumption to two servings per week, while white meat (poultry and fish) have a higher amount of weekly servings.

The current issue is not so much the red meat in general, but the processed red meats such as deli meats, bacon, and so on. Processed meat or any processed food is more detrimental to a person's health.

In this section, I am going to list some of the necessary nutrients that your body will receive when you consume lean unprocessed red meat (beef, pork, lamb). Lean red meats have been found to be fairly neutral with regards to their fatty acid profile, and as a result, their impact on cholesterol levels is more neutral than previously thought.

Lean red meats provide a variety of important micronutrients including zinc, iron, selenium, potassium, B-vitamins, niacin, riboflavin, thiamine, vitamin B-12.

All of these nutrients and more are essential to give your body the best health throughout your life. Particularly, children need a moderate supply of iron in their diets to assist their muscular development and amino blocks.

The link with red meat and cardiovascular disease lies in animal fat, which is saturated fat. Hence, consuming a fair portion of beef with fat trimmings may give you the essential micronutrients, but a lot of saturated fat at the same time. Here's my solution to this situation: as you incorporate the Mediterranean diet into your lifestyle, look for lean cuts of beef. Buy extra lean mince, lean pork chops, and other lean meats such as veal. If you happen to buy red meat with fat on the edges, simply trim the fat off (either before or after cooking, depending on your purpose).

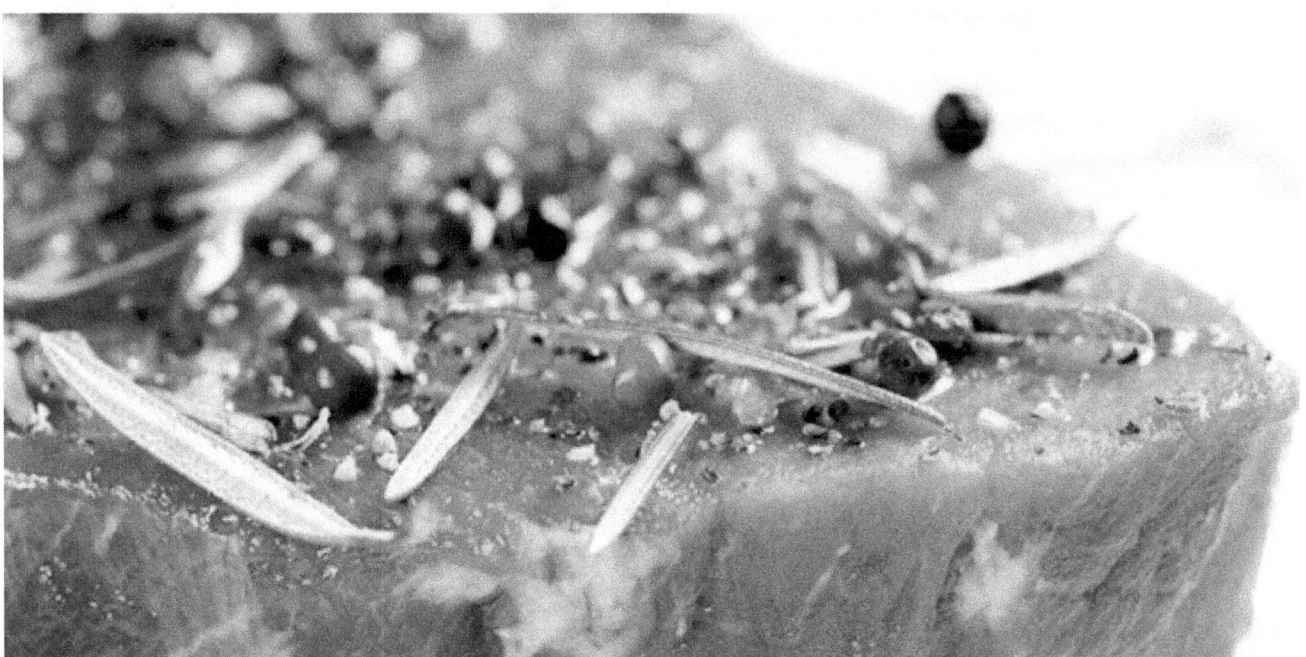

The Mediterranean Food Pyramid

When you signed up for a cookbook on mediterranean food, I am sure you were expecting to see just recipes and a beautiful food presentation on a plate. But this is more than just that. A lot of people have been able to create a lifestyle around mediterranean food because of its importance and benefits. However, the fundamental concept of what exactly constitutes the mediterranean food can be very complicated. Especially because there are several countries that lie within that region. The geographical landscape that covers what the world recognizes as part of the Mediterranean countries includes countries in Europe and Africa. Each of these countries hava a rich cultural heritage that influences their cuisine. What this means in turn is that you would find a lot of differences in what constitutes their diet when you look into each region.

This is why a lot of extensive research was carried out on the subject by experts. And what they arrived at is something called the mediterranean food pyramid. Essentially, this pyramid is a nutritional guide that is made up of all the core ingredients that make up part of the Mediterranean diet group. At the top of the pyramid, you have the types of food that you need the least and then at the bottom of the pyramid, you have the bulk of what is required to be in that group. The interesting thing with this pyramid is that it also directs you on how frequent you need to eat the foods that belong to each group. Some of the foods in the group are very much involved in every meal that you eat while some occasionally show up. We will explore each of these groups in detail so that when you shop for your pantry with the Mediterranean diet in mind, you know exactly what you need.

MEDITERRANEAN DIET

The first layer of the pyramid which is at the top is where you will find foods like your meat as well as white bread, white pasta and the occasional processed sugar. The foods in this group are to be rarely used in the preparation of a meal that is considered Mediterranean. If you are going all-in to get on a diet, this is something that you need to consider because this food groups are said to disrupt the nutritional balance of the meal plan.

The second layer of the pyramid is where you have dairy products such as milk, cheese, yogurt and so on. These provide your daily dairy or calcium quota. They are expected to be included in your meal perhaps once or twice a day at most. If you are a big dairy fan you need to ensure that you stick to portion control because this is also a key aspect in ensuring that you enjoy all the benefits that being on a Mediterranean diet offers.

The third layer is where you have your seafood and poultry produce. You can use them zero to two times a day. This depends on how you structure your diet of course. For instance, when you have produce from the second layer present, you might want to tone down or completely eliminate the addition of poultry produce to that meal. Seafood is an excellent choice because it contains a lot of nutritional benefits that you may not find in other food groups.

The fourth layer of the pyramid offers you nuts and legumes. These are great for snacktime and those in-between meals. However, you would find that some of the recipes we have created here include the addition of nuts to main courses which gives it a very exotic but totally irresistible flavor. Many nuts in this category are said to contain the monosaturated fat which as we mentioned earlier is the good type of fat. You can have nuts in your meal once a day but if they are your absolute favourite food to eat, the maximum number of times you can have them in a day is 3 times.

Next, we have the fruits and vegetables layer which is pretty much very self-descriptive. When it comes to the vegetables, you can have them as many times as possible. The fruits on the other hand, which can also serve as snacks should only be included in your food portion for a maximum of three times a day.

Finally, we have the whole grain and plant oil section. The produce you find in this layer are very crucial to your meal. So, most likely, you might be eating them more than anything else. Since you are going to be using a lot of plant oil, do ensure that you go for the type that isn't processed like olive oil. It is healthy and contains the essential nutrients not to forget the fact that it is also very tasty whether you're using it in salads or in your regular cooking.

On a final note, just in case you are wondering, red wine is absolutely permitted. However, your consumption of it has to be tightly controlled. Perhaps, make two glasses your limit per week. Exceeding this might compromise your Mediterranean diet experience.

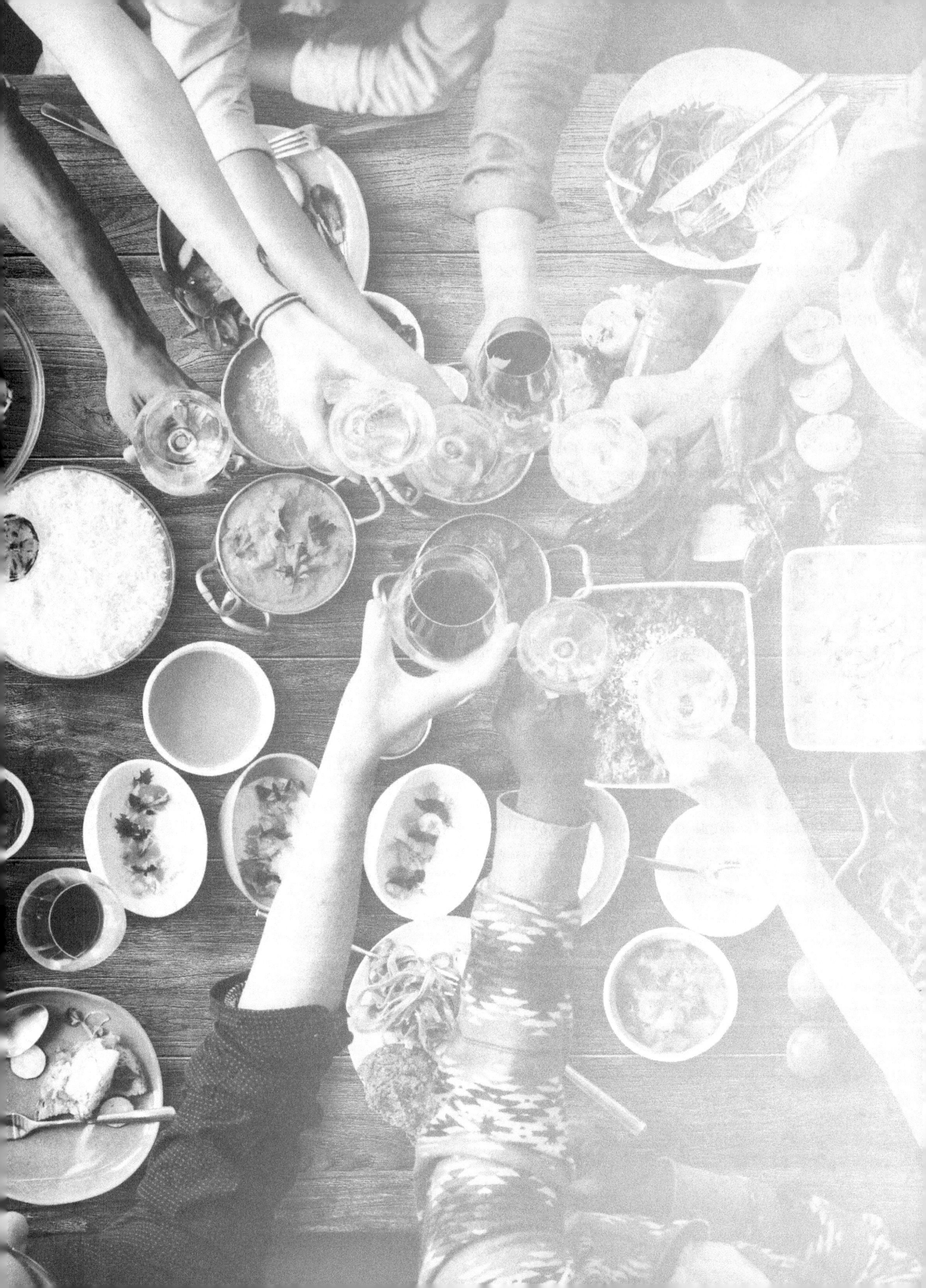

CHAPTER 4

How To Get Started With The Mediterranean Diet

Your goals
Before you get started with this diet, spend some time and come up with the goals you wish to achieve. Your goals will determine your level of motivation whenever you decide to follow a diet. Perhaps you want to lose weight, or maybe want to improve your overall health. Regardless of your goals, it is quintessential that you know what you wish to achieve from the diet. If you don't have any goals, it becomes difficult to stay on track in the long run.

Pick a date
Once you know your goal, you should work on setting a timeline. Select a date you want to start this diet. Don't be in a rush, and don't think that you can get started with this diet right away. It takes a while to prepare your mind and body for the diet you wish to follow. The Mediterranean diet doesn't require any drastic dietary changes. However, if your diet is rich in processed foods and sugars, your body will take time to adjust to the new diet. Therefore, pick a date and ensure you start your diet on that particular date. Don't make any excuses, and don't try to put it off until a later date. If you keep telling yourself that you can start this diet tomorrow, then tomorrow will never come. Take a calendar, mark the date, and get started.

Take the first step
Once you have made up your mind about this diet, then it is time to get started. Don't get scared of the diet, instead, think of it as a stepping-stone towards better health. If you get scared, remind yourself of the goals you wish to achieve from this diet. It will make it easier to keep going.

Clean your pantry
Before you start this diet, it is time to clean your pantry. Go through the Mediterranean diet shopping list given in the next section and make a list of all the ingredients you will require. Once you have this list, it's time to go shopping for groceries. Simultaneously, you're also supposed to get rid of any other items that don't fit the Mediterranean diet eating protocols. So, it is time to get rid of all processed foods, unhealthy carbs, and sugary treats. Think of it as spring-cleaning for

your kitchen. It is quintessential that you do this because if you're surrounded by temptations all the time, the chances of giving in to your urges to eat unhealthy foods will increase. Out of sight, out of mind, is the best approach when it comes to junk food.

Make the transition
Once you follow the steps mentioned up until now, it is time to make the transition. As mentioned in the previous point, if your diet is predominantly rich in processed foods and sugars, it might be a little tricky to shift to any other diet. You might not know this, but a diet rich in sugars is quite addictive to your body. Therefore, there are two ways in which you can change your diet. You can either go cold turkey or make a slow transition to the new diet. Slowly start eliminating all unhealthy foods from your diet while incorporating Mediterranean diet-friendly foods. This way, you are conditioning your mind and body to get used to the new diet. Give yourself at least two to three weeks before you come to any conclusions about this diet.

Support system
You must have a support system in place if you want to stick to this diet in the long run. Let go of the "I will just wing it" attitude. There will be days when you have little to no motivation. This is where your support system comes into the picture. Whenever you feel like you don't have motivation to keep going, you can depend on your support system. Your support system can include your partner, loved ones, friends, or anyone else you want. Talk to them about your reasons for following the diet and tell them what you wish to achieve. By doing this, you are making yourself accountable to someone else. This, in turn, increases your motivation to stick to this diet. You can always get online and get in touch with those who are following the same diet as you.

Be patient
A common mistake a lot of dieters make is that they are always in a hurry. Making any sort of dietary change is not easy, and it takes time. Not just time, but consistency as well. Don't think that you'll be able to shed all those extra pounds overnight. After all, you didn't gain all that extra weight within a day or two. Therefore, you can't expect yourself to get rid of it quickly. Whenever you make a dietary change, you might notice certain fluctuations in your energy levels. This happens because your body is trying to get used to the new diet. So, don't be upset with yourself if you can exercise as vigorously as you used to. Within two to three weeks, your energy levels will stabilize, your body will get used to the new diet, and you will be able to exercise the way you want. Until then, be patient and don't weigh yourself daily. It might be quite tempting to see whether you've lost any weight daily, but it is not practical. There will be days when the scale doesn't fluctuate like you want to. Make it a point to weigh yourself every week. It will help keep track of your progress.

Shopping List
Use this basic shopping list whenever you shop for groceries. Ensure that you stock your pantry with all these ingredients and get rid of any other item, which is not suitable for your diet. Your shopping list must include:
- Veggies like kale, garlic, spinach, arugula, onions, carrots
- Fruits like grapes, oranges, apples and bananas
- Berries like blueberries, strawberries, raspberries
- Frozen veggies
- Grains like whole-grain pasta, whole-grain breads

- Legumes like beans, lentils, chickpeas
- Nuts like walnuts, cashews, almonds
- Seeds like pumpkin seeds and sunflower seeds
- Condiments like turmeric, cinnamon, salt, pepper
- Shrimp and shellfish
- Fish like mackerel, trout, tuna, salmon and sardines
- Cheese, Yogurt and Greek yogurt
- Potatoes and sweet potatoes
- Chicken
- Eggs
- Olives
- Olive oil and avocado oil

If you buy healthy and adequate ingredients, you will most certainly eat the right foods and you will definitely stay on your diet.

Tricks And Tips That Will Make Things Easier

- Keeping in mind that you cannot eat red meat, you can replace it with salmon. It will satisfy your cravings, but it will allow you to stay on your diet.
- Make sure you always have olive oil at hand. You have to forget about using butter if you are on the Mediterranean diet, but you can replace it with the extra virgin olive oil.
- Give up consuming sodas and replace them with some red wine. Cut out the sweet drinks from your diet and try one glass of red wine instead.
- Replace white rice with brown rice. The Mediterranean diet allows you to continue to eat rice but make sure you replace the white rice with brown one. Consume whole grains like buckwheat, corn and quinoa.
- Your snacks should mainly contain fruits. Consume more citrus, melons, berries or grapes. You can also try seeds as a Mediterranean diet snack, but fruits would be a better option.
- Exercise a lot and drink plenty of water. This is a main principle to follow if you are on a Mediterranean diet. It will help you look better and feel amazing. That's a fact!
- Another great idea to keep in mind when you are on such a diet is to make a great shopping list like the one above. It will help you buy the right ingredients. Choose organic products if you can but only if they suit your budget.
- You must keep your body hydrated. Regardless of the dietary changes you make, the one thing you must always concentrate on is proper hydration. When your body is hydrated, all the toxins present within will be flushed out. Not just this, but it also helps improve the health of your skin. You must consume at least eight glasses of water daily. Also, when you're transitioning to this diet or making any dietary changes, hunger pangs are quite common. To keep hunger pangs at bay, ensure that your body is thoroughly hydrated.

Three Reasons Why You Are Not Losing Weight in The Mediterranean Diet

Before we dive into the 4-Week Meal Plan, let's briefly look at some of the reasons why you might not be losing weight even if you are on a Mediterranean Diet.

You're overestimating just how many calories you're burning.

If you don't spend your entire day performing physical labour or are a dynamic athlete, you almost certainly won't lose weight eating 2,000 calories each day unless you're incorporating exercise into the routine. Likewise, simply walking up several flights of stairs to your workplace won't burn enough calories to qualify as a good work out. Many people overestimate the calories they burn per day normally by as much as 25%. Keep track and make use of a journal or an app.

You're concentrating on diet and ignoring exercise.

The Mediterranean diet is more than just a grocery list and a list of recipes. Though it is possible to lose excess weight by modifying diet alone, it is difficult to do it with a sedentary lifestyle. Adding regular physical exercise to any weight loss regimen increases your likelihood of burning more calories than you consume, causing you to slim down even more consistently. To make the Mediterranean diet a highly effective weight loss strategy, make sure to keep the body moving.

You're eating prematurely rather than savoring your meal.

Enjoy your meal by taking enough time to look for fresh ingredients, spend some time cooking with friends or family, and linger in the table.

To be sure you're not overcooking it, pre-portion your nut products in plastic bags or reusable containers to be sure you can enjoy the health advantages without accidentally consuming more than you designed to.

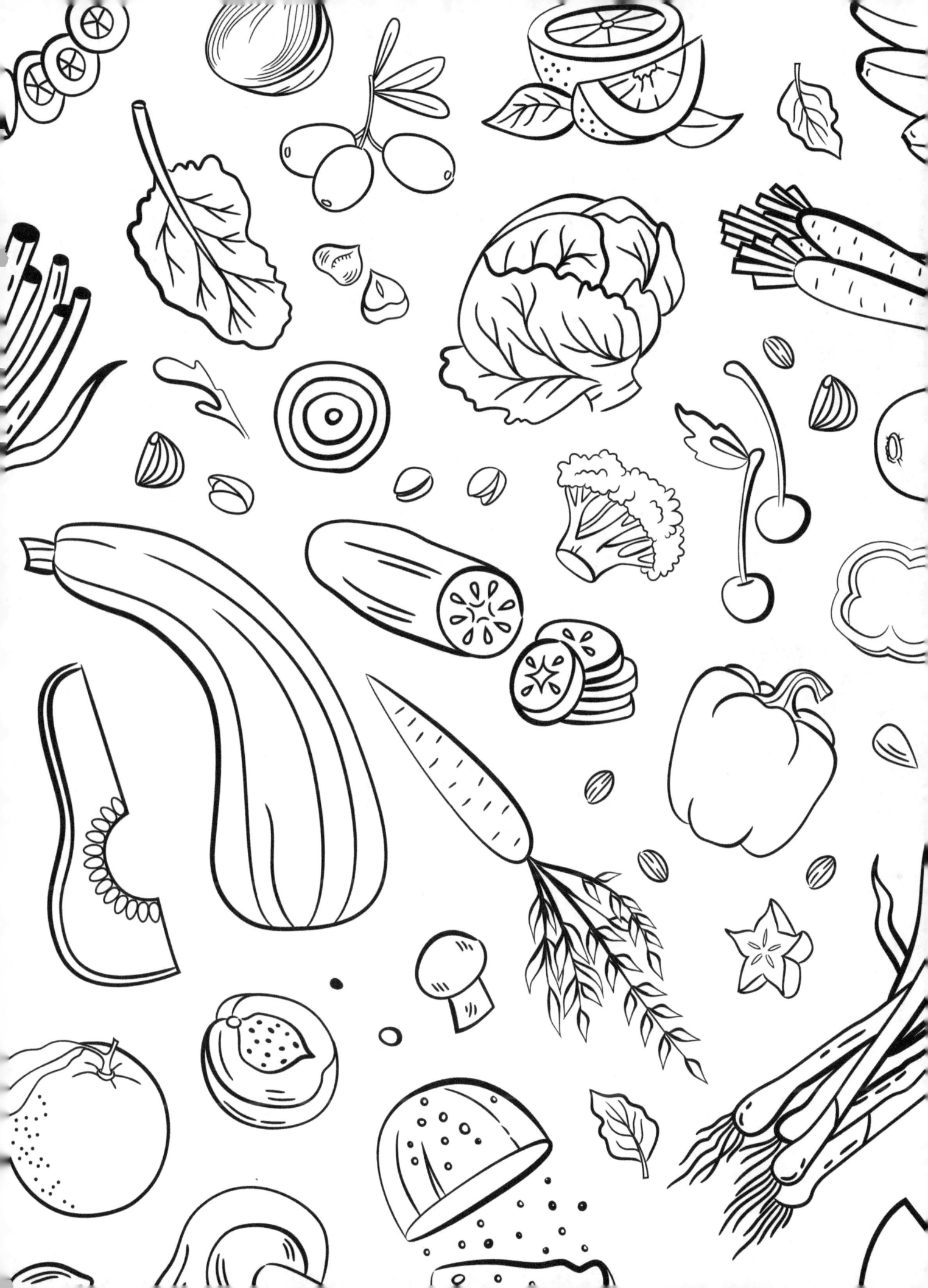

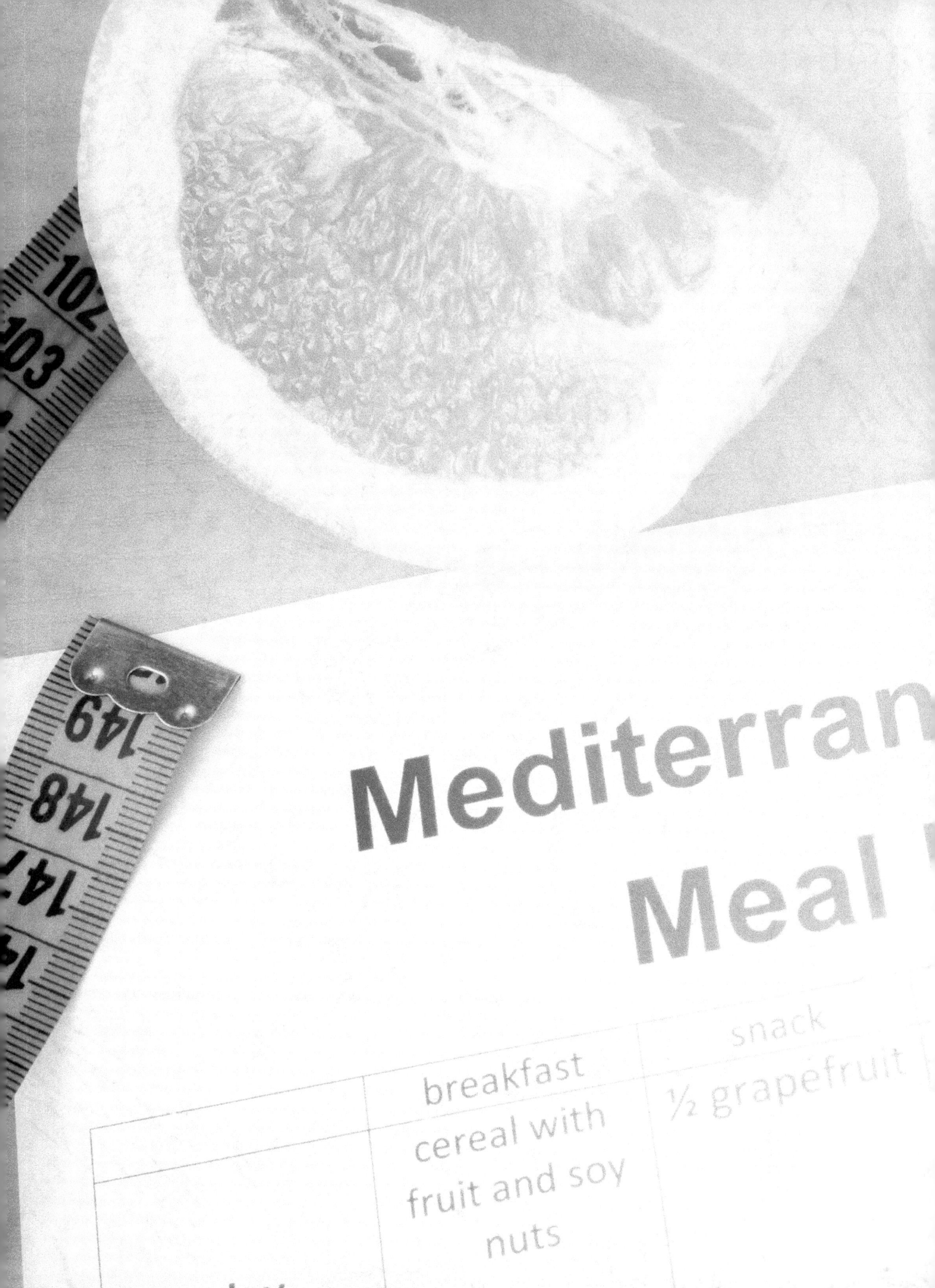

CHAPTER 5

4-Week Meal Plan

In the previous chapters, we have discovered the main traits and the benefits of the Mediterranean diet. We also looked at how you can prepare and fill your pantry with all the necessary ingredients to cook many flavorful and healthy dishes on a daily basis. It's now time to put all of this into practice.

Before we get into the 600+ recipes included in this book, I want to leave you with a simple 4-week meal plan. This plan should be taken as a sample/guideline to help you with your grocery shopping and weekly meal planning. Each daily combination is within 2,000 calories (you can find each recipe's nutritional value in the recipes pages). Feel free to change/add/remove items according to your preference.

NOTE: The number next to each recipe is the recipe's number so that you can easily locate it in this book. Enjoy!

MEDITERRANEAN DIET COOKBOOK

DAY	BREAKFAST	LUNCH	DINNER	DESSERT
1	Banana and Quinoa Casserole (1)	Curry Salmon with Mustard (497)	Mozzarella Bean Pizza (376)	Veggie Fritters (342)
2	Ham Muffins (2)	Fragrant Basmati Rice (130)	Bulgur Lamb Meatballs (345)	Falafel Bites (302)
3	Cheesy Yogurt (3)	Baked Cod Fillets with Ghee Sauce (486)	Rustic Vegetable and Brown Rice Bowl (268)	Healthy Coconut Blueberry Balls (325)
4	Avocado Spread (4)	Vegetable Panini (247)	Grilled Marinated Chicken (413)	Peach Sorbet (574)
5	Artichokes and Cheese Omelet (5)	Mediterranean Pasta with Tomato Sauce and Vegetables (81)	White Pizza with Prosciutto and Arugula (373)	Cucumber Bites (346)
6	Walnut Poached Eggs (6)	Grilled Pesto Chicken (474)	Fish and Veggie Stew (211)	Stuffed Avocado (347)
7	Almond Cream Cheese Bake (7)	Easy Spaghetti Squash (232)	Tuna Salad (228)	Strawberry Sorbet (590)
8	Herbed Fried Eggs (13)	Italian Style Wild Rice (140)	Chicken Fillets with Artichoke Hearts (441)	Wrapped Plums (349)
9	Banana Oats (16)	Fish Soup (214)	Duck Patties (418)	Cucumber Sandwich Bites (350)
10	Avocado and Apple Smoothie (19)	Lamb Stew (455)	Courgette, Fennel, and Orange Salad (251)	Cajun Walnuts And Olives Bowls (362)
11	Avocado Toast (20)	Zucchini Pasta (241)	Quinoa with Almonds and Cranberries (300)	Olives and Cheese Stuffed Tomatoes (352)
12	Mini Frittatas (21)	Easy Seafood French Stew (501)	Cucumber and Nuts Salad (250)	Curry Chicken Drumsticks (420)
13	Berry Oats (22)	Chicken Burgers (417)	Classic Greek Salad (257)	Figs Pie (563)
14	Sun-dried Tomatoes Oatmeal (23)	Cranberry Rice (131)	Broccoli Cheese Burst Pizza (375)	Green Tea and Vanilla Cream (562)

DAY	BREAKFAST	LUNCH	DINNER	DESSERT
15	Quinoa Muffins (24)	Roasted Root Veggies (271)	Baked Sea Bass (529)	Almond Rice Dessert (575)
16	Scrambled Eggs (27)	Tarragon Cod Fillets (542)	Mediterranean Humus Filled Roasted Veggies (249)	Blackberry and Apples Cobbler (560)
17	Baked Omelet Mix (29)	Parmesan Barley Risotto (240)	Lemon Lamb Leg (454)	Lemon Cream (573)
18	Anti-Inflammatory Blueberry Smoothie (30)	Pasta with Veggies (98)	Olives and Lentils Salad (314)	Ricotta Ramekins (587)
19	Cherry - Pomegranate Smoothie Bow (31)	Mediterranean Paella (137)	Pecan Crusted Trout (514)	Cucumber Rolls (351)
20	Breakfast Banana Green Smoothie (32)	Fish and Orzo (528)	Quick Vegetable Kebabs (303)	Savory Pistachio Balls (329)
21	Strawberry Oatmeal Breakfast Smoothie (33)	Mussels Linguine Delight (88)	Summer Veggies in Instant Pot (282)	Buttery Carrot Sticks (361)
22	Veggie Bowl (18)	Eggs with Zucchini Noodles (270)	Halibut and Quinoa Mix (531)	Italian Style Eggplant Chips (66)
23	Slow-cooked Peppers Frittata (17)	Pesto and Lemon Halibut (515)	Chicken Saute (412)	Roasted Almonds (330)
24	Kale and Banana Smoothie (34)	Brown Rice Saute (133)	Yummy Salmon Panzanella (527)	Hot Asparagus Sticks (364)
25	Buttery Pancakes (11)	Leftover Salmon Salad Power Bowls (506)	Chicken Zucchini Boats (426)	Mediterranean Chickpea Snack (44)
26	Cream Olive Muffins (12)	Pan Fried Tuna with Herbs and Nut (512)	Smoked Salmon and Veggies Mix (550)	Creamy Yogurt Banana Bowls (338)
27	Coconut Milk Smoothie (38)	Spring Farro Plate (196)	Mango Chicken Salad (425)	Chia and Berries Smoothie Bowl (581)
28	Quinoa and Eggs Pan (25)	Pasta with Fresh Tomatoes (108)	Baked Trout and Fennel (555)	Tomato Bruschetta (368)

BREAKFAST

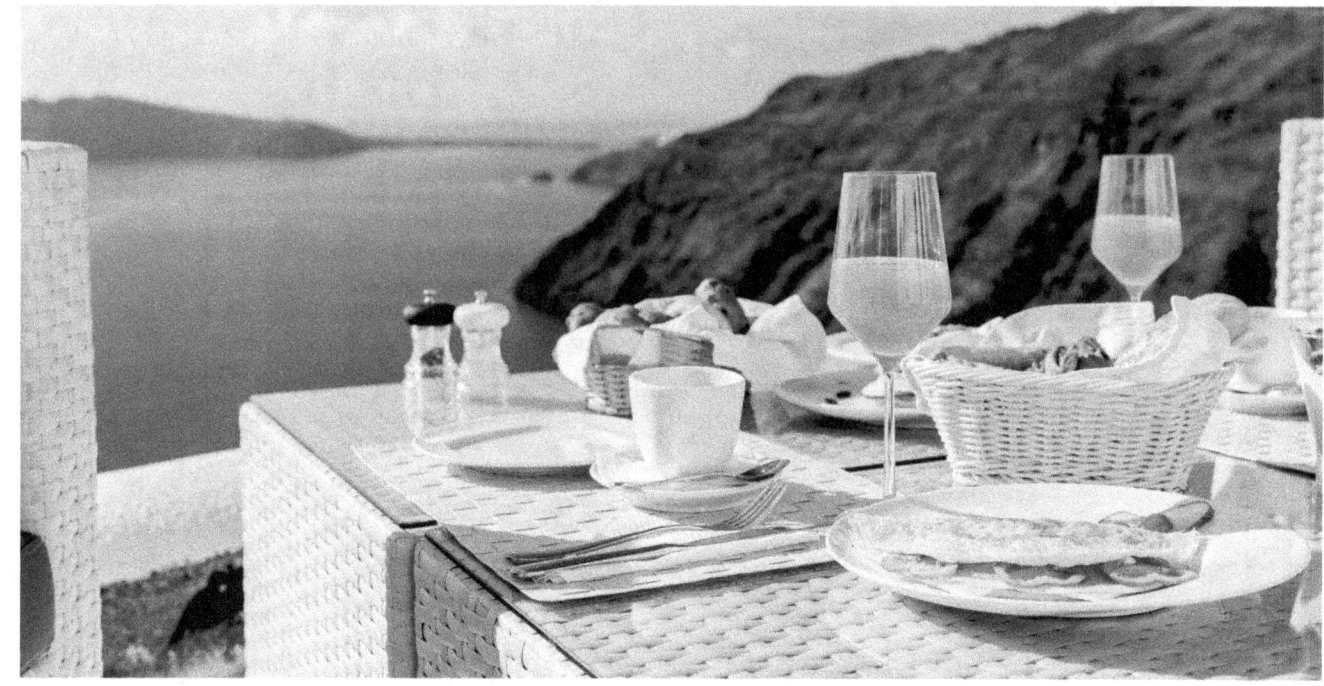

1. Banana and Quinoa Casserole

PREP TIME: 10 mins
COOK TIME: 80 mins
SERVINGS: 8 people

NUTRITION
Calories 213,
Fat 4.1g,
Fiber 4 g,
Carbs 41 g,
Protein 4.5 g

INGREDIENTS

- 3 cups bananas, peeled and mashed
- ¼ cup pure maple syrup
- ¼ cup molasses
- 1 tbsp. cinnamon powder
- 2 tsp. vanilla extract
- 1 tsp. cloves, ground
- 1 tsp. ginger, ground
- ½ tsp. allspice, ground
- 1 cup quinoa
- ¼ cup almonds, chopped
- 2 and ½ cups almond milk

DIRECTIONS

1. In a baking dish, combine the bananas with the maple syrup, molasses and the rest of the ingredients, toss and bake at 350°F for 1 hour and 20 minutes.
2. Divide the mix between plates and serve for breakfast.

2. Ham Muffins

PREP TIME 10 mins
COOK TIME 15 mins
SERVINGS 6 people

INGREDIENTS

- 9 ham slices
- 5 eggs, whisked
- 1/3 cup spinach, chopped
- ¼ cup feta cheese, crumbled
- ½ cup roasted red peppers, chopped
- A pinch of salt and black pepper
- 1 and ½ tbsp. basil pesto
- Cooking spray

DIRECTIONS

1. Grease a muffin tin with cooking spray and line each muffin mould with 1 and ½ ham slices.
2. Divide the peppers and the rest of the ingredients except the eggs, pesto, salt and pepper into the ham cups.
3. In a bowl, mix the eggs with the pesto, salt and pepper, whisk and pour over the peppers mix.
4. Bake the muffins in the oven at 400°F for 15 minutes and serve for breakfast.

NUTRITION
Calories 109 g, Fat 6.7 g, Fiber 1.8 g, Carbs 1.8 g, Protein 9.3 g

3. Cheesy Yogurt

PREP TIME 4 hours 15 mins
COOK TIME 0 mins
SERVINGS 4 people

INGREDIENTS

- 1 cup Greek yogurt
- 1 tbsp. honey
- ½ cup feta cheese, crumbled

DIRECTIONS

1. In a blender, combine the yogurt with the honey and the cheese and pulse well.
2. Divide into bowls and freeze for 4 hours before serving for breakfast.

NUTRITION
Calories 161, Fat 11.5 g, Fiber 9.6 g, Carbs 36.6 g, Protein 15.4 g

4. Avocado Spread

PREP TIME 5 mins

COOK TIME 0 mins

SERVINGS 8 people

NUTRITION
Calories 110,
Fat 10.5 g,
Fiber 3.6 g,
Carbs 5.6 g,
Protein 1.4 g

INGREDIENTS
- 2 avocados, peeled, pitted and roughly chopped
- 1 tbsp. sun-dried tomatoes, chopped
- 2 tbsp. lemon juice
- 3 tbsp. cherry tomatoes, chopped
- ¼ cup red onion, chopped
- 1 tsp. oregano, dried
- 2 tbsp. parsley, chopped
- 4 kalamata olives, pitted and chopped
- A pinch of salt and black pepper

DIRECTIONS
1. Put the avocados in a bowl and mash with a fork.
2. Add the rest of the ingredients, stir to combine and serve as a morning spread.

5. Artichokes and Cheese Omelet

PREP TIME 10 mins

COOK TIME 8 mins

SERVINGS 1 people

NUTRITION
Calories 303,
Fat 17.5 g,
Fiber 9.6 g,
Carbs 6.6 g,
Protein 15.4 g

INGREDIENTS
- 1 tsp. avocado oil
- 1 tbsp. almond milk
- 2 eggs, whisked
- A pinch of salt and black pepper
- 2 tbsp. tomato, cubed
- 2 tbsp. kalamata olives, pitted and sliced
- 1 artichoke heart, chopped
- 1 tbsp. tomato sauce
- 1 tbsp. feta cheese, crumbled

DIRECTIONS
1. In a bowl, combine the eggs with the milk, salt, pepper and the rest of the ingredients except the avocado oil and whisk well.
2. Heat up a pan with the avocado oil over medium-high heat, add the omelet mix, spread into the pan, cook for 4 minutes, flip, cook for 4 minutes more, transfer to a plate and serve.

6. Walnut Poached Eggs

PREP TIME 10 mins
COOK TIME 10 mins
SERVINGS 2 people

NUTRITION
Calories 317,
Fat 36.5 g,
Fiber 3.6 g,
Carbs 17.6 g,
Protein 17.4 g

INGREDIENTS

- 2 slices whole grain bread toasted
- 1 oz sun-dried tomato, sliced
- 1 tbsp. cream cheese
- 1/3 tsp. minced garlic
- 2 slices prosciutto
- 2 eggs
- 1 tbsp. walnuts
- ½ cup fresh basil
- 1 oz Parmesan, grated
- 3 tbsp. olive oil
- ¼ tsp. ground black pepper
- 1 cup water, for cooking

DIRECTIONS

1. Pour water in the saucepan and bring it to boil.
2. Then crack eggs in the boiling water and cook them for 3-4 minutes or until the egg whites are white.
3. Meanwhile, churn together minced garlic and cream cheese.
4. Spread the bread slices with the cream cheese mixture.
5. Top them with the sun-dried tomatoes.
6. Make the pesto sauce: Blend together ground black pepper, Parmesan, olive oil, and basil. When the mixture is homogenous, pesto is cooked.
7. Carefully transfer the poached eggs over the sun-dried tomatoes and sprinkle with pesto sauce.
8. The poached eggs should be hot while serving.

7. Almond Cream Cheese Bake

PREP TIME 10 mins
COOK TIME 2 hours
SERVINGS 4 people

NUTRITION
Calories 352,
Fat 22.5 g,
Fiber 1.6 g,
Carbs 7.6 g,
Protein 10.4 g

INGREDIENTS

- 1 cup cream cheese
- 4 tbsp. honey
- 1 oz almonds, chopped
- ½ tsp. vanilla extract
- 3 eggs, beaten
- 1 tbsp. semolina

DIRECTIONS

1. Put beaten eggs in the mixing bowl.
2. Add cream cheese, semolina, and vanilla extract.
3. Blend the mixture with the help of the hand mixer until it is fluffy.
4. After this, add chopped almonds and mix up the mass well.
5. Transfer the cream cheese mash in the non-sticky baking mold.
6. Flatten the surface of the cream cheese mash well.
7. Preheat the oven to 325°F.
8. Cook the breakfast for 2 hours.
9. The meal is cooked when the surface of the mash is light brown.
10. Chill the cream cheese mash little and sprinkle with honey.

8. Chili Egg Cups

PREP TIME 15 mins
COOK TIME 15 mins
SERVINGS 4 people

NUTRITION

Calories 85,
Fat 6.5 g,
Fiber 0.6 g,
Carbs 0.6 g,
Protein 6.4 g

INGREDIENTS

- 1 tsp. chives, chopped
- 4 eggs
- 1 tsp. tomato paste
- 1 tbsp. Plain yogurt
- ½ tsp. butter, softened
- ¼ tsp. chili flakes
- ½ oz Cheddar cheese, shredded

DIRECTIONS

1. Preheat the oven to 365°F.
2. Brush the muffin molds with the softened butter from inside.
3. Then mix up together Plain yogurt with chili flakes and tomato paste.
4. Crack the eggs in the muffin molds.
5. After this, carefully place the tomato paste mixture over the eggs and top with Cheddar cheese.
6. Sprinkle the eggs with chili flakes and place in the preheated oven.
7. Cook the egg cups for 15 minutes.
8. Then check if the eggs are solid and remove them from the oven.
9. Chill the egg cups till the room temperature and gently remove from the muffin molds.

9. Dill Eggs Mix

PREP TIME 10 mins
COOK TIME 15 mins
SERVINGS 2 people

NUTRITION

Calories 185,
Fat 13.5 g,
Fiber 0.6 g,
Carbs 2.6 g,
Protein 15.4 g

INGREDIENTS

- 2 eggs
- 2 oz Feta cheese
- 1 tsp. fresh dill, chopped
- 1 tsp. butter
- ½ tsp. olive oil
- ¼ tsp. onion powder
- ¼ tsp. chili flakes

DIRECTIONS

1. Toss butter in the skillet.
2. Add olive oil and bring to boil.
3. After this, crack the eggs in the skillet.
4. Sprinkle them with chili flakes and onion powder.
5. Then preheat the oven to 360°F.
6. Transfer the skillet with eggs in the oven and cook for 10 minutes.
7. Then crumble Feta cheese and sprinkle it over the eggs.
8. Bake the eggs for 5 minutes more.

10. Hummus and Tomato Sandwich

PREP TIME
10 mins

COOK TIME
2 mins

SERVINGS
3 people

NUTRITION

Calories 269,
Fat 12.5 g,
Fiber 9.6 g,
Carbs 25.6 g,
Protein 13.4 g

INGREDIENTS

- 6 whole grain bread slices
- 1 tomato
- 3 Cheddar cheese slices
- ½ tsp. dried oregano
- 1 tsp. green chili paste
- ½ red onion, sliced
- 1 tsp. lemon juice
- 1 tbsp. hummus
- 3 lettuce leaves

DIRECTIONS

1. Slice tomato into 6 slices.
2. In the shallow bowl mix up together dried oregano, green chili paste, lemon juice, and hummus.
3. Spread 3 bread slices with the chili paste mixture.
4. After this, place the sliced tomatoes on them.
5. Add sliced onion, Cheddar cheese, and lettuce leaves.
6. Cover the lettuce leaves with the remaining bread slices to get the sandwiches.
7. Preheat the grill to 365°F.
8. Grill the sandwiches for 2 minutes.

11. Buttery Pancakes

PREP TIME
10 mins

COOK TIME
10 mins

SERVINGS
5 people

NUTRITION

Calories 152,
Fat 7.5 g,
Fiber 3.6 g,
Carbs 30.6 g,
Protein 7.4 g

INGREDIENTS

- 1 cup wheat flour, whole-grain
- 1 tsp. baking powder
- 1 tsp. lemon juice
- 3 eggs, beaten
- ¼ cup Splenda
- 1 tsp. vanilla extract
- 1/3 cup blueberries
- 1 tbsp. olive oil
- 1 tsp. butter
- 1/3 cup milk

DIRECTIONS

1. In the mixer bowl, combine together baking powder, wheat flour, lemon juice, eggs, Splenda, vanilla extract, milk, and olive oil.
2. Blend the liquid until it is smooth and homogenous.
3. After this, toss the butter in the skillet and melt it.
4. With the help of the ladle pour the pancake batter in the hot skillet and flatten it in the shape of the pancake.
5. Sprinkle the pancake with the blueberries gently and cook for 1.5 minutes over the medium heat.
6. Then flip the pancake onto another side and cook it for 30 seconds more.
7. Repeat the same steps with all remaining batter and blueberries.
8. Transfer the cooked pancakes in the serving plate.

12. Cream Olive Muffins

PREP TIME
15 mins

COOK TIME
20 mins

SERVINGS
6 people

NUTRITION

Calories 165,
Fat 10.5 g,
Fiber 1.6 g,
Carbs 11.6 g,
Protein 5.4 g

INGREDIENTS

- ½ cup quinoa, cooked
- 2 oz Feta cheese, crumbled
- 2 eggs, beaten
- 3 kalamata olives, chopped
- ¾ cup heavy cream
- 1 tomato, chopped
- 1 tsp. butter, softened
- 1 tbsp. wheat flour, whole grain
- ½ tsp. salt

DIRECTIONS

1. In the mixing bowl whisk eggs and add Feta cheese.
2. Then add chopped tomato and heavy cream.
3. After this, add wheat flour, salt, and quinoa.
4. Then add kalamata olives and mix up the ingredients with the help of the spoon.
5. Brush the muffin molds with the butter from inside.
6. Transfer quinoa mixture in the muffin molds and flatten it with the help of the spatula or spoon if needed.
7. Cook the muffins in the preheated to 355°F oven for 20 minutes.

13. Herbed Fried Eggs

PREP TIME
6 mins

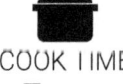
COOK TIME
7 mins

SERVINGS
2 people

NUTRITION

Calories 177,
Fat 14.5 g,
Fiber 0.6 g,
Carbs 0.6 g,
Protein 11.4 g

INGREDIENTS

- 4 eggs
- 1 tbsp. butter
- ½ tsp. chives, chopped
- ½ tsp. fresh parsley, chopped
- 1/3 tsp. fresh dill, chopped
- ¾ tsp. sea salt

DIRECTIONS

1. Toss butter in the skillet and bring it to boil.
2. Then crack the eggs in the coiled butter and sprinkle with sea salt.
3. Cook the eggs with the closed lid for 2 minutes over the medium heat.
4. Then open the lid and sprinkle them with parsley, dill, and chives.
5. Cook the eggs for 3 minutes more over the medium heat.
6. Carefully transfer the cooked meal in the plate. Use the wooden spatula for this step.

14. Chili Scramble

PREP TIME: 15 mins
COOK TIME: 15 mins
SERVINGS: 4 people

NUTRITION
Calories 177,
Fat 7.5 g,
Fiber 1.6 g,
Carbs 4.6 g,
Protein 6.4 g

INGREDIENTS
- 3 tomatoes
- 4 eggs
- ¼ tsp. of sea salt
- ½ chili pepper, chopped
- 1 tbsp. butter
- 1 cup water, for cooking

DIRECTIONS
1. Pour water in the saucepan and bring it to boil.
2. Then remove water from the heat and add tomatoes.
3. Let the tomatoes stay in the hot water for 2-3 minutes.
4. After this, remove the tomatoes from water and peel them.
5. Place butter in the pan and melt it.
6. Add chopped chili pepper and fry it for 3 minutes over the medium heat.
7. Then chop the peeled tomatoes and add into the chili peppers.
8. Cook the vegetables for 5 minutes over the medium heat. Stir them from time to time.
9. After this, add sea salt and crack the eggs
10. Stir (scramble) the eggs well with the help of the fork and cook them for 3 minutes over the medium heat.

15. Couscous and Chickpeas Bowls

PREP TIME: 10 mins
COOK TIME: 6 mins
SERVINGS: 4 people

NUTRITION
Calories 540,
Fat 10.5 g,
Fiber 9.6 g,
Carbs 51.6 g,
Protein 11.4 g

INGREDIENTS
- ¾ cup whole wheat couscous
- 1 yellow onion, chopped
- 1 tbsp. olive oil
- 1 cup water
- 2 garlic cloves, minced
- 15 oz. canned chickpeas, drained and rinsed
- A pinch of salt and black pepper
- 15 oz. canned tomatoes, chopped
- 14 oz. canned artichokes, drained and chopped
- ½ cup Greek olives, pitted and chopped
- ½ tsp. oregano, dried
- 1 tbsp. lemon juice

DIRECTIONS
1. Put the water in a pot, bring to a boil over medium heat, add the couscous, stir, take off the heat, cover the pan, leave aside for 10 minutes and fluff with a fork.
2. Heat up a pan with the oil over medium-high heat, add the onion and sauté for 2 minutes.
3. Add the rest of the ingredients, toss and cook for 4 minutes more.
4. Add the couscous, toss, divide into bowls and serve for breakfast.

16. Banana Oats

PREP TIME
10 mins

COOK TIME
0 mins

SERVINGS
2 people

INGREDIENTS

- 1 banana, peeled and sliced
- 1¾ cup almond milk
- ½ cup cold brewed coffee
- 2 dates, pitted
- 2 tbsp. cocoa powder
- 1 cup rolled oats
- 1 and ½ tbsp. chia seeds

DIRECTIONS

1. In a blender, combine the banana with the milk and the rest of the ingredients, pulse, divide into bowls and serve for breakfast.

NUTRITION

Calories 451
Fat 25.1 g,
Fiber 9.9 g,
Carbs 55.4 g,
Protein 9.3 g

17. Slow-cooked Peppers Frittata

PREP TIME
10 mins

COOK TIME
3 hours

SERVINGS
6 people

INGREDIENTS

- ½ cup almond milk
- 8 eggs, whisked
- Salt and black pepper to the taste
- 1 tsp. oregano, dried
- 1 and ½ cups roasted peppers, chopped
- ½ cup red onion, chopped
- 4 cups baby arugula
- 1 cup goat cheese, crumbled
- Cooking spray

DIRECTIONS

1. In a bowl, combine the eggs with salt, pepper and the oregano and whisk.
2. Grease your slow cooker with the cooking spray, arrange the peppers and the remaining ingredients inside and pour the eggs mixture over them.
3. Put the lid on and cook on Low for 3 hours.
4. Divide the frittata between plates and serve.

NUTRITION

Calories 259,
Fat 20.2,
Fiber 1,
Carbs 4.4,
Protein 16.3

18. Veggie Bowls

PREP TIME 10 mins
COOK TIME 5 mins
SERVINGS 4 people

NUTRITION
Calories 323, Fat 21 g, Fiber 10.9 g, Carbs 24.8 g

INGREDIENTS

- 1 tbsp. olive oil
- 1 lb. asparagus, trimmed and roughly chopped
- 3 cups kale, shredded
- 3 cups Brussels sprouts, shredded
- ½ cup hummus
- 1 avocado, peeled, pitted and sliced
- 4 eggs, soft boiled, peeled and sliced
- For the dressing:
- 2 tbsp. lemon juice
- 1 garlic clove, minced
- 2 tsp. Dijon mustard
- 2 tbsp. olive oil
- Salt and black pepper to the taste

DIRECTIONS

1. Heat up a pan with 2 tbsp. oil over medium-high heat, add the asparagus and sauté for 5 minutes stirring often.
2. In a bowl, combine the other 2 tbsp. oil with the lemon juice, garlic, mustard, salt and pepper and whisk well.
3. In a salad bowl, combine the asparagus with the kale, sprouts, hummus, avocado and the eggs and toss gently.
4. Add the dressing, toss and serve for breakfast.

19. Avocado and Apple Smoothie

PREP TIME 5 mins
COOK TIME 0 mins
SERVINGS 2 people

NUTRITION
Calories 168, Fat 10.1 g, Fiber 6 g, Carbs 21 g, Protein 2.1 g

INGREDIENTS

- 3 cups spinach
- 1 green apple, cored and chopped
- 1 avocado, peeled, pitted and chopped
- 3 tbsp. chia seeds
- 1 tsp. honey
- 1 banana, frozen and peeled
- 2 cups coconut water

DIRECTIONS

1. In your blender, combine the spinach with the apple and the rest of the ingredients, pulse, divide into glasses and serve.

20. Avocado Toast

PREP TIME
10 mins

COOK TIME
0 mins

SERVINGS
2 people

INGREDIENTS

- 1 tbsp. goat cheese, crumbled
- 1 avocado, peeled, pitted and mashed
- A pinch of salt and black pepper
- 2 whole wheat bread slices, toasted
- ½ tsp. lime juice
- 1 persimmon, thinly sliced
- 1 fennel bulb, thinly sliced
- 2 tsp. honey
- 2 tbsp. pomegranate seeds

DIRECTIONS

1. In a bowl, combine the avocado flesh with salt, pepper, lime juice and the cheese and whisk.
2. Spread this onto toasted bread slices, top each slice with the remaining ingredients and serve for breakfast.

NUTRITION

Calories 348,
Fat 20.8 g,
Fiber 12.3 g,
Carbs 38.7 g,
Protein 7.1 g

21. Mini Frittatas

PREP TIME
5 mins

COOK TIME
15 mins

SERVINGS
12 people

INGREDIENTS

- 1 yellow onion, chopped
- 1 cup parmesan, grated
- 1 yellow bell pepper, chopped
- 1 red bell pepper, chopped
- 1 zucchini, chopped
- Salt and black pepper to the taste
- 8 eggs, whisked
- A drizzle of olive oil
- 2 tbsp. chives, chopped

DIRECTIONS

1. Heat up a pan with the oil over medium-high heat, add the onion, the zucchini and the rest of the ingredients except the eggs and chives and sauté for 5 minutes stirring often.
2. Divide this mix on the bottom of a muffin pan, pour the eggs mixture on top, sprinkle salt, pepper and the chives and bake at 350°F for 10 minutes.
3. Serve the mini frittatas for breakfast right away.

NUTRITION

Calories 55,
Fat 3 g,
Fiber 0.7 g,
Carbs 3.2 g,
Protein 4.2 g

22. Berry Oats

INGREDIENTS

- ½ cup rolled oats
- 1 cup almond milk
- ¼ cup chia seeds
- A pinch of cinnamon powder
- 2 tsp. honey
- 1 cup berries, pureed
- 1 tbsp. yogurt

DIRECTIONS

1. In a bowl, combine the oats with the milk and the rest of the ingredients except the yogurt, toss, divide into bowls, top with the yogurt and serve cold for breakfast.

PREP TIME 5 mins
COOK TIME 0 mins
SERVINGS 2 people

NUTRITION
Calories 420,
Fat 30.3 g,
Fiber 7.2 g,
Carbs 35.3 g,
Protein 6.4 g

---

23. Sun-dried Tomatoes Oatmeal

INGREDIENTS

- 3 cups water
- 1 cup almond milk
- 1 tbsp. olive oil
- 1 cup steel-cut oats
- ¼ cup sun-dried tomatoes, chopped
- A pinch of red pepper flakes

DIRECTIONS

1. In a pan, mix the water with the milk, bring to a boil over medium heat.
2. Meanwhile, heat up a pan with the oil over medium-high heat, add the oats, cook them for about 2 minutes and transfer m to the pan with the milk.
3. Stir the oats, add the tomatoes and simmer over medium heat for 23 minutes.
4. Divide the mix into bowls, sprinkle the red pepper flakes on top and serve for breakfast.

PREP TIME 10 mins
COOK TIME 25 mins
SERVINGS 4 people

NUTRITION
Calories 170,
Fat 17.8 g,
Fiber 1.5 g,
Carbs 3.8 g,
Protein 1.5 g

24. Quinoa Muffins

PREP TIME: 10 mins
COOK TIME: 30 mins
SERVINGS: 12 people

NUTRITION
Calories 123,
Fat 5.6g,
Fiber 1.3 g,
Carbs 10.8 g,
Protein 7.5 g

INGREDIENTS

- 1 cup quinoa, cooked
- 6 eggs, whisked
- Salt and black pepper to the taste
- 1 cup Swiss cheese, grated
- 1 small yellow onion, chopped
- 1 cup white mushrooms, sliced
- ½ cup sun-dried tomatoes, chopped

DIRECTIONS

1. In a bowl, combine the eggs with salt, pepper and the rest of the ingredients and whisk well.
2. Divide this into a silicone muffin pan, bake at 350°F for 30 minutes and serve for breakfast.

25. Quinoa and Eggs Pan

PREP TIME: 10 mins
COOK TIME: 23 mins
SERVINGS: 4 people

NUTRITION
Calories 304,
Fat 14 g,
Fiber 3.8 g,
Carbs 27.5 g,
Protein 17.8 g

INGREDIENTS

- 4 bacon slices, cooked and crumbled
- A drizzle of olive oil
- 1 small red onion, chopped
- 1 red bell pepper, chopped
- 1 sweet potato, grated
- 1 green bell pepper, chopped
- 2 garlic cloves, minced
- 1 cup white mushrooms, sliced
- ½ cup quinoa
- 1 cup chicken stock
- 4 eggs, fried
- Salt and black pepper to the taste

DIRECTIONS

1. Heat up a pan with the oil over medium-low heat, add the onion, garlic, bell peppers, sweet potato and the mushrooms, toss and sauté for 5 minutes.
2. Add the quinoa, toss and cook for 1 more minute.
3. Add the stock, salt and pepper, stir and cook for 15 minutes.
4. Divide the mix between plates, top each serving with a fried egg, sprinkle some salt, pepper and crumbled bacon and serve for breakfast.

26. Stuffed Tomatoes

PREP TIME: 10 mins
COOK TIME: 15 mins
SERVINGS: 4 people

INGREDIENTS

- 2 tbsp. olive oil
- 8 tomatoes, insides scooped
- ¼ cup almond milk
- 8 eggs
- ¼ cup parmesan, grated
- Salt and black pepper to the taste
- 4 tbsp. rosemary, chopped

DIRECTIONS

1. Grease a pan with the oil and arrange the tomatoes inside.
2. Crack an egg in each tomato, divide the milk and the rest of the ingredients, introduce the pan in the oven and bake at 375°F for 15 minutes.
3. Serve for breakfast right away.

NUTRITION: Calories 276, Fat 20.3 g, Fiber 4.7 g, Carbs 13.2 g, Protein 13.7 g

27. Scrambled Eggs

PREP TIME: 10 mins
COOK TIME: 10 mins
SERVINGS: 2 people

INGREDIENTS

- 1 yellow bell pepper, chopped
- 8 cherry tomatoes, cubed
- 2 spring onions, chopped
- 1 tbsp. olive oil
- 1 tbsp. capers, drained
- 2 tbsp. black olives, pitted and sliced
- 4 eggs
- A pinch of salt and black pepper
- ¼ tsp. oregano, dried
- 1 tbsp. parsley, chopped

DIRECTIONS

1. Heat up a pan with the oil over medium-high heat, add the bell pepper and spring onions and sauté for 3 minutes.
2. Add the tomatoes, capers and the olives and sauté for 2 minutes more.
3. Crack the eggs into the pan, add salt, pepper and the oregano and scramble for 5 minutes more.
4. Divide the scramble between plates, sprinkle the parsley on top and serve.

NUTRITION: Calories 249, Fat 17 g, Fiber 3.2 g, Carbs 13.3 g, Protein 13.5 g

28. Watermelon "Pizza"

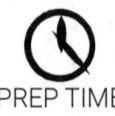
PREP TIME 10 mins

COOK TIME 0 mins

SERVINGS 4 people

NUTRITION
Calories 90,
Fat 3 g,
Fiber 1 g,
Carbs 14 g,
Protein 2 g

INGREDIENTS
- 1 watermelon slice cut 1-inch thick and then from the center cut into 4 wedges resembling pizza slices
- 6 kalamata olives, pitted and sliced
- 1 oz. feta cheese, crumbled
- ½ tbsp. balsamic vinegar
- 1 tsp. mint, chopped

DIRECTIONS
1. Arrange the watermelon "pizza" on a plate, sprinkle the olives and the rest of the ingredients on each slice and serve right away for breakfast.

29. Baked Omelet Mix

PREP TIME 10 mins

COOK TIME 45 mins

SERVINGS 12 people

NUTRITION
Calories 186,
Fat 13 g,
Fiber 1 g,
Carbs 5 g,
Protein 10 g

INGREDIENTS
- 12 eggs, whisked
- 8 oz. spinach, chopped
- 2 cups almond milk
- 12 oz. canned artichokes, chopped
- 2 garlic cloves, minced
- 5 oz. feta cheese, crumbled
- 1 tbsp. dill, chopped
- 1 tsp. oregano, dried
- 1 tsp. lemon pepper
- A pinch of salt
- 4 tsp. olive oil

DIRECTIONS
1. Heat up a pan with the oil over medium-high heat, add the garlic and the spinach and sauté for 3 minutes.
2. In a baking dish, combine the eggs with the artichokes and the rest of the ingredients.
3. Add the spinach mix as well, toss a bit, bake the mix at 375°F for 40 minutes, divide between plates and serve for breakfast.

30. Anti-Inflammatory Blueberry Smoothie

PREP TIME
5 mins

COOK TIME
5 mins

SERVINGS
1 people

NUTRITION

Calories: 340
Protein: 9 g
Fat: 13 g

INGREDIENTS

- Almond milk (1 cup)
- Frozen banana (1)
- Frozen blueberries (2/3-1 cup)
- Leafy greens/spinach (2 handfuls)
- Almond butter (1 tbsp.)
- Cinnamon (.25 tsp.)
- Cayenne pepper (.125-.25 tsp.)
- Optional: Maca powder (1 tsp.)

DIRECTIONS

1. Combine each of the fixings using a high-powered blender.
2. Mix thoroughly until creamy and serve in a chilled glass.

31. Cherry - Pomegranate Smoothie Bow - Gluten-Free & Vegetarian

PREP TIME
5 mins

COOK TIME
5 mins

SERVINGS
4 people

NUTRITION

Calories: 212
Protein: 4 g
Fat: 7 g

INGREDIENTS

- Frozen dark sweet cherries (16 oz. bag)
- 2% Plain Greek yogurt (1.5 cups)
- Pomegranate juice (.75 cup)
- 2% milk (.33 cup (+) more as needed)
- Ground cinnamon (.75 tsp.)
- Vanilla extract (1 tsp.)
- Fresh pomegranate seeds (.5 cup)
- Chopped pistachios (.5 cup)
- Ice cubes (6)

DIRECTIONS

1. Chop the pistachios or purchase (arils) found in the produce section of the market. If you are using the whole fruit, remove the seeds underwater in a container so they will float to the top.
2. Add the fixings into a blender (ice, milk, cinnamon, vanilla, juice, yogurt, and cherries).
3. Pulse until it's creamy smooth. Use a little extra milk to thin the texture to get it to the desired consistency.
4. Pour the prepared smoothie into for dishes and top with two tbsp. of the chopped pistachios and two tbsp. of the seeds. Serve it immediately.

32. Breakfast Banana Green Smoothie

PREP TIME
5 mins

COOK TIME
5 mins

SERVINGS
1 people

INGREDIENTS

- 2 cups baby spinach leaves, or to taste
- 1 banana
- 1 carrot, peeled and cut into large chunks
- ¾ cup plain Fat-free Greek yogurt, or to taste
- ¾ cup ice
- 2 tbsp. honey

DIRECTIONS

1. Put spinach, banana, carrot, yogurt, ice, and honey in a blender; blend until smooth.
2. Enjoy!

NUTRITION

Calories: 212
Protein: 4 g
Fat: 7 g

33. Strawberry Oatmeal Breakfast Smoothie

PREP TIME
5 mins

COOK TIME
5 mins

SERVINGS
2 people

INGREDIENTS

- 1 cup soy milk
- ½ cup rolled oats
- 1 banana, broken into chunks
- 14 frozen strawberries
- ½ tsp. vanilla extract
- 1 ½ tsp. white sugar

DIRECTIONS

1. In a blender, combine soy milk, oats, banana and strawberries. Add vanilla and sugar if desired. Blend until smooth.
2. Pour into glasses and serve.

NUTRITION

Calories: 232
Protein: 4 g
Fat: 5 g

34. Kale and Banana Smoothie

PREP TIME
5 mins

COOK TIME
5 mins

SERVINGS
1 people

NUTRITION

Calories: 221
Protein: 3 g
Fat: 7 g

INGREDIENTS

- 1 banana
- 2 cups chopped kale
- ½ cup light unsweetened soy milk
- 1 tbsp. flax seeds
- 1 tsp. maple syrup

DIRECTIONS

1. Place the banana, kale, soy milk, flax seeds, and maple syrup into a blender. Cover, and puree until smooth. Serve over ice.

35. Summer Stone Fruit Smoothie

PREP TIME
5 mins

COOK TIME
0 mins

SERVINGS
2 people

NUTRITION

Calories: 212
Protein: 4 g
Fat: 7 g

INGREDIENTS

- ½ cup Greek yogurt
- 1 plum, pit removed, flesh roughly chopped
- 1 peach, pit removed, flesh roughly chopped
- 1 nectarine, pit removed, flesh roughly chopped
- ½ cup blueberries, fresh or frozen

DIRECTIONS

1. Combine all ingredients in blender and blend until smooth.
2. Enjoy!

36. Pumpkin Pie Fall Smoothie

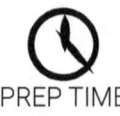
PREP TIME
5 mins

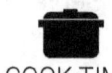
COOK TIME
0 mins

SERVINGS
3 people

NUTRITION

Calories: 231
Protein: 4 g
Fat: 6 g

INGREDIENTS

- 1 cup almond milk
- 1 tsp. agave syrup
- 1 cup pumpkin puree
- 2 tsp. cinnamon
- 1 apple, cored
- Dried cranberries

DIRECTIONS

1. Combine all ingredients except cranberries in blender and blend until smooth.
2. Top with cranberries and enjoy.

37. Green Tart Smoothie

PREP TIME
5 mins

COOK TIME
5 mins

SERVINGS
1 people

NUTRITION

Calories: 214
Protein: 4 g
Fat: 7 g

INGREDIENTS

- 2 cups fresh kale
- 1 cup water
- 2 large stalks of celery, chopped
- ½ cucumber, chopped
- 1/3 grapefruit
- 1 cup frozen pineapple

DIRECTIONS

1. Blend kale and water until smooth.
2. Add remaining ingredients, and blend until smooth.
3. Enjoy!

38. Coconut Milk Smoothie

PREP TIME 10 mins
COOK TIME 0 mins
SERVINGS 1 people

INGREDIENTS

- 1 1/2 cups coconut milk
- 1 frozen banana
- 2 cups raw baby spinach

DIRECTIONS

1. Add everything to a food processor.
2. Blend the ingredients well until smooth.
3. Refrigerate until chilled enough.
4. Serve with your favorite garnish

NUTRITION

Calories: 212
Protein: 4 g
Fat: 7 g

39. Creamy Strawberry Smoothie

PREP TIME 10 mins
COOK TIME 0 mins
SERVINGS 1 people

INGREDIENTS

- 1 banana
- 1/2 cup frozen strawberries
- 1/2 cup frozen mango
- 1/2 cup Greek yogurt
- 1/4 cup coconut milk
- 1/4 tsp. turmeric
- 1/4 tsp. ginger
- 1 tbsp. honey

DIRECTIONS

1. Add everything to a food processor.
2. Blend the ingredients well until smooth.
3. Refrigerate until chilled enough.
4. Serve with your favorite garnish

NUTRITION

Calories: 237
Protein: 4 g
Fat: 3 g

ANTIPASTI, TAPAS, MEZE AND STARTER

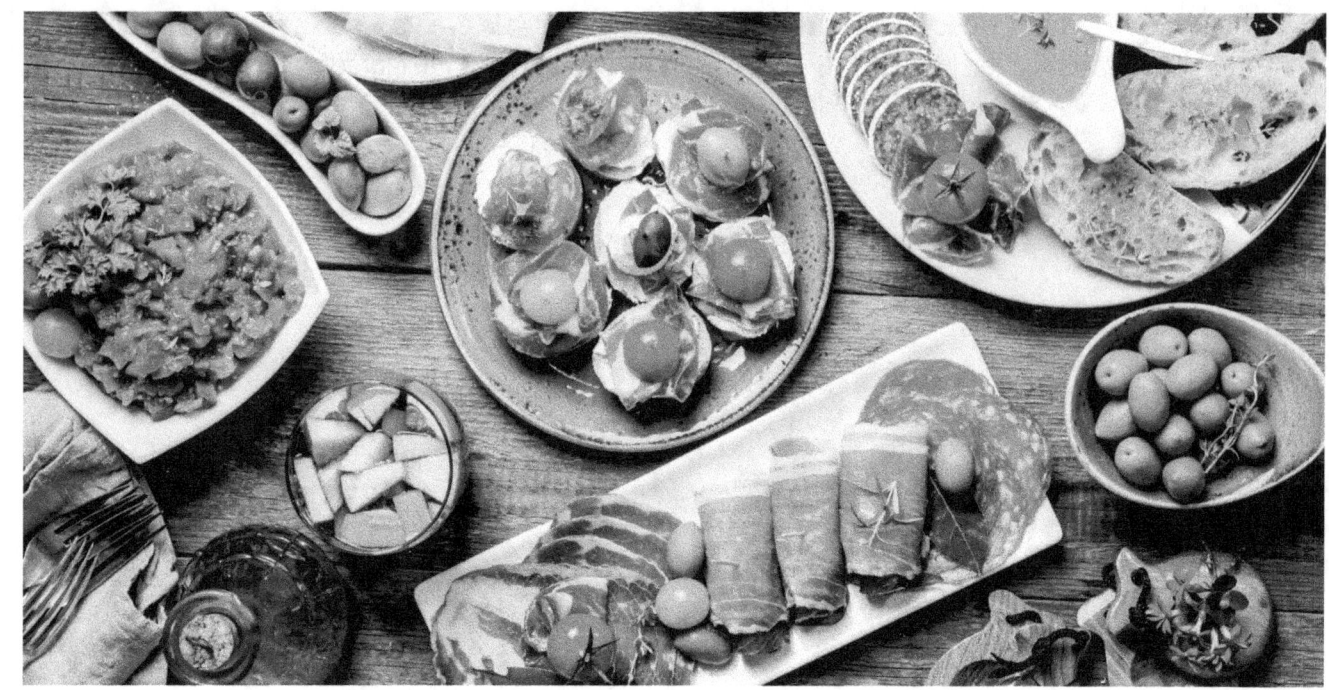

40. Cheddar Potato Crisps

PREP TIME
10 mins

COOK TIME
0 mins

SERVINGS
4 people

NUTRITION

Calories – 494
Fat – 18g
Carbs – 46g
Fiber – 9g
Protein – 24g

INGREDIENTS

- 1 cup Greek yogurt (unsweetened)
- 1/2 cup grated cheddar cheese
- 6 red potatoes, thinly sliced
- 1/2 cup chives
- 3 slices ham
- Cooking oil or spray as required
- Salt and black pepper to taste

DIRECTIONS

1. Take the potatoes; sprinkle with salt and black pepper.
2. Cover and place in the refrigerator for 30 minutes.
3. Heat a grill at medium temperature setting.
4. Spray the potato slices with cooking oil, place over a baking sheet and grill for about 2 minutes.
5. Flip and grill for 2 more minutes. Add the ham slices to the baking sheet and grill for one minute.
6. Add the potato and ham in a serving bowl. Top with the chives, yogurt and grated cheese as desired.

41. Stuffed Sweet Potato

PREP TIME
10 mins

COOK TIME
40 mins

SERVINGS
8 people

NUTRITION

Calories 308,
Fat 2 g,
Fiber 8 g,
Carbs 38 g,
Protein 7 g

INGREDIENTS

- 8 sweet potatoes, pierced with a fork
- 14 oz. canned chickpeas, drained and rinsed
- 1 small red bell pepper, chopped
- 1 tbsp. lemon zest, grated
- 2 tbsp. lemon juice
- 3 tbsp. olive oil
- 1 tsp. garlic, minced
- 1 tbsp. oregano, chopped
- 2 tbsp. parsley, chopped
- A pinch of salt and black pepper
- 1 avocado, peeled, pitted and mashed
- ¼ cup water
- ¼ cup tahini paste

DIRECTIONS

1. Arrange the potatoes on a baking sheet lined with parchment paper, bake them at 400°F for 40 minutes, cool them down and cut a slit down the middle in each.
2. In a bowl, combine the chickpeas with the bell pepper, lemon zest, half of the lemon juice, half of the oil, half of the garlic, oregano, half of the parsley, salt and pepper, toss and stuff the potatoes with this mix.
3. In another bowl, mix the avocado with the water, tahini, the rest of the lemon juice, oil, garlic and parsley, whisk well and spread over the potatoes.
4. Serve cold for breakfast.

42. Rosemary Bulgur Appetizer

PREP TIME
25 mins

COOK TIME
0 mins

SERVINGS
6 people

NUTRITION

Calories – 182
Fat – 6g
Carbs – 28g
Fiber – 4g|
Protein – 8g

INGREDIENTS

- ½ cup couscous
- 2 tbsp. olive oil
- 1 ¾ cup onions, chopped
- 2 cups vegetable broth
- 1 cup bulgur
- 1 tbsp. chives, chopped
- 1 tbsp. parsley, chopped
- ¼ tsp. rosemary, chopped

DIRECTIONS

1. Over medium stove flame; heat the oil in a skillet or saucepan (preferably medium size).
2. Sauté the onions until softened and translucent, stir in between.
3. Add the bulgur and 1 ½ cups vegetable broth; simmer the mixture until the bulgur is tender.
4. Remove it from the heat and fluff with a fork.
5. In another skillet or saucepan, heat the remaining vegetable broth and simmer. Add the oil and couscous. Stir and cook this until your couscous is tender. Fluff it with a fork.
6. In a mixing bowl, combine the bulgur and couscous. Add the rosemary, chives and parsley on top. Season it with black pepper and salt.
7. Serve as an appetizer or light meal.

43. Cauliflower Fritters

PREP TIME
10 mins

COOK TIME
50 mins

SERVINGS
4 people

NUTRITION

Calories 333,
Fat 12.6 g,
Fiber 12.8 g,
Carbs 44.7 g,
Protein 13.6 g

INGREDIENTS

- 30 oz. canned chickpeas, drained and rinsed
- 2 and ½ tbsp. olive oil
- 1 small yellow onion, chopped
- 2 cups cauliflower florets chopped
- 2 tbsp. garlic, minced
- A pinch of salt and black pepper

DIRECTIONS

1. Spread half of the chickpeas on a baking sheet lined with parchment pepper, add 1 tbsp. oil, season with salt and pepper, toss and bake at 400°F for 30 minutes.
2. Transfer the chickpeas to a food processor, pulse well and put the mix into a bowl.
3. Heat up a pan with the ½ tbsp. oil over medium-high heat, add the garlic and the onion and sauté for 3 minutes.
4. Add the cauliflower, cook for 6 minutes more, transfer this to a blender, add the rest of the chickpeas, pulse, pour over the crispy chickpeas mix from the bowl, stir and shape medium fritters out of this mix.
5. Heat up a pan with the rest of the oil over medium-high heat, add the fritters, cook them for 3 minutes on each side and serve for breakfast.

44. Mediterranean Chickpea Snack

PREP TIME
30 mins

COOK TIME
0 mins

SERVINGS
2 people

NUTRITION

Calories – 321
Fat – 8g
Carbs – 42g
Fiber – 12g
Protein – 22g

INGREDIENTS

- ½ tsp. garlic powder
- 1 can (10 oz.) chickpeas, rinsed and drained
- ½ tsp. dried basil
- 1 tsp. extra-virgin olive oil
- ¼ tsp. sea salt
- 1 tsp. Nutritional Yeast
- ¼ tsp. red pepper flakes

DIRECTIONS

1. Preheat the oven to 450°F. Line a baking pan with a parchment paper. Grease it with some refined coconut oil or avocado oil (You can also use cooking spray)
2. Combine the chickpeas, seasonings, and oil in a mixing bowl.
3. Arrange the chickpeas in the pan. Roast the chickpeas for about 10 minutes. Toss and keep roasting for 10 more minutes.
4. Serve warm.

45. Avocado Chickpea Pizza

PREP TIME 20 mins
COOK TIME 20 mins
SERVINGS 2 people

NUTRITION
Calories 416,
Fat 24.5 g,
Fiber 9.6 g,
Carbs 36.6 g,
Protein 15.4 g

INGREDIENTS

- 1 and ¼ cups chickpea flour
- A pinch of salt and black pepper
- 1 and ¼ cups water
- 2 tbsp. olive oil
- 1 tsp. onion powder
- 1 tsp. garlic, minced
- 1 tomato, sliced
- 1 avocado, peeled, pitted and sliced
- 2 oz. gouda, sliced
- ¼ cup tomato sauce
- 2 tbsp. green onions, chopped

DIRECTIONS

1. In a bowl, mix the chickpea flour with salt, pepper, water, the oil, onion powder and the garlic, stir well until you obtain a dough, knead a bit, put in a bowl, cover and leave aside for 20 minutes.
2. Transfer the dough to a working surface, shape a bit circle, transfer it to a baking sheet lined with parchment paper and bake at 425°F for 10 minutes.
3. Spread the tomato sauce over the pizza, also spread the rest of the ingredients and bake at 400°F for 10 minutes more.
4. Cut and serve for breakfast.

46. Pita Wedges with Almond Bean Dip

PREP TIME 10 mins
COOK TIME 10 mins
SERVINGS 5 people

NUTRITION
Calories – 356
Fat – 21g
Carbs – 23g
Fiber – 6g
Protein – 6g

INGREDIENTS

- 8 oz. beet, cubed
- 5 garlic cloves, peeled
- ¼ cup almond, slivered
- 15 ½ oz. garbanzo beans
- ¾ cup extra-virgin olive oil
- 1 ½ tbsp. red wine vinegar
- Whole-wheat pita wedges to serve

DIRECTIONS

1. In a saucepan or deep skillet, boil the beet in sufficient quantity of water until it is tender. Drain, peel, cut in cubes and blend in a food processor.
2. Add the garbanzo beans, almonds, oil, and garlic and blend everything well until smooth. Add the red wine and blend for one more minute.
3. Season with black pepper and salt. Chill in the refrigerator. Serve with pita wedges.

47. Ginger Antipasti

PREP TIME
10 mins

COOK TIME
0 mins

SERVINGS
6 people

INGREDIENTS

- 1 tsp. ginger powder
- 1 cup fresh parsley, chopped
- 1 tbsp. apple cider vinegar
- 3 tbsp. avocado oil
- 2 oz celery stalk, chopped

DIRECTIONS

1. Mix all ingredients in the bowl and leave for 5 minutes in the fridge.

NUTRITION

Calories 16g
Protein 0.5g
Carbs 1.5g
Fat 1g

48. Mediterranean Chickpea Spread

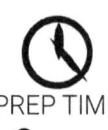
PREP TIME
8 mins

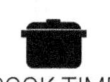
COOK TIME
5 mins

SERVINGS
2 people

INGREDIENTS

- 2 cups chickpeas (canned or pre-soaked and cooked)
- 2 tbsp. lemon juice
- 1/2 tsp. cumin
- 2 cloves garlic, minced
- 4 tsp. olive oil
- Salt to taste
- Ground cinnamon (optional)

DIRECTIONS

1. In a mixing bowl, add the chickpeas; mash thoroughly using a fork (you can also use a blender).
2. Add the olive oil, garlic and lemon juice. Combine well; top with some cinnamon.
3. Serve with vegetable sticks, whole-wheat crackers, or whole-wheat pita wedges.

NUTRITION

Calories – 412
Fat – 11g
Carbs – 34g
Fiber – 14g
Protein – 20g

49. Rosemary Beets

PREP TIME 10 mins
COOK TIME 4 mins
SERVINGS 6 people

INGREDIENTS

- 1-lb. beets, sliced, peeled
- 2 tbsp. lemon juice
- 1 tsp. dried rosemary
- ¼ tsp. garlic powder
- 1 tbsp. olive oil

DIRECTIONS

1. Sprinkle the beets with lemon juice, rosemary, garlic powder, and olive oil.
2. Then preheat the grill to 400°F.
3. Place the sliced beet in the grill and cook it for 2 minutes per side.

NUTRITION

56 Calories
1.3g Protein
7.9g Carbs
2.5g Fat
1.6g Fiber

50. Scallions Dip

PREP TIME 5 mins
COOK TIME 15 mins
SERVINGS 4 people

INGREDIENTS

- 1 cup spinach, chopped
- 2 oz scallions, chopped
- ¼ cup plain yogurt
- ¼ tsp. chili powder
- 1 tsp. olive oil

DIRECTIONS

1. Melt the olive oil in the saucepan.
2. Add spinach and scallions.
3. Saute the greens for 10 minutes.
4. Then add chili powder and plain yogurt. Stir well and cook it for 5 minutes more.
5. Then blend the mixture with the help of the immersion blender.

NUTRITION

27 Calories
1.4g Protein
2.5g Carbs
1.4g Fat
0.6g Fiber

51. Dill Tapas

PREP TIME
5 mins

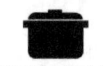
COOK TIME
0 mins

SERVINGS
8 people

NUTRITION

77 Calories
4.5g Protein
6.7g Carbs
3.4g Fat
0.8g Fiber

INGREDIENTS

- ½ tsp. garlic powder
- 2 cups plain yogurt
- ½ cup dill, chopped
- ¼ tsp. ground black pepper
- 2 pecans, chopped
- 2 tbsp. lemon juice

DIRECTIONS

1. Put all ingredients in the bowl and stir well with the help of the spoon.

52. Sour Cream Dip

PREP TIME
10 mins

COOK TIME
0 mins

SERVINGS
8 people

NUTRITION

138 Calories
1.4g Protein
5g Carbs
13.4g Fat
3.4g Fiber

INGREDIENTS

- 4 oz yogurt
- ¼ tsp. chili flakes
- ¼ tsp. salt
- 2 avocados, peeled, pitted
- 1 tsp. olive oil
- ½ tsp. lemon juice
- 2 tbsp. fresh parsley, chopped

DIRECTIONS

1. Put all ingredients in the blender and blend until smooth.
2. Store the dip in the closed vessel in the fridge for up to 5 days.

53. Arugula Antipasti

INGREDIENTS

- 2 oz chives, chopped
- 1 cup arugula, chopped
- 2 cups chickpeas, canned
- 1 jalapeno pepper, chopped
- 1 tbsp. avocado oil
- 1 tsp. lemon juice

DIRECTIONS

1. Put all ingredients in the bowl and stir well.

PREP TIME 5 mins
COOK TIME 0 mins
SERVINGS 8 people

NUTRITION

188 Calories
10g Protein
30.9g Carbs
3.3g Fat
9.1g Fiber

---

54. Goat Cheese Dip

INGREDIENTS

- 3 oz goats cheese, soft
- 2 oz plain yogurt
- 2 oz chives, chopped
- 1 tbsp. lemon juice
- ¼ tsp. ground black pepper
- 2 bell peppers

DIRECTIONS

1. Grill the bell peppers for 3-4 minutes per side.
2. Then peel the peppers and remove seeds.
3. Then put bell peppers in the blender.
4. Add all remaining ingredients, blend them well and transfer in the ramekins.

PREP TIME 10 mins
COOK TIME 8 mins
SERVINGS 4 people

NUTRITION

92 Calories
5.9g Protein
6.5g Carbs
4.9g Fat
1.2g Fiber

55. Mozzarella Dip

PREP TIME
10 mins

COOK TIME
20 mins

SERVINGS
10 people

NUTRITION

46 Calories
2.5g Protein
5.4g Carbs
2.2g Fat
2.6g Fiber

INGREDIENTS

- 1-lb. artichoke hearts, diced
- ¾ cup spinach, chopped
- 1 cup mozzarella cheese, grated
- 1 tsp. Italian seasonings
- ½ tsp. garlic powder
- ¼ cup organic almond milk

DIRECTIONS

1. Put all ingredients in the saucepan, stir well, and close the lid.
2. Saute the meal on low heat for 20 minutes. Stir it from time to time.
3. Then chill the dip well.

56. Spicy Salsa

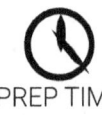
PREP TIME
40 mins

COOK TIME
0 mins

SERVINGS
16 people

NUTRITION

16 Calories
0.4g Protein
1.8g Carbs
1g Fat
0.6g Fiber

INGREDIENTS

- 3 cups tomatoes, chopped
- 1 tsp. salt
- 1 tsp. white pepper
- ½ cup red onion, chopped
- 1 cup fresh cilantro, chopped
- 1 jalapeno pepper, chopped
- 1 tbsp. olive oil
- 1 tbsp. apple cider vinegar

DIRECTIONS

1. Put all ingredients in the salad bowl and mix well.
2. Leave the cooked salsa for 30 minutes in the fridge.

57. Cheese Spread

PREP TIME
10 mins

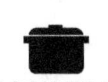
COOK TIME
8 mins

SERVINGS
6 people

INGREDIENTS

- ½ cup cream cheese
- 1 pickle, grated
- 1 oz fresh dill, chopped
- ¼ tsp. ground paprika

DIRECTIONS

1. Carefully mix cream cheese with dill and ground paprika.
2. Then add a grated pickle and gently mix the spread.

NUTRITION

81 Calories
2.5g Protein
3.4g Carbs
7g Fat
0.8g Fiber

58. Prosciutto Beans

PREP TIME
10 mins

COOK TIME
0 mins

SERVINGS
8 people

INGREDIENTS

- 2 cups canned cannellini beans, drained
- 1 tbsp. scallions, diced
- 3 tbsp. olive oil
- ¼ tsp. chili flakes
- 1 tbsp. lemon juice
- 3 oz beef, chopped, cooked

DIRECTIONS

1. Put all ingredients in the bowl and stir well.

NUTRITION

219 Calories
14.1g Protein
27.7g Carbs
6.3g Fat
11.5g Fiber

59. Carrot Chips

PREP TIME
5 mins

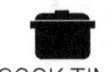
COOK TIME
10 mins

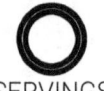
SERVINGS
6 people

INGREDIENTS

- 2 carrots, thinly sliced
- 1 tsp. salt
- 1 tsp. olive oil

DIRECTIONS

1. Line the baking tray with baking paper.
2. Then arrange the sliced carrot in one layer.
3. Sprinkle the vegetables with olive oil and salt.
4. Bake the carrot chips for 10 minutes or until the vegetables are crunchy.

NUTRITION

15 Calories
0.2g Protein
2g Carbs
0.8g Fat
0.5g Fiber

60. Antipasti Salad

PREP TIME
10 mins

COOK TIME
0 mins

SERVINGS
4 people

INGREDIENTS

- ½ cup green olives, pitted and sliced
- 1 cucumber, spiralized
- 1 cup cherry tomatoes, halved
- 4 oz Feta cheese, crumbled
- 2 tbsp. olive oil

DIRECTIONS

1. Put green olives, spiralized cucumber, and cherry tomatoes in the bowl.
2. Add olive oil and stir well.
3. Then top the salad with Feta.

NUTRITION

185 Calories
4.9g Protein
6.9g Carbs
16.3g Fat
0.9g Fiber

61. Black Olives Spread

INGREDIENTS

- 3 cups black olives, pitted
- ½ cup chickpeas, canned
- 1 tsp. Italian seasonings
- 3 tbsp. sunflower oil
- ½ tsp. ground black pepper

DIRECTIONS

1. Put all ingredients in the blender and blend until smooth.

PREP TIME 10 mins
COOK TIME 0 mins
SERVINGS 10 people

NUTRITION

122 Calories
2.3g Protein
8.7g Carbs
9.3g Fat
3.1g Fiber

62. Bell Pepper Antipasti

INGREDIENTS

- 5 bell peppers
- 1 tbsp. olive oil
- 3 tbsp. avocado oil
- ½ tsp. salt
- 2 garlic cloves, minced
- 3 tbsp. fresh cilantro, chopped

DIRECTIONS

1. Pierce the bell peppers with the help of a knife and sprinkle with olive oil.
2. Grill the vegetables at 400F for 2 minutes per side.
3. Then peel them and remove seeds.
4. Put the grilled bell peppers in the blender and add all remaining ingredients.
5. Blend the mixture well.

PREP TIME 10 mins
COOK TIME 4 mins
SERVINGS 6 people

NUTRITION

63 Calories
1.2g Protein
8.2g Carbs
3.5g Fat
1.7g Fiber

63. Hummus Rings

PREP TIME
10 mins

COOK TIME
0 mins

SERVINGS
4 people

INGREDIENTS

- ½ cup hummus
- 2 cucumbers

DIRECTIONS

1. Roughly slice the cucumbers and remove the cucumber flesh.
2. Then fill every cucumber ring with hummus.

NUTRITION

74 Calories
3.5g Protein
9.9g Carbs
3.2g Fat
2.6g Fiber

64. Fish Strips

PREP TIME
10 mins

COOK TIME
0 mins

SERVINGS
4 people

INGREDIENTS

- 1 cucumber, sliced
- 1 tsp. apple cider vinegar
- 2 tbsp. plain yogurt
- 1 tsp. dried dill
- 3 oz salmon, smoked, sliced

DIRECTIONS

1. Arrange the sliced cucumber in the plate in one layer.
2. Then sprinkle them with apple cider vinegar, plain yogurt, and dried dill.
3. Then top the cucumbers with sliced salmon.

NUTRITION

35 Calories
4.6g Protein
0.8 Carbs
1.4g Fat
0.1g Fiber

65. Vegetable Balls

PREP TIME
10 mins

COOK TIME
5 mins

SERVINGS
8 people

INGREDIENTS

- 2 eggplants, grilled
- 2 tbsp. olive oil
- 1 garlic clove, minced
- 1 egg, beaten
- ½ cup oatmeal, ground
- ½ tsp. ground black pepper
- 2 oz Parmesan, grated

DIRECTIONS

1. Blend the eggplants until smooth.
2. Then mix up blended eggplants with garlic, egg, oatmeal, ground black pepper, and Parmesan.
3. Make the small balls.
4. Heat the skillet with olive oil and put the eggplant balls inside.
5. Roast them for on high heat for 1 minute per side.

NUTRITION

115 Calories
5g Protein,
2g Carbs
6.2g Fat
5.4g Fiber

66. Italian Style Eggplant Chips

PREP TIME
10 mins

COOK TIME
5 mins

SERVINGS
10 people

INGREDIENTS

- 2 eggplants, thinly sliced
- 1 tsp. ground black pepper
- 1 tsp. Italian seasonings
- 1 tbsp. olive oil

DIRECTIONS

1. Rub the eggplant sliced with ground black pepper and Italian seasonings.
2. Then sprinkle the vegetable sliced with olive oil.
3. Grill the eggplant sliced for 2 minutes per side at 400F or until the vegetables are crunchy.

NUTRITION

41 Calories
1.1g Protein
6.6g Carbs
1.8g Fat
3.9g Fiber

67. Lentil Dip

PREP TIME
10 mins

COOK TIME
0 mins

SERVINGS
7 people

NUTRITION

131 Calories
9.8g Protein
17.1g Carbs
2.7g Fat
8.5g Fiber

INGREDIENTS

- 1 cup green lentils, cooked
- 1 tbsp. apple cider vinegar
- 1 tomato, chopped
- 1 tsp. olive oil
- 2 oz Parmesan, grated

DIRECTIONS

1. Mix up all ingredients in the bowl and blend gently with the help of the immersion blender.

68. Cheese Baby Potatoes

PREP TIME
10 mins

COOK TIME
20 mins

SERVINGS
2 people

NUTRITION

136 Calories
7.7g Protein
4.5g Carbs
9.7g Fat
0.4g Fiber

INGREDIENTS

- 4 baby potatoes
- 2 oz Cheddar cheese, shredded
- ¼ tsp. garlic powder
- 1 tsp. avocado oil

DIRECTIONS

1. Cut the baby potatoes into halves and sprinkle with garlic powder and avocado oil.
2. Bake the potatoes for 10 minutes at 365F.
3. Then top them with Cheddar cheese and bake for 10 minutes more.

69. Tuna Paste

INGREDIENTS

- 7 oz tuna, canned
- 2 tbsp. cream cheese
- 1 tbsp. chives, chopped

DIRECTIONS

1. Put all ingredients in the bowl and stir well with the help of the fork.

PREP TIME: 5 mins
COOK TIME: 0 mins
SERVINGS: 6 people

NUTRITION

73 Calories
9g Protein
0.1g Carbs
3.8g Fat
0g Fiber

70. Zucchini Chips

INGREDIENTS

- 2 zucchinis, thinly sliced
- 1 oz Parmesan, grated

DIRECTIONS

1. Line the baking tray with baking paper.
2. Put the zucchini in the tray in one layer and top with Parmesan.
3. Bake the chips for 12 minutes at 375F.

PREP TIME: 5 mins
COOK TIME: 12 mins
SERVINGS: 10 people

NUTRITION

15 Calories
1.4g Protein
1.4g Carbs
0.7g Fat
0.4g Fiber

71. Crunchy Chickpeas

PREP TIME
5 mins

COOK TIME
10 mins

SERVINGS
2 people

INGREDIENTS

- ¼ cup chickpeas, canned
- 1 tbsp. avocado oil
- 1 tsp. ground paprika

DIRECTIONS

1. Line the baking tray with baking paper.
2. Mix up chickpeas with ground paprika and avocado oil and transfer the mixture in the tray. Flatten it gently.
3. Bake the chickpeas for 10 minutes at 400F. Stir them every 2 minutes.

NUTRITION

103 Calories
5.1g Protein
16.1g Carbs
2.5g Fat
5.1g Fiber

---

72. Stuffed Dates

PREP TIME
5 mins

COOK TIME
0 mins

SERVINGS
4 people

INGREDIENTS

- 4 dates, pitted
- 4 walnuts

DIRECTIONS

1. Fill the dates with walnuts.

NUTRITION

75 Calories
1.5g Protein
7g Carbs
5g Fat
1.4g Fiber

73. Almond Gazpacho

PREP TIME 15 mins
COOK TIME 0 mins
SERVINGS 4 people

INGREDIENTS
- ½ cup almonds
- 1 cup cucumbers, chopped
- ½ tsp. minced garlic
- 3 oz water, warm
- 2 oz chives, chopped
- 1 tbsp. sunflower oil
- ¼ cup fresh dill, chopped
- ¼ cup plain yogurt

DIRECTIONS
1. Put all ingredients in the blender and blend until smooth.
2. Cool the cooked gazpacho in the fridge for 10-15 minutes.

NUTRITION
127 Calories
4.6g Protein
7g Carbs
9.9g Fat
2.4g Fiber

74. Turkey Chowder

PREP TIME 5 mins
COOK TIME 20 mins
SERVINGS 2 people

INGREDIENTS
- ½ cup ground turkey
- ¼ cup leek, chopped
- 1 tsp. dried rosemary
- 1 cup of water
- 1 cup plain yogurt
- 1 tsp. olive oil

DIRECTIONS
1. Roast the ground turkey with olive oil in the pan for 10 minutes. Stir well.
2. Then add all remaining ingredients and close the lid.
3. Cook the chowder for 10 minutes more on the medium heat.

NUTRITION
277 Calories
29.8g Protein
10.6g Carbs
13g Fat
0.5g Fiber

PASTA AND COUSCOUS

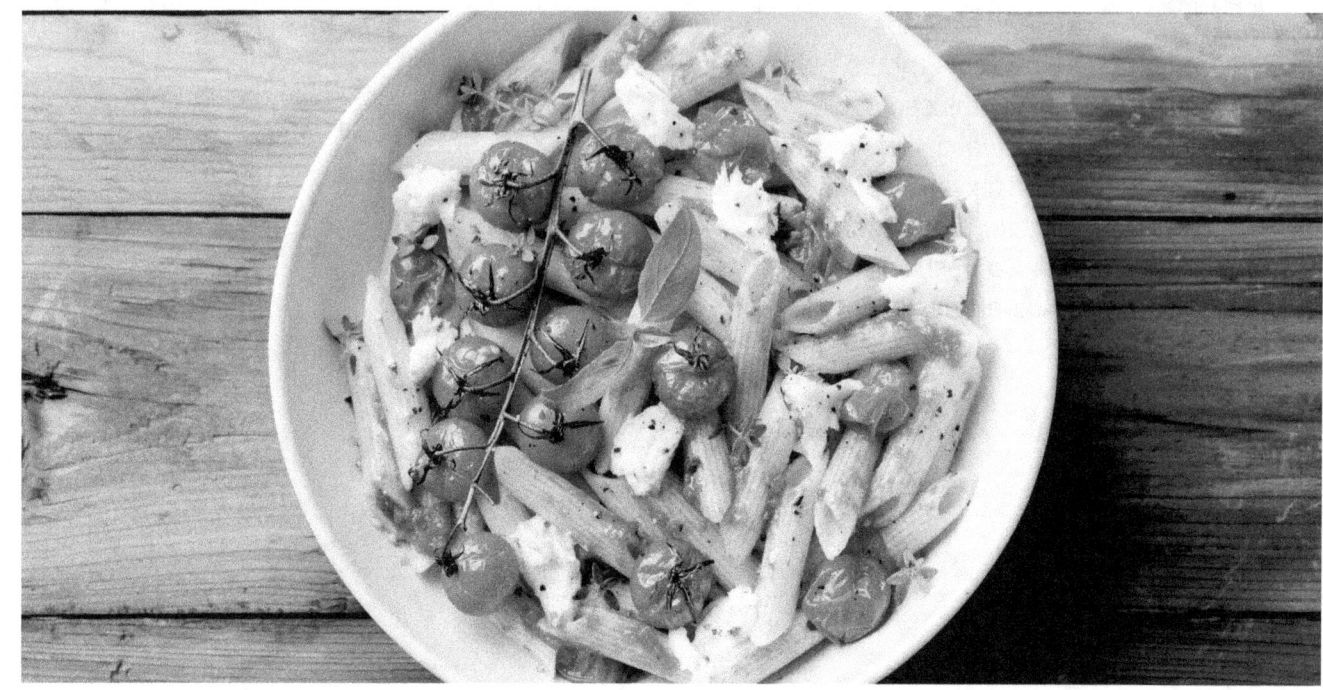

75. Herb-Topped Focaccia

PREP TIME
20 mins

COOK TIME
2 hours

SERVINGS
10 people

NUTRITION

Calories: 53;
Protein: 12.3g;
Carbs: 3.4g;
Fat: 6.3g

INGREDIENTS

- 1 tbsp. dried rosemary or 3 tbsp. minced fresh rosemary
- 1 tbsp. dried thyme or 3 tbsp. minced fresh thyme leaves
- ½ cup extra-virgin olive oil
- 1 tsp. sugar
- 1 cup warm water
- 1 (¼-oz.) packet active dry yeast
- 2½ cups flour, divided
- 1 tsp. salt

DIRECTIONS

1. In a small bowl, combine the rosemary and thyme with the olive oil.
2. In a large bowl, whisk together the sugar, water, and yeast. Let stand for 5 minutes.
3. Add 1 cup of flour, half of the olive oil mixture, and the salt to the mixture in the large bowl. Stir to combine.
4. Add the remaining 1½ cups flour to the large bowl. Using your hands, combine dough until it starts to pull away from the sides of the bowl.
5. Put the dough on a floured board or countertop and knead 10 to 12 times. Place the dough in a well-oiled bowl and cover with plastic wrap. Put it in a warm, dry space for 1 hour.
6. Oil a 9-by-13-inch baking pan. Turn the dough onto the baking pan, and using your hands gently push the dough out to fit the pan.
7. Using your fingers, make dimples into the dough. Evenly pour the remaining half of the olive oil mixture over the dough. Let the dough rise for another 30 minutes.
8. Preheat the oven to 450°F. Place the dough into the oven and let cook for 18 to 20 minutes, until you see it turn a golden brown.

76. Caramelized Onion Flatbread with Arugula

PREP TIME: 10 mins
COOK TIME: 25 mins
SERVINGS: 4 people

NUTRITION
Calories: 63;
Protein: 12.3g;
Carbs: 3.4g;
Fat: 6.3g

INGREDIENTS
- 4 tbsp. extra-virgin olive oil, divided
- 2 large onions, sliced into ¼-inch-thick slices
- 1 tsp. salt, divided
- 1 sheet puff pastry
- 1 (5-oz.) package goat cheese
- 8 oz. arugula
- ½ tsp. freshly ground black pepper

DIRECTIONS
1. Preheat the oven to 400°F.
2. In a large skillet over medium heat, cook 3 tbsp. olive oil, the onions, and ½ tsp. of salt, stirring, for 10 to 12 minutes, until the onions are translucent and golden brown.
3. To assemble, line a baking sheet with parchment paper. Lay the puff pastry flat on the parchment paper. Prick the middle of the puff pastry all over with a fork, leaving a ½-inch border.
4. Evenly distribute the onions on the pastry, leaving the border.
5. Crumble the goat cheese over the onions. Put the pastry in the oven to bake for 10 to 12 minutes, or until you see the border become golden brown.
6. Remove the pastry from the oven, set aside. In a medium bowl, add the arugula, remaining 1 tbsp. of olive oil, remaining ½ tsp. of salt, and ½ tsp. black pepper; toss to evenly dress the arugula.
7. Cut the pastry into even squares. Top the pastry with dressed arugula and serve.

77. Quick Shrimp Fettuccine

PREP TIME: 10 mins
COOK TIME: 10 mins
SERVINGS: 4 people

NUTRITION
Calories: 83;
Protein: 12.3g;
Carbs: 3.4g;
Fat: 6.3g

INGREDIENTS
- 8 oz. fettuccine pasta
- ¼ cup extra-virgin olive oil
- 3 tbsp. garlic, minced
- 1 lb. large shrimp (21-25), peeled and deveined
- 1/3 cup lemon juice
- 1 tbsp. lemon zest
- ½ tsp. salt
- ½ tsp. freshly ground black pepper

DIRECTIONS
1. Bring a large pot of salted water to a boil. Add the fettuccine and cook for 8 minutes.
2. In a large saucepan over medium heat, cook the olive oil and garlic for 1 minute.
3. Add the shrimp to the saucepan and cook for 3 minutes on each side. Remove the shrimp from the pan and set aside.
4. Add the lemon juice and lemon zest to the saucepan, along with the salt and pepper.
5. Reserve ½ cup of the pasta water and drain the pasta.
6. Add the pasta water to the saucepan with the lemon juice and zest and stir everything together. Add the pasta and toss together to evenly coat the pasta. Transfer the pasta to a serving dish and top with the cooked shrimp. Serve warm.

78. Simple Pesto Pasta

PREP TIME
10 mins

COOK TIME
10 mins

SERVINGS
4 people

NUTRITION

Calories: 113;
Protein: 12.3g;
Carbs: 3.4g;
Fat: 6.3g

INGREDIENTS

- 1 lb. spaghetti
- 4 cups fresh basil leaves, stems removed
- 3 cloves garlic
- 1 tsp. salt
- ½ tsp. freshly ground black pepper
- ¼ cup lemon juice
- ½ cup pine nuts, toasted
- ½ cup grated Parmesan cheese
- 1 cup extra-virgin olive oil

DIRECTIONS

1. Bring a large pot of salted water to a boil. Add the spaghetti to the pot and cook for 8 minutes.
2. Put basil, garlic, salt, pepper, lemon juice, pine nuts, and Parmesan cheese in a food processor bowl with chopping blade and purée.
3. While the processor is running, slowly drizzle the olive oil through the top opening. Process until all the olive oil has been added.
4. Reserve ½ cup of the pasta water. Drain the pasta and put it into a bowl. Immediately add the pesto and pasta water to the pasta and toss everything together. Serve warm.

79. Flat Meat Pies

PREP TIME
20 mins

COOK TIME
15 mins

SERVINGS
4 people

NUTRITION

Calories: 53;
Protein: 12.3g;
Carbs: 3.4g;
Fat: 6.3g

INGREDIENTS

- ½ lb. ground beef
- 1 small onion, finely chopped
- 1 medium tomato, finely diced and strained
- ½ tsp. salt
- ½ tsp. freshly ground black pepper
- 2 sheets puff pastry

DIRECTIONS

1. Preheat the oven to 400°F.
2. In a medium bowl, combine the beef, onion, tomato, salt, and pepper. Set aside.
3. Line 2 baking sheets with parchment paper. Cut the puff pastry dough into 4-inch squares and lay them flat on the baking sheets.
4. Scoop about 2 tbsp. of beef mixture onto each piece of dough. Spread the meat on the dough, leaving a ½-inch edge on each side.
5. Put the meat pies in the oven and bake for 12 to 15 minutes until edges are golden brown.

80. Meaty Baked Penne

PREP TIME: 10 mins
COOK TIME: 40 mins
SERVINGS: 6 people

NUTRITION
Calories: 173;
Protein: 12.3g;
Carbs: 3.4g;
Fat: 6.3g

INGREDIENTS

- 1 lb. penne pasta
- 1 lb. ground beef
- 1 tsp. salt
- 1 (25-oz.) jar marinara sauce
- 1 (1-lb.) bag baby spinach, washed
- 3 cups shredded mozzarella cheese, divided

DIRECTIONS

1. Bring a large pot of salted water to a boil, add the penne, and cook for 7 minutes. Reserve 2 cups of e pasta water and drain the pasta.
2. Preheat the oven to 350°F.
3. In a large saucepan over medium heat, cook the ground beef and salt. Brown the ground beef for about 5 minutes.
4. Stir in marinara sauce, and 2 cups of pasta water. Let simmer for 5 minutes.
5. Add a handful of spinach at a time into the sauce, and cook for another 3 minutes.
6. To assemble, in a 9-by-13-inch baking dish, add the pasta and pour the pasta sauce over it. Stir in 1½ cups of the mozzarella cheese. Cover the dish with foil and bake for 20 minutes.
7. After 20 minutes, remove the foil, top with the rest of the mozzarella, and bake for another 10 minutes. Serve warm.

81. Mediterranean Pasta with Tomato Sauce and Vegetables

PREP TIME: 15 mins
COOK TIME: 25 mins
SERVINGS: 8 people

NUTRITION
Calories: 154
Protein: 6 g
Fat: 2 g
Carbs: 28 g

INGREDIENTS

- 8 oz. linguine or spaghetti, cooked
- 1 tsp. garlic powder
- 1 (28 oz.) can whole peeled tomatoes, drained and sliced
- 1 tbsp. olive oil
- 1 (8 oz.) can tomato sauce
- ½ tsp. Italian seasoning
- 8 oz. mushrooms, sliced
- 8 oz. yellow squash, sliced
- 8 oz. zucchini, sliced
- ½ tsp. sugar
- ½ cup grated Parmesan cheese

DIRECTIONS

1. In a medium saucepan, mix tomato sauce, tomatoes, sugar, Italian seasoning, and garlic powder. Bring to boil on medium heat. Reduce heat to low. Cover and simmer for 20 minutes.
2. In a large skillet, heat olive oil on medium-high heat.
3. Add squash, mushrooms, and zucchini. Cook, stirring, for 4 minutes or until tender-crisp.
4. Stir vegetables into the tomato sauce.
5. Place pasta in a serving bowl.
6. Spoon vegetable mixture over pasta and toss to coat.
7. Top with grated Parmesan cheese.

82. Very Vegan Patras Pasta

PREP TIME
5 mins

COOK TIME
10 mins

SERVINGS
6 people

INGREDIENTS

- 4-quarts salted water
- 10-oz. gluten-free and whole-grain pasta
- 5-cloves garlic, minced
- 1-cup hummus
- Salt and pepper
- 1/3-cup water
- ½-cup walnuts
- ½-cup olives
- 2-tbsp dried cranberries (optional)

DIRECTIONS

1. Bring the salted water to a boil for cooking the pasta.
2. In the meantime, prepare for the hummus sauce. Combine the garlic, hummus, salt, and pepper with water in a mixing bowl. Add the walnuts, olive, and dried cranberries, if desired. Set aside.
3. Add the pasta in the boiling water. Cook the pasta following the manufacturer's specifications until attaining an al dente texture. Drain the pasta.
4. Transfer the pasta to a large serving bowl and combine with the sauce.

NUTRITION

Calories: 329
Protein: 12 g
Fat: 13 g
Carbs: 43 g

83. Cheesy Spaghetti with Pine Nuts

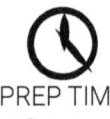
PREP TIME
10 mins

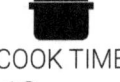
COOK TIME
10 mins

SERVINGS
4 people

INGREDIENTS

- 8 oz. spaghetti
- 4 tbsp. (½ stick) unsalted butter
- 1 tsp. freshly ground black pepper
- ½ cup pine nuts
- 1 cup fresh grated Parmesan cheese, divided

DIRECTIONS

1. Bring a large pot of salted water to a boil. Add the pasta and cook for 8 minutes.
2. In a large saucepan over medium heat, combine the butter, black pepper, and pine nuts. Cook for 2 to 3 minutes or until the pine nuts are lightly toasted.
3. Reserve ½ cup of the pasta water. Drain the pasta and put it into the pan with the pine nuts.
4. Add ¾ cup of Parmesan cheese and the reserved pasta water to the pasta and toss everything together to evenly coat the pasta.
5. To serve, put the pasta in a serving dish and top with the remaining ¼ cup of Parmesan cheese.

NUTRITION

Calories: 238;
Protein: 12.3g;
Carbs: 3.4g;
Fat: 6.3g

84. Creamy Garlic-Parmesan Chicken Pasta

PREP TIME: 5 mins
COOK TIME: 25 mins
SERVINGS: 6 people

NUTRITION
Calories: 153;
Protein: 12.3g;
Carbs: 3.4g;
Fat: 6.3g

INGREDIENTS

- 2 boneless, skinless chicken breasts
- 3 tbsp. extra-virgin olive oil
- 1½ tsp. salt
- 1 large onion, thinly sliced
- 3 tbsp. garlic, minced
- 1 lb. fettuccine pasta
- 1 cup heavy (whipping) cream
- ¾ cup freshly grated Parmesan cheese, divided
- ½ tsp. freshly ground black pepper

DIRECTIONS

1. Bring a large pot of salted water to a simmer.
2. Cut the chicken into thin strips.
3. In a large skillet over medium heat, cook the olive oil and chicken for 3 minutes.
4. Next add the salt, onion, and garlic to the pan with the chicken. Cook for 7 minutes.
5. Bring the pot of salted water to a boil and add the pasta, then let it cook for 7 minutes.
6. While the pasta is cooking, add the cream, ½ cup of Parmesan cheese, and black pepper to the chicken; simmer for 3 minutes.
7. Reserve ½ cup of the pasta water. Drain the pasta and add it to the chicken cream sauce.
8. Add the reserved pasta water to the pasta and toss together. Let simmer for 2 minutes. Top with the remaining ¼ cup Parmesan cheese and serve warm.

85. Artichoke Chicken Pasta

PREP TIME: 20 mins
COOK TIME: 5 mins
SERVINGS: 4 people

NUTRITION
Calories – 486
Fat – 10g
Carbs – 42g
Fiber – 9g
Protein – 37g

INGREDIENTS

- 2 cloves garlic, crushed
- 2 lemons, wedged
- 2 tbsp. lemon juice
- 14 oz. artichoke hearts, chopped
- 1-lb. chicken breast fillet, diced
- ½ cup feta cheese, crumbled
- 1 tbsp. olive oil
- 16 oz. whole-wheat (gluten-free) pasta of your choice
- 3 tbsp. parsley, chopped
- ½ cup red onion, chopped
- 2 tsp. oregano
- 1 tomato, chopped
- Ground black pepper and salt, to taste

DIRECTIONS

1. Pour the water into a deep saucepan and boil it. Add the pasta and some salt; cook it as per package directions. Drain the water and set aside the pasta.
2. Over medium stove flame, heat the oil in a skillet or saucepan (preferably of medium size).
3. Sauté the onions and garlic until softened and translucent, stir in between.
4. Add the chicken and cook until it is no longer pink.
5. Mix in the tomatoes, artichoke hearts, parsley, feta cheese, oregano, lemon juice and the cooked pasta.
6. Combine well and cook for 3-4 minutes, stirring frequently.
7. Season with black pepper and salt. Garnish with lemon wedges and serve warm.

86. Spinach Beef Pasta

PREP TIME
30 mins

COOK TIME
10 mins

SERVINGS
4 people

NUTRITION

Calories – 334
Fat – 13g
Carbs – 36g
Fiber – 6g
Protein – 16g

INGREDIENTS

- 1 ¼ cups uncooked orzo pasta
- ¾ cup baby spinach
- 2 tbsp. olive oil
- 1 ½ lb. beef tenderloin
- ¾ cup feta cheese
- 2 quarts water
- 1 cup cherry tomatoes, halved
- ¼ tsp. salt

DIRECTIONS

1. Rub the meat with pepper and cut into small cubes.
2. Over medium stove flame; heat the oil in a deep saucepan (preferably of medium size).
3. Add and stir-fry the meat until it is evenly brown.
4. Add the water and boil the mixture; stir in the orzo and salt.
5. Cook the mixture for 7-8 minutes. Add the spinach and cook until it wilts.
6. Add the tomatoes and cheese; combine and serve warm.

87. Asparagus Parmesan Pasta

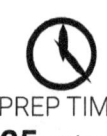
PREP TIME
25 mins

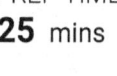
COOK TIME
4 mins

SERVINGS
2 people

NUTRITION

Calories – 402
Fat – 31g
Carbs – 33g
Fiber – 6g
Protein – 44g

INGREDIENTS

- 1 tsp. extra-virgin olive oil
- 1 tsp. lemon juice
- ¾ cup whole milk
- ½ bunch asparagus, trimmed and cut into small pieces
- ½ cup parmesan cheese, grated
- 2 tbsp. garlic, minced
- 2 tbsp. almond flour
- 2 tsp. whole grain mustard
- 4 oz. whole-wheat penne pasta
- 1 tsp. tarragon, minced
- Ground black pepper and salt, to taste

DIRECTIONS

1. Pour the water into a deep saucepan and boil it. Add the pasta and some salt; cook it as per package directions. Drain the water and set aside the pasta.
2. Take another pan, pour 8 cups of water and let it come to boiling. Add the asparagus and boil until it is soft. Drain and set aside.
3. In a mixing bowl, combine the milk, flour, mustard, black pepper and salt. Set aside.
4. Over medium stove flame, heat the oil in a skillet or saucepan (preferably of medium size).
5. Sauté the garlic until softened and fragrant, stirring in between.
6. Add the milk mixture and let it simmer. Add the tarragon, lemon juice and lemon zest; mix to combine.
7. Add the cooked pasta, asparagus, and simmer until the sauce thickens, stirring frequently.
8. Top with parmesan cheese and serve warm.

88. Mussels Linguine Delight

PREP TIME: 20 mins
COOK TIME: 10 mins
SERVINGS: 4 people

NUTRITION
Calories – 634
Fat – 15g
Carbs – 36g
Fiber – 7g
Protein – 39g

INGREDIENTS

- 1 lb. mussels, cleaned and debearded
- 1 tbsp. olive oil
- ½ tsp. oregano
- ½ tsp. basil, chopped
- 1 clove garlic, minced
- 1 lemon, wedges
- 8 oz. whole-wheat linguine pasta
- 1 pinch pepper flakes, crushed
- 1 (14.5 oz.) can tomatoes, crushed
- ¼ cup white wine

DIRECTIONS

1. Pour the water into a deep saucepan and boil it. Add the pasta and some salt; cook it as per package directions. Drain the water and set aside the pasta.
2. Over a medium stove flame; heat the oil in a skillet or saucepan (preferably medium size).
3. Sauté the garlic until softened and fragrant, stir in between.
4. Add the tomatoes, basil, pepper flakes and oregano. Reduce the heat and simmer the mix.
5. Add the mussels, wine and increase the heat. Cook for 3-5 minutes.
6. Wait for the mussels to cook and open. Mix in the pasta.
7. Garnish with the parsley; serve with some lemon wedges on the side.

89. Arugula Pasta Soup

PREP TIME: 15 mins
COOK TIME: 5 mins
SERVINGS: 6 people

NUTRITION
Calories – 317
Fat – 7g
Carbs – 32g
Fiber – 6g
Protein – 38g

INGREDIENTS

- 7 oz. chickpeas, rinsed
- 4 eggs, lightly beaten
- 2 tbsp. lemon juice
- 3 cups arugula, chopped
- 6 tbsp. parmesan cheese
- 6 cups chicken broth
- 1 pinch of nutmeg
- 1 bunch scallions, sliced (greens and whites sliced separately)
- 1 1/3 cups whole-wheat pasta shells
- 2 cups water
- Ground black pepper, to taste

DIRECTIONS

1. In a cooking pot or deep saucepan, combine the pasta, scallion whites, chickpeas, water, broth and nutmeg.
2. Heat the mixture; cover and bring to a boil.
3. Take off the lid and simmer the mixture for about 4 minutes. Add the arugula and cook until it is wilted.
4. Mix in the eggs and season with black pepper and salt.
5. Mix in the lemon juice and scallion greens. Top with the parmesan cheese; serve warm.

90. Pasta with garlic and Hoat Pepper

PREP TIME
25 mins

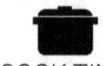
COOK TIME
4 mins

SERVINGS
4 people

INGREDIENTS

- 400g Spaghetti
- 8 tbsp. Extra virgin olive oil
- 4 cloves garlic, chopped
- 1 Chili pepper
- Coarse salt

DIRECTIONS

1. Put the water to boil, when it comes to a boil add salt and dip the spaghetti.
2. Meanwhile, in a saucepan heat the oil with the garlic deprived of the inner and chopped germ and the chopped peppers. Be careful: the flame should be sweet and the garlic should not darken.
3. Halfway through cooking, remove the spaghetti and continue cooking in the pan with the oil and garlic, adding the cooking water as if it were a risotto.
4. When cooked, serve the spaghetti.

NUTRITION

Calories 201, Fat 4.3g, Protein 5.8g, Carbs 20.1g

---

91. Stuffed Pasta Shells

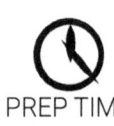
PREP TIME
15 mins

COOK TIME
10 mins

SERVINGS
4 people

INGREDIENTS

- 5 Cups Marinara Sauce
- 15 Oz. Ricotta Cheese
- 1 ½ Cups Mozzarella Cheese, Grated
- ¾ Cup Parmesan Cheese, Grated
- 2 tbsp. Parsley, Fresh & Chopped
- ¼ Cup Basil Leaves, Fresh & Chopped
- 8 Oz. Spinach, Fresh & Chopped
- ½ tsp. Thyme
- Sea Salt & Black Pepper to Taste
- 1 lb. Ground Beef
- 1 Cup Onions, Chopped
- 4 Cloves Garlic, Diced
- 2 tbsp. Olive Oil, Divided
- 12 Oz. Jumbo Pasta Shells

DIRECTIONS

1. Start by cooking your pasta shells by following your package instructions. Once they're cooked, then set them to the side.
2. Press sauté and then add in half of your olive oil. Cook your garlic and onions, which should take about four minutes. Your onions should be tender, and your garlic should be fragrant.
3. Add your ground beef in, seasoning it with thyme, salt, and pepper, cooking for another four minutes.
4. Add in your basil, parsley, spinach and marinara sauce.
5. Cover your pot, and cook for five minutes on low pressure.
6. Use a quick release, and top with cheeses.
7. Press sauté again, making sure that it stays warm until your cheese melts.
8. Take a tbsp. of the mixture, stuffing it into your pasta shells.
9. Top with your remaining sauce before serving warm.

NUTRITION

Calories: 710
Protein: 45.2 g
Fat: 23.1 g
Carbs: 70 g

92. Homemade Pasta Bolognese

PREP TIME: 20 mins
COOK TIME: 10 mins
SERVINGS: 4 people

NUTRITION
Calories: 1091
Fat: 54.7g
Carbs: 92.8g
Protein: 74g

INGREDIENTS
- Minced meat 17 oz.
- Pasta 12 oz.
- Sweet red onion 1 piece
- Garlic 2 cloves
- Vegetable oil 1 tbsp.
- Tomato paste 3 tbsp.
- Grated Parmesan Cheese 2 oz.
- Bacon 3 pieces

DIRECTIONS
1. Fry finely chopped onions and garlic in a frying pan in vegetable oil until a characteristic smell.
2. Add minced meat and chopped bacon to the pan. Constantly break the lumps with a spatula and mix so that the minced meat is crumbly.
3. When the mince is ready, add tomato paste, grated Parmesan to the pan, mix, reduce heat and leave to simmer.
4. At this time, boil the pasta. I don't salt water, because for me tomato paste and sauce as a whole turn out to be quite salty.
5. When the pasta is ready, discard it in a colander, arrange it on plates, add meat sauce with tomato paste on top of each serving.

93. Asparagus Pasta

PREP TIME: 10 mins
COOK TIME: 25 mins
SERVINGS: 6 people

NUTRITION
Calories: 307
Protein: 18 g
Fat: 14 g
Carbs: 33 g

INGREDIENTS
- 8 Oz. Farfalle Pasta, Uncooked
- 1 ½ Cups Asparagus, Fresh, Trimmed & Chopped into 1 Inch Pieces
- 1 Pint Grape Tomatoes, Halved
- 2 tbsp. Olive Oil
- Sea Salt & Black Pepper to Taste
- 2 Cups Mozzarella, Fresh & Drained
- 1/3 Cup Basil Leaves, Fresh & Torn
- 2 tbsp. Balsamic Vinegar

DIRECTIONS
1. Start by heating the oven to 400°F, and then get out a stockpot. Cook your pasta per package instructions, and reserve ¼ cup of pasta water.
2. Get out a bowl and toss the tomatoes, oil, asparagus, and season with salt and pepper. Spread this mixture on a baking sheet, and bake for fifteen minutes. Stir twice in this time.
3. Remove your vegetables from the oven, and then add the cooked pasta to your baking sheet. Mix with a few tbsp. of pasta water so that your sauce becomes smoother.
4. Mix in your basil and mozzarella, drizzling with balsamic vinegar. Serve warm.

94. Penne Bolognese Pasta

PREP TIME 15 mins

COOK TIME 20 mins

SERVINGS 2 people

NUTRITION

Calories: 435
Protein: 18 g
Fat: 14 g
Carbs: 33 g

INGREDIENTS

- Penne pasta 7 oz.
- Beef 5 oz.
- Parmesan Cheese 1 oz.
- Celery Stalk 1 oz.
- Shallots 26 g
- Carrot 1.5 oz.
- Garlic 1 clove
- Thyme 1 g
- Tomatoes in own juice 6 oz.
- Parsley 3 g
- Oregano 1 g
- Butter 20 g
- Dry white wine 50 ml
- Olive oil 40 ml

DIRECTIONS

1. Pour the penne into boiling salted water and cook for 9 minutes.
2. Roll the beef through a meat grinder.
3. Dice onion, celery, carrots and garlic in a small cube.
4. Fry the chopped vegetables in a heated frying pan in olive oil with minced meat for 4–5 minutes, salt and pepper.
5. Add oregano to the fried minced meat and vegetables, pour 50 ml of wine, add the tomatoes along with the juice and simmer for 10 minutes until the tomatoes are completely softened.
6. Add the boiled penne and butter to the sauce and simmer for 1-2 minutes, stirring continuously.
7. Put in a plate, sprinkle with grated Parmesan and chopped parsley, decorate with a sprig of thyme and serve.

95. Quick Pasta Bolognese

PREP TIME 10 mins

COOK TIME 25 mins

SERVINGS 2 people

NUTRITION

Calories: 710
Protein: 18 g
Fat: 14 g
Carbs: 33 g

INGREDIENTS

- Ground beef 17 oz.
- Garlic 2 cloves
- Tomato paste 3 tbsp.
- Tomatoes 14 oz.
- Beef broth 150 ml
- A mixture of Italian herbs 1 tsp.
- Penne pasta 14 oz.
- Basil leaves to taste
- Fresh mushrooms to taste

DIRECTIONS

1. Prepare the paste following the instructions on the packaging.
2. Heat the oil in a pan, sauté the minced meat for 5 minutes, then add the mushrooms and fry for another 3 minutes. Add garlic and tomato paste and simmer for 2 minutes. Add tomatoes, broth or wine, dried herbs and spices. Bring to a boil and simmer for 10 minutes.
3. Drain the water from the pasta, mix it with the sauce, sprinkle with basil leaves on top.

96. Pilaf with Cream Cheese

PREP TIME
10 mins

COOK TIME
30 mins

SERVINGS
4 people

NUTRITION

Calories: 364g
Protein: 5g
Fat: 30g
Carbs: 20g

INGREDIENTS

- 2 Cups Yellow Long Grain Rice, Parboiled
- 1 Cup Onion
- 4 Green Onions
- 3 tbsp. Butter
- 3 tbsp. Vegetable Broth
- 2 tsp. Cayenne Pepper
- 1 tsp. Paprika
- ½ tsp. Cloves, Minced
- 2 tbsp. Mint Leaves, Fresh & Chopped
- 1 Bunch Fresh Mint Leaves to Garnish
- 1 tbsp. Olive Oil
- Sea Salt & Black Pepper to Taste
- Cheese Cream:
- 3 tbsp. Olive Oil
- Sea Salt & Black Pepper to Taste
- 9 Oz. Cream Cheese

DIRECTIONS

1. Start by heating your oven to 360°F, and then get out a pan. Heat your butter and olive oil together, and cook your onions and spring onions for two minutes.
2. Add in your salt, pepper, paprika, cloves, vegetable broth, rice and remaining seasoning. Sauté for three minutes.
3. Cover with foil, and bake for another half hour. Allow it to cool.
4. Mix in the cream cheese, cheese, olive oil, salt and pepper. Serve your pilaf garnished with fresh mint leaves.

97. Herbed Pasta

PREP TIME
15 mins

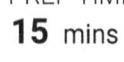
COOK TIME
15 mins

SERVINGS
4 people

NUTRITION

Calories 301
Fat 8.9 g
Carbs 47.7 g
Fiber 6.7 g
Protein 8.5 g

INGREDIENTS

- 1 (8-oz.) package linguini pasta
- 2 tbsp. olive oil
- 1 tbsp. garlic, minced
- 1 tbsp. dried oregano, crushed
- 1 tbsp. dried basil, crushed
- 1 tsp. dried thyme, crushed
- 2 cups plum tomatoes, chopped

DIRECTIONS

1. In a large pan of lightly salted boiling water, add the pasta and cook for about 8-10 minutes or according to package's directions.
2. Drain the pasta well.
3. In a large skillet, heat oil over medium heat and sauté the garlic for about 1 minute.
4. Stir in herbs and sauté for about 1 minute more.
5. Add the pasta and cook for about 2-3 minutes or until heated completely.
6. Fold in tomatoes and remove from heat. Serve hot.

98. Pasta with Veggies

PREP TIME
15 mins

COOK TIME
20 mins

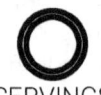
SERVINGS
6 people

NUTRITION

Calories 446
Fat 15.1 g
Carbs 62.2 g
Fiber 4.6 g
Protein 15.2 g

INGREDIENTS

- 3 tomatoes
- 1-lb. farfalle pasta
- ¼ cup olive oil
- 1-lb. fresh mushrooms, sliced
- 3 garlic cloves, minced
- 1 tsp. dried oregano, crushed
- 1 (2-oz.) can black olives, drained
- ¾ cup feta cheese, crumbled

DIRECTIONS

1. In a large pan of the salted boiling water, add the tomatoes and cook for about 1 minute.
2. With a slotted spoon, transfer the tomatoes into a bowl of ice water.
3. In the same pan of the boiling water, add the pasta and cook for about 8-10 minutes.
4. Drain the pasta well.
5. Meanwhile, peel the blanched tomatoes and then chop them.
6. In a large skillet, heat oil over medium heat and sauté the mushrooms and garlic for about 4-5 minutes.
7. Add the tomatoes and oregano and cook for about 3-4 minutes.
8. Divide the pasta onto serving plates and top with mushroom mixture.
9. Garnish with olives and feta and serve.

99. Pasta with Chicken & Veggies

PREP TIME
15 mins

COOK TIME
10 mins

SERVINGS
7 people

NUTRITION

Calories 429
Fat 17.1 g
Carbs 43.1 g
Fiber 2.7 g
Protein 26.3 g

INGREDIENTS

- 3 tbsp. olive oil
- 1-lb. boneless, skinless chicken breast, sliced diagonally
- 1 (8½-oz.) jar sun-dried tomatoes, julienned
- 2 tbsp. garlic, minced
- 1-lb. angel hair pasta
- 1 (8½-oz.) can water-packed artichoke hearts, quartered and drained
- ½ cup kalamata olive, pitted
- ¼ cup fresh basil
- 6 oz. feta cheese, crumbled
- ¼ cup heavy cream
- 1 tsp. dried oregano
- Salt and ground black pepper, as required

DIRECTIONS

1. In a skillet, heat the oil over medium heat and sear the chicken strips for about 5-6 minutes or until browned completely.
2. Add the sun-dried tomatoes and garlic and sauté for about 2 minutes.
3. Meanwhile, in a large pan of the salted boiling water, add the pasta and cook for about 5-6 minutes.
4. Drain the pasta well.
5. In the skillet, add the artichoke hearts, olives, basil and feta cheese and sauté for about 1 minute.
6. Add the cream and stir to combine.
7. Stir in the oregano, salt and black pepper and remove from the heat.
8. In a large serving bowl, add the pasta and chicken mixture and toss to coat well.
9. Serve immediately.

100. Pasta with Shrimp & Spinach

PREP TIME 15 mins
COOK TIME 10 mins
SERVINGS 4 people

NUTRITION
Calories 457
Fat 19.1 g
Carbs 38.9 g
Fiber 1.7 g
Protein 32.5 g

INGREDIENTS

- 1 cup sour cream
- ½ cup feta cheese, crumbled
- 3 garlic cloves, chopped
- 2 tsp. dried basil, crushed
- ¼ tsp. red pepper flakes, crushed
- 8 oz. fettuccine pasta
- 1 (10-oz.) packages frozen spinach, thawed
- 12 oz. medium shrimp, peeled and deveined
- Salt and ground black pepper, as required

DIRECTIONS

1. In a large serving bowl, add the sour cream, feta, garlic, basil, red pepper flakes and salt and mix well.
2. Set aside until using.
3. In a large pan of the lightly salted boiling water, add the fettucine and cook for about 10 minutes or according to the package's directions.
4. After 8 minutes, stir in the spinach and shrimp and cook for about 2 minutes.
5. Drain the pasta mixture well.
6. Add the hot pasta mixture into the bowl of the sour cream mixture and gently, toss to coat.
7. Serve immediately.

101. Carbonara Pasta With Champignons

PREP TIME 10 mins
COOK TIME 25 mins
SERVINGS 2 people

NUTRITION
Calories: 767
Protein: 18 g
Fat: 32 g
Carbs: 33 g

INGREDIENTS

- Spaghetti 9 oz.
- Bacon 7 oz.
- Cream 20% 7 oz.
- Parmesan Cheese 3.5 oz.
- Egg yolk 4 pieces
- Garlic 5 cloves
- Champignons 5 oz.
- Olive oil 10 ml
- Salt to taste
- Ground black pepper to taste

DIRECTIONS

1. Prepare the ingredients.
2. Cut the bacon into strips, chop the garlic finely, chop the mushrooms.
3. Fry the garlic in a pan, then the mushrooms and bacon.
4. Grate the parmesan.
5. Put egg yolks in a plate, salt, pepper and beat.
6. Add cream and grated cheese to the yolks, mix.
7. Boil spaghetti to al dente (about a minute less than indicated on the packet).
8. Put the spaghetti in a pan, add the sauce, bacon and mushrooms.

102. Spaghetti Carbonara With Red Onion

PREP TIME
15 mins

COOK TIME
25 mins

SERVINGS
4 people

NUTRITION

Calories: 307
Protein: 18 g
Fat: 14 g
Carbs: 33 g

INGREDIENTS

- Spaghetti 9 oz.
- Butter 3/4 oz.
- Garlic 2 cloves
- Red onion 1 head
- Bacon 2 oz.
- Cream 20% 200 ml
- Grated Parmesan Cheese 2 oz.
- 4 eggs
- Salt to taste
- Ground black pepper to taste

DIRECTIONS

1. Boil water in a large saucepan and cook the pasta until al dente. Usually for this you need to cook it for a minute less than indicated on the pack.
2. While the pasta is boiling, melt the butter in a pan and fry finely chopped onion, garlic and bacon on it. To softness and to a distinct garlic and fried bacon smell.
3. Remove the pan from the heat and beat four egg yolks with cream and grated Parmesan in a deep bowl. Salt and pepper the mixture, whisk again.
4. In the prepared spaghetti, pour the pieces of bacon fried with onions and garlic. Pour in a mixture of cream, yolks and parmesan, mix. And serve immediately, sprinkled with freshly grated cheese and black pepper

103. Cuttlefish Pasta With Carbonara Sauce

PREP TIME
15 mins

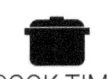
COOK TIME
30 mins

SERVINGS
3 people

NUTRITION

Calories: 593
Protein: 18 g
Fat: 14 g
Carbs: 33 g

INGREDIENTS

- Pasta 7 oz.
- Smoked bacon 5 oz.
- Grated Parmesan Cheese 2 oz.
- Champignons 7 oz.
- Cream 200 ml
- Egg yolk 1 piece
- Garlic 3 cloves
- Butter 2 tbsp.
- Ground black pepper pinch
- Ground nutmeg pinch

DIRECTIONS

1. Boil spaghetti. At this time, fry the garlic and bacon in butter for three minutes.
2. Add the mushroom slices to the bacon, mix and fry for eight to ten minutes. During this time, the spaghetti will cook, drain from them and add to the mushrooms and bacon.
3. The final stage - cream, egg yolk, ground black pepper, ground nutmeg and grated cheese. Beat all this and pour spaghetti, fry for five minutes and serve.

104. Spaghetti Carbonara

PREP TIME
10 mins

COOK TIME
25 mins

SERVINGS
2 people

NUTRITION

Calories: 702
Protein: 18 g
Fat: 14 g
Carbs: 33 g

INGREDIENTS

- Spaghetti 160 g
- Pancetta 4 oz.
- Hard cheese 2 oz.
- Egg yolk 2 pieces
- Salt to taste
- Freshly ground black pepper to taste

DIRECTIONS

1. Bring well-salted water to a boil. Cook spaghetti to al dente. Save a little broth from the paste; you may need it. Drain the rest.
2. While preparing the pasta, heat the pan and fry the pancetta on it until golden, remove from heat.
3. In a small bowl, beat the yolks with grated cheese until smooth.
4. Return the pan with the pancetta to a small fire, add about 50 ml of the broth from the pasta, throw the spaghetti there and mix well until the boiling stops. Most of the water should boil.
5. Remove the pan from the heat and add the yolks with cheese and mix quickly until the yolks thicken. If the sauce seems too thick, add a little more paste broth. Pepper and salt to taste, serve.

105. Chanterelle Pasta

PREP TIME
15 mins

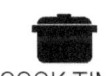
COOK TIME
30 mins

SERVINGS
4 people

NUTRITION

Calories: 360
Protein: 18 g
Fat: 16 g
Carbs: 32 g

INGREDIENTS

- Chanterelles 7 oz.
- Tagliatelle pasta 7 oz.
- Tomato Sauce 7 oz.
- Garlic 2 cloves
- Olive oil 20 ml
- Dry white wine 30 ml
- Butter 10 g
- Parmesan Cheese 2 oz.
- Salt to taste
- Ground black pepper to taste

DIRECTIONS

1. Heat olive oil in a pan with a thick bottom, add a couple of whole cloves of garlic, add chanterelles (pre-washed and well-dried).
2. Fry the chanterelles 5-7 minutes until golden brown, pour in white wine, evaporate.
3. Then pour the tomato sauce and simmer for about 5 minutes. At the end, add butter, salt and pepper.
4. Add the paste cooked al-dente to the sauce and mix. Serve garnished with sliced parmesan and parsley.

106. Pasta "Verochka"

PREP TIME
5 mins

COOK TIME
20 mins

SERVINGS
2 people

NUTRITION

Calories: 687
Protein: 18 g
Fat: 14 g
Carbs: 33 g

INGREDIENTS

- Spaghetti 10 oz.
- Cream 33% 200 ml
- Lightly salted trout 3.5 oz.
- Grated Parmesan Cheese 2 oz.
- Dried oregano to taste
- Dried basil to taste

DIRECTIONS

1. Boil spaghetti - or other suitable pasta - until cooked, following the time indicated on the package. You do not need to salt water - the salt will give the fish.
2. Meanwhile, finely chop the red fish - not necessarily trout, any. And its quantity may be different - if only the fish had no more pasta.
3. Heat the cream in a pan (it is better to take Fatter) and add fish to them. Keep on fire, stirring constantly and, most importantly, not boiling. When the fish loses color, you can remove the pan from the heat.
4. Throw the prepared pasta into a colander and add to the sauce. Or add the sauce to the paste - as anyone is more familiar and convenient. Add oregano and basil, mix.
5. Sprinkle the paste spread on the plates with grated Parmesan.

107. Pasta e Patate

PREP TIME
15 mins

COOK TIME
30 mins

SERVINGS
3 people

NUTRITION

Calories: 615
Protein: 18 g
Fat: 29 g
Carbs: 33 g

INGREDIENTS

- Bacon 5 oz.
- Onions 3 oz.
- Spaghetti 8 oz.
- Potato 14 oz.
- Parmesan Cheese 3 oz.
- Olive oil 30 ml
- Freshly ground black pepper to taste
- Salt to taste

DIRECTIONS

1. Fry the bacon in a dry skillet. Add olive oil and fry finely chopped onions, not until golden brown.
2. Add chopped potatoes to the onion, fry and add water to the onion. Cook until al dente, 5-10 minutes.
3. Break the spaghetti, toss it to the potatoes, add water, continue cooking until the spaghetti is ready. Pour a little water over the entire cooking process so that a little liquid is left in the finale, sufficient to make a sauce.
4. In the finale add grated parmesan, olive oil, freshly ground black pepper, mix well

108. Pasta with Fresh Tomatoes

INGREDIENTS

- Tagliatelle pasta 7 oz.
- Tomatoes 1 piece
- 5 black olives
- Garlic 2 cloves
- Olive oil 50 ml

DIRECTIONS

1. Boil the pasta in salted boiling water.
2. Simultaneously in 1 tbsp. of olive oil, lightly fry the garlic and sliced olives.
3. Dice the fresh tomatoes and add to the garlic and olives. Cooking tomatoes is not necessary, they should only warm up.
4. Slightly salt and pepper the sauce.
5. Drain the water and combine the pasta with the sauce.
6. Put the pasta in a plate and lightly pour olive oil.

PREP TIME 15 mins
COOK TIME 30 mins
SERVINGS 3 people

NUTRITION
Calories: 667
Protein: 18 g
Fat: 52 g
Carbs: 33 g

---

109. Spaghetti Carbonara With Chicken

INGREDIENTS

- Durum wheat spaghetti 10 oz.
- Cream 100 ml
- Garlic 2 cloves
- Chicken egg 3 pieces
- Basil to taste
- Sesame seeds 15 g
- Salt to taste
- Olive oil 3 tbsp.
- Parmesan Cheese 2 oz.
- Chicken fillet 7 oz.

DIRECTIONS

1. Finely chop the chicken fillet and fry in olive oil until tender.
2. Peel the garlic, chop finely and add to the chicken. Fry it all together for 1-2 minutes. Then add cream, salt to taste. Stew on low heat so that the cream does not curl.
3. Add a spoonful of olive oil to boiling water, salt to taste to taste. Cooking spaghetti to al dente.
4. Cooking the sauce. To do this, beat the eggs, then add basil, salt, sesame and grated parmesan.
5. Once the spaghetti is ready, we discard them in a colander, then - in a pan with chicken and garlic, pour everything in the resulting sauce and simmer for another 2-3 minutes over low heat.

PREP TIME 5 mins
COOK TIME 30 mins
SERVINGS 2 people

NUTRITION
Calories: 624
Protein: 18 g
Fat: 28 g
Carbs: 33 g

110. Carbonara With Fettuccine

PREP TIME
10 mins

COOK TIME
25 mins

SERVINGS
4 people

NUTRITION

Calories: 916
Protein: 18 g
Fat: 41 g
Carbs: 33 g

INGREDIENTS

- Fettuccine Pasta 17 oz.
- Bacon 8 slices
- 4 eggs
- Grated Parmesan Cheese 2 oz.
- Cream 315 ml

DIRECTIONS

1. Cut the bacon into thin strips and fry in a pan over medium heat until crisp. Lay on a paper towel.
2. Put the pasta in a pot of boiling salted water and cook until cooked. Drain and return to pan.
3. While the pasta is boiling, beat the eggs with cream and parmesan until smooth. Add the bacon and mix well. Pour the sauce into a hot paste and mix well.
4. Return to a frying pan to a very small fire and simmer a little less than 1 minute until the sauce thickens slightly.

111. Fast Spaghetti Carbonara

PREP TIME
5 mins

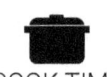
COOK TIME
30 mins

SERVINGS
3 people

NUTRITION

Calories: 847
Protein: 18 g
Fat: 49 g
Carbs: 33 g

INGREDIENTS

- Spaghetti 3 oz.
- Bacon 1.5 oz.
- Cream 35% 50 ml
- Chicken egg 1 piece
- Dry white wine 20 ml
- Grana padano cheese 0.8 oz.

DIRECTIONS

1. We put spaghetti in boiling water, cook for 12 minutes, put it in a sieve.
2. At the chicken egg, we separate the yolk from the Protein, mix the yolks with animal cream, grana padano cheese, and pepper.
3. Cut the bacon with a large plate into large plates, fry in butter, add dry white wine and olive oil.
4. Into the fried bacon with wine and oil we introduce ready-made spaghetti, add the mass with egg and cream, mix quickly

112. Pasta with Greens

PREP TIME
35 mins

COOK TIME
− mins

SERVINGS
8 people

NUTRITION

Calories: 296
Fat: 9.7 g
Carbs: 44.6 g
Protein: 9.6 g

INGREDIENTS

- Swiss chard – 1 bunch (remove the stems)
- Oil packed sun-dried tomatoes – ½ cup (chopped)
- Green olives – ½ cup (chopped and pitted)
- Fresh parmesan cheese – ¼ cup (grated)
- Dry fusilli pasta – 1 (16 oz.) package
- Olive oil – 2 tbsp.
- Kalamata olives – ½ cup (chopped and pitted)
- Garlic – 1 clove (minced)

Tip: You can substitute the pasta with another any other that you like.

DIRECTIONS

1. Cook pasta in lightly salted water for 10 to 12 minutes until al dente then drain.
2. Put the chard in a microwave safe bowl, fill with water until it is about ½ filled with water. Cook on high in the microwave for about 5 minutes until the chard is limp then drain.
3. Over medium heat, heat the oil in a skillet. Stir in the oil, the sun-dried tomatoes, green olives, kalamata olives and garlic.
4. Mix in the chard the cook and stir until the mixture is tender.
5. Toss with the pasta and sprinkle with parmesan cheese to serve.

113. Harvest Pasta

PREP TIME
35 mins

COOK TIME
4 mins

SERVINGS
6 people

NUTRITION

Calories: 392
Fat: 8.8 g
Carbs: 64.9 g
Protein: 13.4 g

INGREDIENTS

- Kalamata olives – 1/3 cup (pitted)
- Garlic – 2 cloves (minced)
- White sugar – 1 tbsp. or more to taste
- Dried oregano – 1 tsp.
- Vegetarian burger crumbs – ¾ cup
- Diced tomatoes – 2 (14.5 oz.) cans
- Bottled roasted red peppers – 1/3 cup (chopped)
- Balsamic vinegar – 1 ½ tbsp.
- Olive oil – 2 tbsp.
- Black pepper to taste
- Penne pasta – 1 lb.

Tip: You can also use a stick blender to puree the sauce in the pot until it is smooth.

DIRECTIONS

1. In a large saucepan, stir the olives, garlic, sugar, oregano, tomatoes, red pepper, vinegar. Bring this to simmer for about 20 to 30 minutes over medium high-heat before reducing to medium-low and let simmer until the sauce starts to thicken.
2. In a large pot, pour lightly salted water and boil over high heat. Once the water is boiling, put in the penne pasta and leave to boil.
3. Cook the pasta uncovered for about 11 minutes and remember to stir occasionally until the pasta is al-dente. After this drain.
4. Once the tomato sauce is done, pour it into the blender no more than halfway full. Hold down the lid and carefully start the blender using a few pulses to get the sauce moving before leaving it on to puree. Afterwards, puree until the mixture is smooth, then return to the pot.
5. Stir in the burger crumbs and simmer until it is hot. Then pour the finished sauce over the penne pasta to serve.

114. Pollo Mediterranean

PREP TIME
25 mins

COOK TIME
10 mins

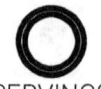
SERVINGS
4 people

NUTRITION

Calories: 392
Fat: 19.7 g
Carbs: 9.2 g
Protein: 38 g

INGREDIENTS

- Olive oil – 2 tbsp.
- Garlic – 3 cloves (minced)
- Ground black pepper – ½ tsp.
- Sun-dried tomatoes packed in oi – ¼ cup (chopped and drained)
- Dry white wine – ½ cup
- Chicken tenders – 12 (sliced into strips)
- Salt – ½ tsp.
- Italian seasoning – 1 tbsp.
- Green olives – 2 tbsp. (sliced)
- Fresh parsley – 2 tbsp. (chopped)
- Sour cream – ½ cup
- Salt – ½ tsp.
- Milk – 1 cup
- Cornstarch – 1 ½ tsp.
- Water – ¼ cup

DIRECTIONS

1. In a skillet and over medium heat, heat olive oil. Place chicken and garlic in the pan. Season with pepper, Italian seasoning and ½ tsp. of salt.
2. Stir in the olives, wine, parsley, tomatoes and olives then reduce heat to a low and continue cooking until the chicken is no longer pink at the center. Remove and place chicken on a late with the sauce still in the pan. Stir into the remaining sauce ½ tsp. of sauce.
3. In a small bowl, whisk cornstarch and water together. Increase heat to the medium and whisk in the cornstarch mixture. Continue stirring until the sauce has thickened. Serve the sauce with chicken.

115. Pasta Fagioli Soup

PREP TIME
25 mins

COOK TIME
35 mins

SERVINGS
6 people

NUTRITION

Calories: 288;
Fat: 3.6 g;
Carbs: 48.5 g;
Protein: 15.8 mg;

INGREDIENTS

- Water – 3 cups
- Crisp cooked bacon – 8 slices (crumbled)
- Dried parsley- 1 tbsp.
- Garlic – 1 tbsp. (minced)
- Garlic powder – 1 tsp.
- Ground black pepper – ½ tsp.
- Salt- 1 ½ tsp.
- Dried basil – ½ tsp.
- Tomato sauce – 1 (8 oz.) can
- Seashell pasta – ½ lb.
- Great Northern beans – 2 (14 oz.) cans (undrained)
- Chicken broth – 2 (14.5 oz.) can
- Diced tomatoes – 1 (29 oz.) can
- Chopped spinach – 1(14 oz.) can (drained)

DIRECTIONS

1. Combine all the other ingredients apart from pasta in a large stock pot to cook and boil. Let simmer for about 40 minutes.
2. Add pasta and cook with the pot uncovered until the pasta is tender. This should take approximately 10 minutes.
3. Serve.

Tip: You can substitute half of the canned ingredients for better nutritional outcomes.

116. Pasta al Mediterraneo

PREP TIME: 25 mins
COOK TIME: 15 mins
SERVINGS: 6 people

NUTRITION
Calories: 519
Fat: 22 g
Carbs: 59.5 g
Protein: 24.2 g

INGREDIENTS

- Perciatelli pasta – 1 lb.
- Pine nuts – 3 tbsp. (lightly roasted)
- Fresh parsley – 2 tbsp. (chopped)
- Lemon – 1 (juiced)
- Can tuna – 2 (5 oz.) package (drained)
- Kalamata olives – 12 (pitted and sliced)
- Garlic – 1 clove (crushed)
- Fresh basil – 4 oz. (chopped)
- Olive oil – 6 tbsp.
- Feta cheese – 2 oz. (optional)

DIRECTIONS

1. Cook pasta in a large bowl of slightly salted water until al dente. Meanwhile, mix in a large bowl, olives, garlic, basil, tuna, pine nuts, parsley and crumbled feta cheese.
2. Drain the pasta. If the plan is to serve cold, then rinse the pasta with cold water until it is no longer hot. In a large bowl, place pasta together with lemon juice and olive oil. Stir into the pasta mixture, the tuna mixture.
3. Serve hot or cold.

Tip: If possible, use fresh lemon juice instead of bottled ones.

117. Tomato Basil Penne Pasta

PREP TIME: 45 mins
COOK TIME: 20 mins
SERVINGS: 4 people

NUTRITION
Calories: 502;
Fat: 24.8 g;
Carbs: 47.1 g;
Protein: 24.1 g;

INGREDIENTS

- Basil oil – 1 tbsp.
- Garlic – 3 cloves (minced)
- Pepper jack cheese – 1 cup
- Parmesan cheese – ¼ cup (grated)
- Basil oil – 1 tbsp.
- Grape tomatoes – 1 pint (halved)
- Mozzarella cheese – 1cup (shredded)
- Fresh basil – 1 tbsp. (minced)

DIRECTIONS

1. Over high heat, bring a large pot of water to boil. Cook pasta in the boiling water for about 11 minutes until al dente, then drain.
2. In a large skillet and over medium-high heat, heat the basil and olive oil. Cook garlic in oil until soft. Afterwards, add tomatoes, reduce the heat to a medium and leave to dimmer for 10 minutes.
3. Stir in the mozzarella, parmesan cheese and pepper jack. When the cheese begins to melt, mix in the cooked penne pasta. Season with fresh basil.

Tip: If basil oil is unavailable, use 2 tbsp. of olive oil.

118. Whole Wheat Pasta Toss

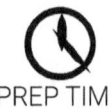

PREP TIME
25 mins

COOK TIME
30 mins

SERVINGS
8 people

NUTRITION

Calories: 367
Fat: 14.7 g
Carbs: 47.4 g
Protein: 12.9 g

INGREDIENTS

- Olive oil – 1/3 cup
- Marinated artichoke hearts – 1 (8 oz.) jar (drained)
- Kalamata olives – ¼ cup (pitted and quartered)
- Feta cheese – ½ cup (crumbled)
- Whole wheat penne pasta – 1 (1 lb.) package
- Garlic – 4 large cloves (pressed)
- Pickled red peppers – 7 (cut into strips)
- Fresh spinach leaves – 2 cups

DIRECTIONS

1. Fill a large bowl with lightly salted water and bring to boil. Put in the penne and continue to boil. Cook the pasta uncovered, stirring occasionally for 8 minutes or until al dente, then drain.
2. In a large non-stick skillet and over medium heat, heat olive oil, the cook and stir in garlic into the hot oil for about 30 seconds until it is fragrant, for about 5 minutes. Gently fold the spinach into the mixture and stir just until slightly wilted and dark green.
3. Remove the mixture from heat and stir in the penne pasta until it is thoroughly combined; lightly toss pasta mixture in with the feta steam, cover the skillet with a lid and let the vegetables and pasta steam for about 10 minutes before serving.

119. Quick Mediterranean Pasta

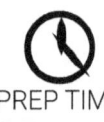

PREP TIME
25 mins

COOK TIME
10 mins

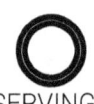

SERVINGS
6 people

NUTRITION

Calories: 178
Fat: 3.1 g
Carbs: 31.4 g
Protein: 5.5 g

INGREDIENTS

- Breadcrumbs – ¼ cup
- Dried basil – 1 tsp.
- Spaghetti – 8 oz.
- Dried oregano – 1 tsp.
- Olive oil – 1 tbsp.

DIRECTIONS

1. Boil slightly salted water in a large pot, put spaghetti in it and cook until al dente. Rinse and cool with water, then drain well.
2. Mix the breadcrumbs, basil, oregano and cooked pasta in a large bowl. Pour as much olive oil as you would like over the mixture and serve.

120. Mediterranean Fish and Pasta Stew

PREP TIME
20 mins

COOK TIME
30 mins

SERVINGS
4 people

NUTRITION

Calories: 237
Fat: 4.2 g
Carbs: 26.2 g
Protein: 25.3 g

INGREDIENTS

- Onions – 2 (chopped)
- Crushed tomatoes – 1 (28 oz.) can
- Fresh parsley – ½ cup (chopped)
- Worcestershire sauce – 2 tbsp.
- Paprika – 1 tsp.
- Dry pasta – 3 oz.
- Garlic – 4 cloves (minced)
- Olive oil – 1 tbsp.
- Water – 6 cups
- Fresh cilantro – ½ cup (chopped)
- Ground cinnamon – 1 tsp.
- Cod fillets – 1 ½ lb. (cubed)
- Salt to taste
- Ground black pepper – 1 tbsp.

DIRECTIONS

1. In a large pot, sauté the onions and garlic in the olive oil for 5 minutes over medium heat while stirring constantly.
2. Add tomatoes with the liquid, parsley, water and cilantro. Bring the mixture to boil and reduce heat to low and simmer for about 15 minutes.
3. Stir in the Worcestershire sauce, paprika, cinnamon and fish, the simmer over medium heat for 10 minutes. Add the pasta and simmer for about 8 minutes more or until the pasta is tender.
4. Season with salt and ground pepper to taste.

121. Parsley Pesto Paste

PREP TIME
5 mins

COOK TIME
15 mins

SERVINGS
4 people

NUTRITION

Calories 266
Fat 25g
Carbs 6g
Protein 8g

INGREDIENTS

- 2 cups of parsley leaves
- 1/2 cup of grated parmesan cheese
- Two cloves of garlic
- 1/2 cup lemon juice
- 1/4 cup olive oil
- 1/3 cup pine nut
- Table salt to taste

DIRECTIONS

1. Put all ingredients except the parmesan cheese in a food processor then pulse until smooth.
2. Remove from the blender, add grated parmesan and gently stir.
3. Serve.

122. Potato in Tomato Paste

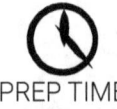
PREP TIME
25 mins

COOK TIME
30 mins

SERVINGS
4 people

NUTRITION

Calories 312,
Fat 14g, Carbs 43g, Protein 6g

INGREDIENTS

- Four large cubed potatoes
- 1 Tbsp aromatic dry spices mix
- One onion, chopped
- 4 Tbsp Olive oil
- Black pepper
- One minced garlic clove
- 1 cup tomato paste
- 1 cup of water
- Chopped parsley,
- Salt

DIRECTIONS

1. Heat the olive oil in a pan over medium heat and sauté the onion until translucent.
2. Add the potatoes, the spice mixture and continue to sauté.
3. Add the garlic, tomato paste, diced tomato, water, salt and pepper, and stir.
4. Cover the pot and cook for half an hour over low heat.
5. Serve with fresh coriander.

123. Hummus

PREP TIME
15 mins

COOK TIME
10 mins

SERVINGS
4 people

NUTRITION

Calories 77
Fat 4.3 g
Carbs 8.1g
Protein 2.6 g

INGREDIENTS

- 1/2 cup tahini
- 1 tsp salt
- Two cloves garlic halved
- 1 tbsp olive oil
- 2 cup canned garbanzo beans, drained
- 1/2 cup lemon juice
- 1 tbsp paprika
- 1 tsp parsley

DIRECTIONS

1. Pulse the garlic, lemon juice, garbanzos, salt, and tahini in a food processor until smooth.
2. Add this to a bowl with olive oil, paprika, and parsley.
3. Enjoy.

124. Hollandaise Sauce

PREP TIME 10 mins
COOK TIME 5 mins
SERVINGS 1 people

INGREDIENTS

- One lemon (Zested and juiced)
- One tsp garlic powder
- 1/2 tsp cayenne pepper
- 1/2 cup cashew butter
- Two tsp Dijon mustard
- 1/2 cup of warm water
- 1/2 tsp ground turmeric

DIRECTIONS

1. In a food processor, put all ingredients, and then pulse until smooth.
2. Put it in a sealed container and refrigerate it for up to three days.
3. Enjoy.

NUTRITION

Calories 150
Protein 6 g
Fat 12 g
Carbs 10 g

---

125. Creamy Tahini Dip

PREP TIME 5 mins
COOK TIME 4 mins
SERVINGS 4 people

INGREDIENTS

- Half a lemon (Juiced)
- One crushed garlic clove
- Salt
- 1/2 cup tahini
- 2 cups of water
- Fresh parsley, chopped
- Black pepper

DIRECTIONS

1. Put the tahini, salt, lemon juice, garlic, and a little water in a bowl then stir until the tahini becomes white and smooth.
2. Sprinkle the parsley and black pepper and serve.
3. Enjoy.

NUTRITION

Calories 93
Protein 2.6 g
Fat 8.1 g
Carbs 4.4 g

126. Basil Lime Dip

PREP TIME
5 mins

COOK TIME
10 mins

SERVINGS
16 people

INGREDIENTS

- Ten garlic cloves, crushed
- 1/4 cup brown rice syrup
- 8 oz. hemp oil
- One tsp of sea salt
- One pinch xanthan gum
- 1 1/2 cups chopped basil,
- Six tbsp key lime juice

DIRECTIONS

1. In an airtight jar, put all the ingredients except the xanthan gum, and then shake to well.
2. Put the mixture plus the xanthan, into a blender and pulse.
3. Return the mixture in the jar.
4. Enjoy.

NUTRITION

Calories 143
Cholesterol 0 mg
Fat 14 g
Carbs 6 g

127. Cilantro Dip

PREP TIME
5 mins

COOK TIME
4 mins

SERVINGS
7 people

INGREDIENTS

- 12 cloves of garlic
- 4 cups cilantro leaves
- One tsp salt
- 1/2 tsp ground black pepper
- 1 cup olive oil

DIRECTIONS

1. Add all ingredients to a blender and pulse until velvety.
2. You can put in the refrigerator for up to two days.
3. Enjoy.

NUTRITION

Calories 230;
Fat 20.5 g;
Carbs 7.1 g;
Protein 5 g

128. Tahini Sauce

INGREDIENTS

- Four mashed garlic cloves
- Salt to taste
- 1 cup tahini paste
- 1/2 cup lemon juice
- Seven tbsp water

DIRECTIONS

1. Put all ingredients in a bowl and whisk until well combined.
2. Refrigerate up to 5 days.
3. Enjoy.

PREP TIME: 7 mins
COOK TIME: 5 mins
SERVINGS: 6 people

NUTRITION
Calories 77;
Fat 6.6 g;
Carbs 3.2 g;
Protein 2.3 g

---

129. Arugula Salsa

INGREDIENTS

- 30 Kalamata olives, pitted, quartered
- Three tbsp olive oil
- One chopped red bell pepper
- One chopped yellow bell pepper
- Two tsp fennel seeds, crushed
- 1 cup baby arugula, chopped

DIRECTIONS

1. Heat oil in a pan over medium heat.
2. Add fennel seeds and sauté until fragrant.
3. Add bell peppers and sauté until they are soft.
4. Transfer into a bowl.
5. Add salt, pepper, and arugula and stir until arugula wilts.
6. Enjoy.

PREP TIME: 5 mins
COOK TIME: 20 mins
SERVINGS: 6 people

NUTRITION
Calories 16;
Fat 0.1 g;
Carbs 3.9 g;
Protein 0.6 g

RICE AND GRAINS

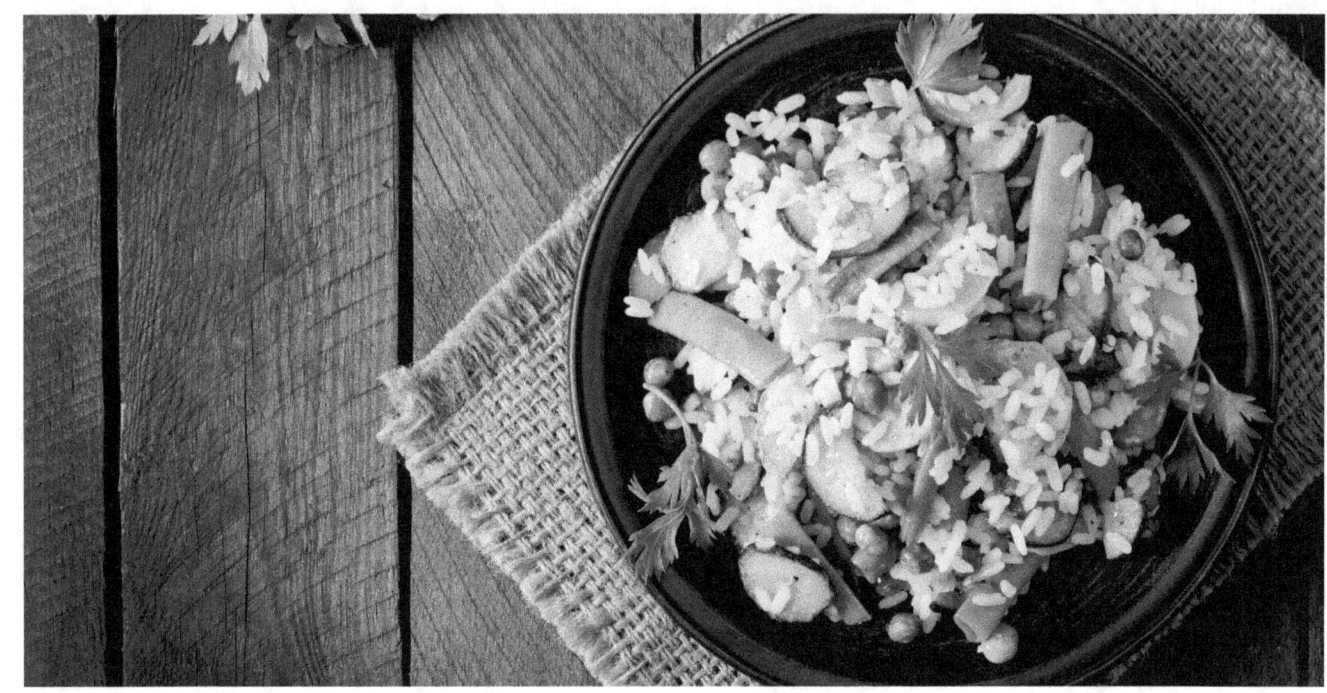

130. Fragrant Basmati Rice

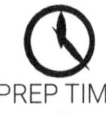
PREP TIME
5 mins

COOK TIME
17 mins

SERVINGS
6 people

NUTRITION

Calories: 334;
Protein: 12.3g;
Carbs: 19.4g;
Fat: 6.3g

INGREDIENTS

- 1 cup long-grain rice
- 1 tbsp. olive oil
- 1 tsp. dried rosemary
- 2 ½ cup water

DIRECTIONS

1. Heat the olive oil in the saucepan.
2. Add rice and roast it for 2 minutes. Stir it constantly.
3. Then add rosemary and water.
4. Stir the rice and close the lid.
5. Cook it for 15 minutes or until it soaks all water.

131. Cranberry Rice

PREP TIME: 5 mins
COOK TIME: 20 mins
SERVINGS: 4 people

INGREDIENTS
- ¼ cup basmati rice
- 1 cup of organic almond milk
- 2 oz dried cranberries
- ¼ tsp. ground cinnamon

DIRECTIONS
1. Put all ingredients in the saucepan, stir, and close the lid.
2. Cook the rice on low heat for 20 minutes

NUTRITION
Calories: 153;
Protein: 12.3g;
Carbs: 3.4g;
Fat: 6.3g

132. Italian Style Wild Rice

PREP TIME: — mins
COOK TIME: 20 mins
SERVINGS: 6 people

INGREDIENTS
- 1 cup wild rice
- 3 cups chicken stock
- 1 tsp. Italian seasonings
- 2 oz Feta, crumbled
- 1 tbsp. olive oil

DIRECTIONS
1. Mix wild rice with olive oil and chicken stock.
2. Close the lid and cook it for 25 minutes over the medium-low heat.
3. Then add Italian seasonings and crumbled feta.
4. Stir the rice.

NUTRITION
Calories: 253;
Protein: 15.3g;
Carbs: 3.4g;
Fat: 6.3g

133. Brown Rice Saute

PREP TIME
5 mins

COOK TIME
20 mins

SERVINGS
3 people

NUTRITION

Calories: 237;
Protein: 12.3g;
Carbs: 3.4g;
Fat: 6.3g

INGREDIENTS

- 3 oz brown rice
- 9 oz chicken stock
- 1 tsp. curry powder
- 1 onion, diced
- 4 tbsp. olive oil

DIRECTIONS

1. Heat olive oil in the saucepan.
2. Add onion and cook it until light brown.
3. Add brown rice, curry powder, and chicken stock.
4. Close the lid and saute the rice for 15 minutes.

134. Pesto Rice

PREP TIME
8 mins

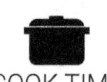
COOK TIME
15 mins

SERVINGS
4 people

NUTRITION

Calories: 353;
Protein: 12.3g;
Carbs: 3.4g;
Fat: 6.3g

INGREDIENTS

- ½ cup of basmati rice
- 1.5cup of water
- 2 tbsp. pesto sauce

DIRECTIONS

1. Simmer the rice water for 15 minutes on the low heat or until the rice soaks all liquid.
2. Then mix cooked tice with pesto sauce.

135. Rice Salad

PREP TIME 10 mins

COOK TIME 0 mins

SERVINGS 4 people

NUTRITION
Calories: 153;
Protein: 12.3g;
Carbs: 18.4g;
Fat: 6.3g

INGREDIENTS

- ½ cup long-grain rice, cooked
- ½ cup corn kernels, cooked
- 1 tomato, chopped
- 1 tsp. chili flakes
- ¼ cup plain yogurt
- 1 cucumber pickle

DIRECTIONS

1. Grate the cucumber pickle and mix it with cooked rice, corn kernels, tomato, chili flakes, and plain yogurt.

136. Rice Meatballs

PREP TIME 10 mins

COOK TIME 15 mins

SERVINGS 20 people

NUTRITION
Calories: 183;
Protein: 12.3g;
Carbs: 17g
Fat: 6.3g

INGREDIENTS

- ¼ cup Cheddar cheese, shredded
- 1 tsp. ground black pepper
- 1 cup of basmati rice, cooked
- ¼ cup ground chicken
- 1 tsp. olive oil

DIRECTIONS

1. In the mixing bowl, mix Cheddar cheese, ground black pepper, rice, and ground chicken.
2. Then make the balls from the mixture.
3. Heat the olive oil well and put the rice balls in the hot oil.
4. Roast the balls for 1 minute per side on high heat.
5. Then transfer the balls in the oven and bake them for 20 minutes at 360F.

137. Mediterranean Paella

PREP TIME
10 mins

COOK TIME
30 mins

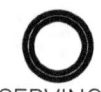
SERVINGS
6 people

NUTRITION

Calories: 223;
Carbs: 21g;
Protein: 12.3g;
Fat: 6.3g

INGREDIENTS

- 1 cup risotto rice
- 2 oz yellow onion, diced
- ½ tsp. ground paprika
- 1 cup tomatoes, chopped
- 1 cup shrimps, peeled
- 1 tsp. olive oil
- 3 cups of water

DIRECTIONS

1. Heat olive oil in the saucepan.
2. Add onion and cook it for 2 minutes.
3. Then stir well, add shrimps, ground paprika, tomatoes, and stir well.
4. Cook the ingredients for 5 minutes.
5. Add water and risotto rice. Stir well, close the lid, and cook the meal for 20 minutes on low heat.

138. Fast Chicken Rice

PREP TIME
10 mins

COOK TIME
20 mins

SERVINGS
5 people

NUTRITION

Calories: 213;
Protein: 12.3g;
Carbs: 14g;
Fat: 6.3g

INGREDIENTS

- 1 cup basmati rice
- 3 tbsp. avocado oil
- 2.5 cups chicken stock
- ½ tsp. dried dill
- 10 oz chicken breast, skinless, boneless, chopped

DIRECTIONS

1. Mix oil with rice and roast it in the saucepan for 5 minutes over the low heat.
2. Then add chicken and chicken stock.
3. Add dill, stir the ingredients and cook the meal on medium heat for 15 minutes or until all ingredients are cooked.

139. Rice Jambalaya

PREP TIME: 5 mins
COOK TIME: 30 mins
SERVINGS: 8 people

INGREDIENTS
- 1 cup tomatoes, chopped
- 1 cup bell pepper, chopped
- ¼ cup carrot, chopped
- 1 tsp. cayenne pepper
- 4 cups chicken stock
- 1 cup of basmati rice
- 2 tbsp. olive oil
- ½ cup chickpeas, cooked

DIRECTIONS
1. Melt the olive oil and add carrot, bell pepper, and tomatoes.
2. Cook the vegetables for 10 minutes on medium heat.
3. Then add chicken stock, chickpeas, and rice.
4. Add cayenne pepper and stir the meal.
5. Close the lid and cook it for 20 minutes on low heat.

NUTRITION
Calories: 263;
Protein: 10.3g;
Carbs: 3.4g;
Fat: 6.3g

140. Jasmine Rice with Scallions

PREP TIME: 10 mins
COOK TIME: 10 mins
SERVINGS: 6 people

INGREDIENTS
- 3 tbsp. olive oil
- 1 cup jasmine rice
- 2 tbsp. scallions, chopped
- ½ tsp. ground black pepper
- 2 tsp. lemon juice

DIRECTIONS
1. Cook the rice according to the directions of the manufacturer.
2. Then add scallions, olive oil, ground black pepper, and lemon juice.
3. Carefully stir the meal.

NUTRITION
Calories: 189;
Protein: 12.3g;
Carbs: 17g;
Fat: 6.3g

141. Cremini Mushrooms Pilaf

PREP TIME
10 mins

COOK TIME
25 mins

SERVINGS
6 people

NUTRITION

Calories: 193;
Protein: 12.3g;
Carbs:18g
Fat: 6.3g

INGREDIENTS

- 2 cups of water
- ½ cup white onion, diced
- 1 cup cremini mushrooms, chopped
- 1 cup of basmati rice
- ¼ tsp. lime zest, grated
- 2 oz goat cheese, crumbled
- 2 tbsp. olive oil

DIRECTIONS

1. Put rice in the saucepan.
2. Add water and cook for 15 minutes over the low heat.
3. Then roast the mushrooms with olive oil, lime zest, and white onion in the skillet until they are light brown.
4. Add the cooked mushrooms in the cooked rice. Stir well.
5. Top the meal with crumbled goat cheese.

142. Vegetable Rice

PREP TIME
10 mins

COOK TIME
30 mins

SERVINGS
6 people

NUTRITION

Calories: 187;
Protein: 12.3g;
Carbs:14g
Fat: 4.3g

INGREDIENTS

- 2 cups wild rice
- 1 tsp. Italian seasonings
- 1 tbsp. olive oil
- ¼ cup carrot, diced
- ½ cup snap peas, frozen
- 5 cups of water

DIRECTIONS

1. Mix 4 cups of water and wild rice in the saucepan.
2. Cook the rice for 15 minutes or until the rice soaks all liquid.
3. Then heat the olive oil in the separated saucepan.
4. Add carrot and roast it until light brown.
5. Add snap peas, water, and rice.
6. Stir well and close the lid.
7. Cook the rice for 10 minutes.

143. Tomato Rice

PREP TIME 10 mins

COOK TIME 20 mins

SERVINGS 4 people

NUTRITION

Calories: 53;
Protein: 12.3g;
Carbs: 13g;
Fat: 6.3g

INGREDIENTS

- 1 cup basmati rice
- 3 cups chicken stock
- 1 tsp. ground coriander
- ¼ tsp. dried thyme
- 2 tbsp. olive oil
- 2 tbsp. tomato paste

DIRECTIONS

1. Roast the rice with olive oil in the saucepan for 5 minutes. Stir it.
2. Then add thyme, coriander, and tomato paste.
3. Add water, mix the rice mixture, and close the lid.
4. Cook the rice for 15 minutes over the medium heat.

144. Rice with Grilled Tomatoes

PREP TIME 10 mins

COOK TIME 20 mins

SERVINGS 6 people

NUTRITION

Calories: 83;
Protein: 12.3g;
Carbs: 13g
Fat: 6.3g

INGREDIENTS

- 1 cup of basmati rice
- cups chicken stock
- 1 tsp. olive oil
- 2 tomatoes, roughly sliced

DIRECTIONS

1. Sprinkle the tomatoes with olive oil and grill in the preheated to 400F grill for 1 minute per side.
2. Then cook rice with chicken stock for 15 minutes.
3. Transfer the cooked rice in the bowls and top with grilled tomatoes.

145. Rice and Meat Salad

PREP TIME
10 mins

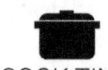
COOK TIME
0 mins

SERVINGS
6 people

INGREDIENTS

- 1 cup white cabbage, shredded
- 1 cup long grain rice, cooked
- 8 oz beef steak, cooked, cut into the strips
- 1/3 cup plain yogurt
- 1 tsp. salt
- 1 tsp. chives, chopped

DIRECTIONS

1. Put cabbage and rice in the big bowl.
2. Add white rice and meat strips.
3. Then add plain yogurt, chives, and salt.
4. Stir the salad until homogenous.

NUTRITION

Calories: 123;
Protein: 14.3g;
Carbs: 12.8g;
Fat: 6.3g

146. Rice Bowl

PREP TIME
10 mins

COOK TIME
0 mins

SERVINGS
6 people

INGREDIENTS

- 1 cup of basmati rice, cooked
- 4 oz beef sirloin, grilled
- ½ cup tomatoes, chopped
- 2 tbsp. soy sauce
- 1 tsp. ground paprika
- 2 oz scallions, sliced

DIRECTIONS

1. Put the cooked rice in the serving bowls.
2. Add beef sirloin, tomatoes, and scallions.
3. Then sprinkle the meal with soy sauce and ground paprika.

NUTRITION

Calories: 63;
Protein: 12.3g;
Carbs: 13.7g;
Fat: 6.3g

147. Zucchini Rice

PREP TIME: 10 mins
COOK TIME: 25 mins
SERVINGS: 2 people

INGREDIENTS
- ½ cup of long grain rice
- 1 cup chicken stock
- 1 zucchini, cubed
- 1 tbsp. olive oil
- 1 tsp. curry powder
- 1 tbsp. raisins

DIRECTIONS
1. Mix rice and chicken stock in the saucepan and cook for 15 minutes or until the rice soaks the liquid.
2. Then heat the olive oil.
3. Add zucchini in the oil and roast for 5 minutes.
4. After this, sprinkle the zucchini with curry powder, add raisins and rice.
5. Carefully mix the rice and cook for 5 minutes.

NUTRITION
Calories: 113;
Protein: 12.3g;
Carbs: 14g;
Fat: 4.3g

148. Rice Soup

PREP TIME: 10 mins
COOK TIME: 20 mins
SERVINGS: 4 people

INGREDIENTS
- 3 cups chicken stock
- ½ lb. chicken breast, shredded
- 1 tbsp. chives, chopped
- 1 egg, whisked
- ½ white onion, diced
- 1 bell pepper, chopped
- 1 tbsp. olive oil
- ¼ cup arborio rice
- ½ tsp. salt
- 1 tbsp. fresh cilantro, chopped

DIRECTIONS
1. Pour olive oil in the stock pan and preheat it.
2. Add onion and bell pepper. Roast the vegetables for 3-4 minutes. Stir them from time to time.
3. After this, add rice and stir well.
4. Cook the ingredients for 3 minutes over the medium heat.
5. Then add chicken stock and stir the soup well.
6. Add salt and bring the soup to boil.
7. Add shredded chicken breast, cilantro, and chives. Add egg and stir it carefully.
8. Close the lid and simmer the soup for 5 minutes over the medium heat.
9. Remove the cooked soup from the heat.

NUTRITION
Calories 176,
Fat 7.6g,
Carbs: 9g,
Protein 15.2g

149. Rice with Prunes

PREP TIME
5 mins

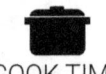
COOK TIME
20 mins

SERVINGS
7 people

INGREDIENTS

- 1.5 cup basmati rice
- 3 tbsp. organic canola oil
- 5 prunes, chopped
- ¼ cup cream cheese
- 3.5 cups water
- ½ tsp. salt

DIRECTIONS

1. Mix water and basmati rice in the saucepan and boil for 15 minutes on low heat.
2. Then add cream cheese, salt, and prunes.
3. Stir the rice carefully and bring it to boil.
4. Add organic canola oil and cook for 1 minute more.

NUTRITION

Calories: 83;
Protein: 12.3g;
Carbs: 12g;
Fat: 6.3g

150. Rice and Fish Cakes

PREP TIME
10 mins

COOK TIME
10 mins

SERVINGS
6 people

INGREDIENTS

- 6 oz salmon, canned, shredded
- 1 egg, beaten
- ¼ cup of basmati rice, cooked
- 1 tsp. dried cilantro
- ½ tsp. chili flakes
- 1 tbsp. organic canola oil

DIRECTIONS

1. Mix salmon with egg, basmati rice, dried cilantro, and chili flakes.
2. Heat the organic canola oil in the skillet.
3. Make the small cakes from the salmon mixture and put in the hot oil.
4. Roast the cakes for 2 minutes per side or until they are light brown.

NUTRITION

Calories: 123;
Protein: 12.3g;
Carbs: 7g;
Fat: 6.3g

151. Salsa Rice

PREP TIME: 10 mins
COOK TIME: 15 mins
SERVINGS: 6 people

NUTRITION
Calories: 109;
Protein: 12.3g;
Carbs: 7.4g;
Fat: 6.3g

INGREDIENTS
- 9 oz long grain rice
- 4 cups chicken stock
- 1 cup of salsa
- 2 tbsp. avocado oil

DIRECTIONS
1. Mix chicken stock and rice in the saucepan.
2. Cook the rice for 15 minutes on medium heat.
3. Then cool it to the room temperature and mix with avocado oil and salsa.

152. Seafood Rice

PREP TIME: 10 mins
COOK TIME: 30 mins
SERVINGS: 4 people

NUTRITION
Calories: 73;
Protein: 12.3g;
Carbs: 3.4g;
Fat: 6.3g

INGREDIENTS
- ½ cup seafood mix, frozen
- ½ cup of long grain rice
- 3 cups of water
- 1 tbsp. olive oil
- ½ tsp. ground coriander

DIRECTIONS
1. Boil the rice with water for 15-18 minutes or until it soaks all water.
2. Then heat olive oil in the saucepan.
3. Add seafood mix and ground coriander. Cook the ingredients for 10 minutes on low heat.
4. Then add rice, stir well, and cook for 5 minutes more.

153. Vegetarian Pilaf

PREP TIME
10 mins

COOK TIME
30 mins

SERVINGS
6 people

NUTRITION

Calories: 123;
Protein: 10.3g;
Carbs: 2.4g;
Fat: 6.3g

INGREDIENTS

- 1 cup of long grain rice
- 2 cups of water
- 1 carrot, grated
- 2 tbsp. olive oil
- 1 tbsp. dried dill
- ½ tsp. dried mint
- ½ tsp. salt

DIRECTIONS

1. Boil rice with water for 15 minutes on medium heat.
2. Meanwhile, melt the olive oil and add the carrot.
3. Roast the carrot for 10 minutes or until it is soft.
4. Then add dried dill, mint, and cooked rice.
5. Carefully stir the pilaf and cook for 5 minutes.

154. Rice Rolls

PREP TIME
15 mins

COOK TIME
35 mins

SERVINGS
6 people

NUTRITION

Calories: 69;
Protein: 12.3g;
Carbs: 3.4g;
Fat: 6.3g

INGREDIENTS

- 4 white cabbage leaves
- 4 oz ground chicken
- ½ tsp. garlic powder
- ¼ cup of long grain rice, cooked
- ½ cup chicken stock
- ½ cup tomatoes, chopped

DIRECTIONS

1. In the bowl, mix ground chicken, garlic powder, and rice.
2. Then put the rice mixture on every cabbage leaf and roll.
3. Arrange the rice rolls in the saucepan.
4. Add chicken stock and tomatoes and close the lid.
5. Cook the rice rolls for 35 minutes on low heat.

155. Rice Stew with Squid

PREP TIME 10 mins
COOK TIME 30 mins
SERVINGS 6 people

INGREDIENTS
- 5 oz long grain rice
- 4 oz squid, sliced
- 1 jalapeno pepper, chopped
- ½ cup tomatoes, chopped
- 1 onion, diced
- 2 cups chicken stock
- 1 tbsp. avocado oil

DIRECTIONS
1. Roast the onion with avocado oil in the skillet for 3-4 minutes or until the onion is light brown.
2. Add squid, jalapeno pepper, and tomatoes.
3. Cook the ingredients for 7 minutes.
4. Then cook rice with water for 15 minutes.
5. Add cooked rice in the squid mixture, stir, and cook for 3 minutes more.

NUTRITION
Calories: 153;
Protein: 12.3g;
Carbs: 3.4g;
Fat: 6.3g

156. Creamy Millet

PREP TIME 10 mins
COOK TIME 10 mins
SERVINGS 6 people

INGREDIENTS
- ½ cup millet
- 1 oz cream cheese
- ¼ tsp. salt
- 1.5 cup hot water

DIRECTIONS
1. Mix hot water and millet in the saucepan.
2. Boil it for 8 minutes on low heat.
3. Add cream cheese and salt.
4. Carefully stir the cooked millet.

NUTRITION
Calories: 53;
Protein: 12.3g;
Carbs: 3.4g;
Fat: 6.3g

157. Oatmeal Cakes

PREP TIME
15 mins

COOK TIME
7 mins

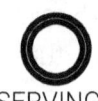
SERVINGS
4 people

NUTRITION

Calories: 63;
Protein: 12.3g;
Carbs: 3.4g;
Fat: 6.3g

INGREDIENTS

- ½ cup oatmeal
- 1 egg, beaten
- 1 carrot, grated
- 1 tbsp. olive oil
- 1 tsp. flax meal

DIRECTIONS

1. Put oatmeal, egg, grated carrot, and flax meal in the blender. Blend the mixture well.
2. Then heat olive oil in the skillet.
3. Make the medium size cakes from the oatmeal mixture and cook for 3 minutes per side on medium heat.

158. Yogurt Buckwheat

PREP TIME
5 mins

COOK TIME
13 mins

SERVINGS
2 people

NUTRITION

Calories: 69;
Protein: 12.3g;
Carbs: 3.4g;
Fat: 6.3g

INGREDIENTS

- ½ cup buckwheat
- 1.5 cup chicken stock
- 1 tbsp. plain yogurt

DIRECTIONS

1. Put all ingredients in the saucepan and close the lid.
2. Cook the meal for 13 minutes on low heat or until the buckwheat soaks all liquid.
3. Carefully stir the cooked meal.

159. Halloumi Buckwheat Bowl

PREP TIME: 10 mins
COOK TIME: 15 mins
SERVINGS: 4 people

INGREDIENTS
- 1 cup buckwheat
- cups chicken stock
- 4 oz halloumi cheese
- 1 tbsp. olive oil
- ½ tsp. dried thyme

DIRECTIONS
1. Mix chicken stock and buckwheat in the saucepan, bring to boil and cook for 7 minutes on medium heat.
2. After this, sprinkle the halloumi cheese with olive oil and dried thyme.
3. Grill it for 2 minutes per side or until the cheese is light brown.
4. Then put the cooked buckwheat in the bowls.
5. Chop the cheese roughly and top the buckwheat with it.

NUTRITION
Calories: 93; Protein: 12.3g; Carbs: 3.4g; Fat: 6.3g

160. Aromatic Green Millet

PREP TIME: 10 mins
COOK TIME: 7 mins
SERVINGS: 5 people

INGREDIENTS
- 1 cup millet
- 2 cups of water
- 4 tbsp. pesto sauce
- ¼ tsp. cayenne pepper

DIRECTIONS
1. Mix water and millet in the saucepan and boil for 7 minutes.
2. Then add cayenne pepper and pesto sauce.
3. Stir the millet until homogenous and green.

NUTRITION
Calories: 205; Protein: 5.3g; Carbs: 4.4g; Fat: 7.3g

161. Quinoa with Pumpkin

PREP TIME
5 mins

COOK TIME
20 mins

SERVINGS
6 people

INGREDIENTS

- ½ cup pumpkin, cubed
- 1 tbsp. lemon juice
- 1 tsp. liquid honey
- 1 cup quinoa
- 2 cups of water
- ¼ cup of organic almond milk

DIRECTIONS

1. Put almond milk and pumpkin in the saucepan.
2. Add lemon juice and water.
3. Cook the pumpkin for 10 minutes.
4. Then add quinoa and cook the meal for 10 minutes.
5. Remove the cooked meal from the heat, add liquid honey, and stir well.

NUTRITION

Calories: 177;
Protein: 6.3g;
Carbs: 4.7g;
Fat: 5.3g

162. Almond Quinoa

PREP TIME
5 mins

COOK TIME
4 mins

SERVINGS
4 people

INGREDIENTS

- 1 cup quinoa
- 2 cups of water
- 1 cup organic almond milk
- ½ cup strawberries, sliced
- 1 tbsp. honey

DIRECTIONS

1. Pour water and milk in the saucepan and bring to boil.
2. Add quinoa and cook it for 12 minutes.
3. Then cool the cooked quinoa and add honey. Stir.
4. Transfer the quinoa in the bowls and top with strawberries.

NUTRITION

Calories: 193;
Protein: 6.3g;
Carbs: 3.4g;
Fat: 3.3g

163. Spring Rolls with Quinoa

PREP TIME: 10 mins
COOK TIME: 1 min
SERVINGS: 8 people

INGREDIENTS
- 8 rice pepper wraps
- 1 cup quinoa, cooked
- 1 carrot, cut into strips
- 1 cup lettuce leaves
- 1 tbsp. olive oil

DIRECTIONS
1. Make the rice pepper wraps wet.
2. Then put the cooked quinoa on every rice pepper wrap.
3. Add carrot and lettuce leaves and wrap them into the rolls.
4. Brush every roll with olive oil and put it in the hot skillet.
5. Roast the spring rolls for 20 seconds per side.

NUTRITION
Calories: 257; Protein: 6.3g; Carbs: 3.4g; Fat: 6.3g

---

164. Mushroom Quinoa Skillet

PREP TIME: 10 mins
COOK TIME: 25 mins
SERVINGS: 6 people

INGREDIENTS
- 1 cup mushrooms, sliced
- ½ cup of water
- 1 tbsp. olive oil
- 1 tsp. Italian seasonings
- ½ cup quinoa
- ½ cup organic almond milk
- ¼ tsp. dried thyme

DIRECTIONS
1. Roast mushrooms with olive oil in the saucepan for 10 minutes.
2. Then stir them well, add Italian seasonings, dried thyme, and quinoa.
3. Add almond milk and water.
4. Close the lid and simmer the meal for 15 minutes. Stir it from time to time to avoid burning.

NUTRITION
Calories: 12; Protein: 3.3g; Carbs: 3.4g; Fat: 6.3g

165. Strawberry Quinoa Bowl

PREP TIME
15 mins

COOK TIME
0 mins

SERVINGS
8 people

INGREDIENTS

- 2 ½ cup quinoa, cooked
- ¼ cup strawberries, roughly chopped
- ½ cup fresh spinach, chopped
- 2 pecans, chopped
- 1 tbsp. balsamic vinegar
- 1 tsp. avocado oil

DIRECTIONS

1. Mix quinoa, fresh spinach, and pecans in the big bowl.
2. Then add strawberries and avocado oil.
3. Gently shake the mixture and transfer in the serving bowls.
4. Sprinkle every serving with a small amount of balsamic vinegar.

NUTRITION

Calories: 283;
Protein: 8.3g;
Carbs: 3.4g;
Fat: 6.3g

166. Quinoa Meatballs

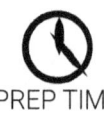
PREP TIME
15 mins

COOK TIME
30 mins

SERVINGS
6 people

INGREDIENTS

- ½ cup quinoa, cooked
- ½ cup ground pork
- 1 tbsp. chives, chopped
- 1 egg, beaten
- 1 tbsp. sesame seeds
- 1 tsp. chili flakes
- 1 cup tomato juice

DIRECTIONS

1. In the bowl mi quinoa, ground pork, chives, egg, sesame seeds, and chili flakes.
2. Then make the small meatballs and put them in the baking pan.
3. Top the meatballs with tomato juice and cook in the preheated to 375F oven for 30 minutes.

NUTRITION

Calories: 177;
Protein: 16.3g;
Carbs: 3.4g;
Fat: 6.3g

167. Stir-Fried Farro

PREP TIME
10 mins

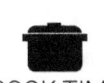
COOK TIME
8 mins

SERVINGS
4 people

NUTRITION

Calories: 196;
Protein: 6.3g;
Carbs: 3.4g;
Fat: 6.3g

INGREDIENTS

- 1 cup farro, cooked
- 1 egg, beaten
- 1 tbsp. olive oil
- ½ tsp. chili flakes

DIRECTIONS

1. Heat olive oil and egg beaten egg.
2. Cook it for 1 minute and then stir it carefully.
3. Add cooked farro and chili flakes.
4. Fry the meal for 7 minutes. Stir it from time to time.

168. Quick Farro Skillet

PREP TIME
10 mins

COOK TIME
15 mins

SERVINGS
6 people

NUTRITION

Calories: 147;
Protein: 4.3g;
Carbs: 4.1g;
Fat: 5.9g

INGREDIENTS

- 2 oz fresh spinach, chopped
- 2 oz asparagus, chopped
- 1/3 cup farro, cooked
- 1 tbsp. olive oil
- ½ tsp. curry powder

DIRECTIONS

1. Line the skillet with baking paper.
2. Put all ingredients in the prepared skillet, flatten them gently and transfer in the preheated to 365°F oven.
3. Cook the meal for 15 minutes.

169. Bulgur Bowl

PREP TIME
10 mins

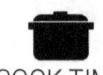
COOK TIME
0 mins

SERVINGS
4 people

INGREDIENTS

- 6 oz salmon, boiled, chopped
- ½ cup bulgur, cooked
- 1 cup fresh cilantro, chopped
- 1 cup tomato, chopped
- 3 tbsp. lemon juice
- 1 tbsp. olive oil

DIRECTIONS

1. Put salmon, bulgur, cilantro, and tomato in the bowl.
2. Add lemon juice and olive oil.
3. Shake the mixture well and transfer in the serving bowls.

NUTRITION

Calories: 153;
Protein: 12.3g;
Carbs: 6.4g;
Fat: 11.4g

170. Boiled Bulgur with Kale

PREP TIME
10 mins

COOK TIME
11 mins

SERVINGS
6 people

INGREDIENTS

- 1 cup bulgur
- cups water
- 1 cup kale
- ½ zucchini, chopped
- ½ tsp. allspices
- 6 tbsp. olive oil
- 2 oz goat cheese, crumbled

DIRECTIONS

1. Mix water and bulgur in the saucepan and cook boil for 11 minutes.
2. Then cool the bulgur and mix it with chopped kale, zucchini, allspices, and olive oil.
3. Transfer the bulgur meal in the serving bowls and top with goat cheese.

NUTRITION

Calories: 251;
Protein: 6.3g;
Carbs: 3.4g;
Fat: 6.3g

171. Chicken and Rice Soup

PREP TIME 10 mins
COOK TIME 20 mins
SERVINGS 6 people

INGREDIENTS
- 4 cups chicken stock
- 1 cup of water
- 1-lb. chicken breast, shredded
- 1 cup of rice, cooked
- 3 egg yolks
- 3 tbsp. lemon juice
- 1/3 cup fresh parsley, chopped
- ½ tsp. salt
- ¼ tsp. ground black pepper

DIRECTIONS
1. Pour water and chicken stock in the saucepan and bring to boil.
2. Then pour one cup of the hot liquid in the food processor.
3. Add cooked rice, egg yolks, lemon juice, and salt. Blend the mixture until smooth.
4. After this, transfer the smooth rice mixture into the saucepan with remaining chicken stock liquid.
5. Add shredded chicken breast, parsley, and ground black pepper.
6. Boil the soup for 5 minutes more.

NUTRITION
Calories 235,
Fat 4.8,
Carbs 25.9,
Protein 20.2

172. Tomato Bulgur

PREP TIME 5 mins
COOK TIME 20 mins
SERVINGS 3 people

INGREDIENTS
- ½ cup bulgur
- 1 onion, diced
- 3 tbsp. tomato paste
- ½ tsp. salt
- 2 tbsp. olive oil
- 1 cup of water

DIRECTIONS
1. Melt the olive oil in the saucepan.
2. Add diced onion and cook it until light brown.
3. Then add bulgur and tomato paste. Stir the ingredients.
4. Add water and cook the meal for 15 minutes.

NUTRITION
186 Calories,
4g Protein,
24.2g Carbs,
9.5g Fat

173. Bulgur Mix

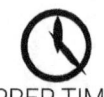
PREP TIME
10 mins

COOK TIME
0 mins

SERVINGS
3 people

NUTRITION

176 Calories,
8.3g Protein,
33.4g Carbs,
1.8g Fat

INGREDIENTS

- ½ cup bulgur, cooked
- ¼ cup corn kernels, cooked
- ¼ cup chickpeas, cooked
- ¼ cup snap peas, cooked
- 4 tbsp. plain yogurt

DIRECTIONS

1. Put all ingredients in the big bowl and carefully stir.

174. Aromatic Baked Brown Rice

PREP TIME
10 mins

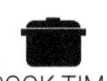
COOK TIME
20 mins

SERVINGS
6 people

NUTRITION

Calories: 302
Protein: 8 g
Fat: 14 g
Carbs: 23 g

INGREDIENTS

- ½ cup minced fresh parsley
- ¾ cup jarred roasted red peppers, rinsed, patted dry, and chopped
- 1 cup chicken or vegetable broth
- 1½ cups long-grain brown rice, rinsed
- 2 onions, chopped fine
- 2¼ cups water
- 4 tsp. extra-virgin olive oil
- Grated Parmesan cheese
- Lemon wedges
- Salt and pepper

DIRECTIONS

1. Place the oven rack in the centre of the oven and pre-heat your oven to 375°F. Heat oil in a Dutch oven on moderate heat until it starts to shimmer. Put in onions and 1 tsp. salt and cook, stirring intermittently, till they become tender and well browned, 12 to 14 minutes.
2. Mix in water and broth and bring to boil. Mix in rice, cover, and move pot to oven. Bake until rice becomes soft and liquid is absorbed, 65 to 70 minutes.
3. Remove pot from oven. Sprinkle red peppers over rice, cover, and allow to sit for about five minutes. Put in parsley to rice and fluff gently with fork to combine. Sprinkle with salt and pepper to taste. Serve with grated Parmesan and lemon wedges.

175. Aromatic Barley Pilaf

PREP TIME: 10 mins
COOK TIME: 10 mins
SERVINGS: 6 people

NUTRITION
Calories: 222
Protein: 18 g
Fat: 14 g
Carbs: 22 g

INGREDIENTS

- ¼ cup minced fresh parsley
- 1 small onion, chopped fine
- 1½ cups pearl barley, rinsed
- 1½ tsp. lemon juice
- 1½ tsp. minced fresh thyme or ½ tsp. dried
- 2 garlic cloves, minced
- 2 tbsp. minced fresh chives
- 2½ cups water
- 3 tbsp. extra-virgin olive oil
- Salt and pepper

DIRECTIONS

1. Heat oil in a big saucepan on moderate heat until it starts to shimmer. Put in onion and ½ tsp. salt and cook till they become tender, approximately five minutes. Mix in barley, garlic, and thyme and cook, stirring often, until barley is lightly toasted and aromatic, approximately three minutes.
2. Mix in water and bring to simmer. Decrease heat to low, cover, and simmer until barley becomes soft and water is absorbed, 20 to 40 minutes.
3. Remove from the heat, lay clean dish towel underneath lid and let pilaf sit for about ten minutes. Put in parsley, chives, and lemon juice to pilaf and fluff gently with fork to combine. Sprinkle with salt and pepper to taste. Serve.

176. Basmati Rice Pilaf Mix

PREP TIME: 10 mins
COOK TIME: 15 mins
SERVINGS: – people

NUTRITION
Calories: 234
Protein: 8 g
Fat: 11 g
Carbs: 33 g

INGREDIENTS

- ¼ cup currants
- ¼ cup sliced almonds, toasted
- ¼ tsp. ground cinnamon
- ½ tsp. ground turmeric
- 1 small onion, chopped fine
- 1 tbsp. extra-virgin olive oil
- 1½ cups basmati rice, rinsed
- 2 garlic cloves, minced
- 2¼ cups water
- Salt and pepper

DIRECTIONS

1. Heat oil in a big saucepan on moderate heat until it starts to shimmer. Put in onion and ¼ tsp. salt and cook till they become tender, approximately five minutes. Put in rice, garlic, turmeric, and cinnamon and cook, stirring often, until grain edges begin to turn translucent, approximately three minutes.
2. Mix in water and bring to simmer. Decrease heat to low, cover, and simmer gently until rice becomes soft and water is absorbed, 16 to 18 minutes.
3. Remove from the heat, drizzle currants over pilaf. Cover, laying clean dish towel underneath lid, and let pilaf sit for about ten minutes. Put in almonds to pilaf and fluff gently with fork to combine. Sprinkle with salt and pepper to taste. Serve.

177. Brown Rice Salad with Asparagus, Goat Cheese, and Lemon

PREP TIME
10 mins

COOK TIME
15 mins

SERVINGS
2 people

NUTRITION

Calories: 242
Protein: 18 g
Fat: 8 g
Carbs: 12 g

INGREDIENTS

- ¼ cup minced fresh parsley
- ¼ cup slivered almonds, toasted
- 1 lb. asparagus, trimmed and cut into 1-inch lengths
- 1 shallot, minced
- 1 tsp. grated lemon zest plus 3 tbsp. juice
- 1½ cups long-grain brown rice
- 2 oz. goat cheese, crumbled (½ cup)
- 3½ tbsp. extra-virgin olive oil
- Salt and pepper

DIRECTIONS

1. Bring 4 quarts water to boil in a Dutch oven. Put in rice and 1½ tsp. salt and cook, stirring intermittently, until rice is tender, about half an hour. Drain rice, spread onto rimmed baking sheet, and drizzle with 1 tbsp. lemon juice. Allow it to cool completely, about fifteen minutes.
2. Heat 1 tbsp. oil in 12-inch frying pan on high heat until just smoking. Put in asparagus, ¼ tsp. salt, and ¼ tsp. pepper and cook, stirring intermittently, until asparagus is browned and crisp-tender, about 4 minutes; move to plate and allow to cool slightly.
3. Beat remaining 2½ tbsp. oil, lemon zest and remaining 2 tbsp. juice, shallot, ½ tsp. salt, and ½ tsp. pepper together in a big container.
4. Put in rice, asparagus, 2 tbsp. goat cheese, 3 tbsp. almonds, and 3 tbsp. parsley. Gently toss to combine and allow to sit for about ten minutes. Sprinkle with salt and pepper to taste.
5. Move to serving platter and drizzle with remaining 2 tbsp. goat cheese, remaining 1 tbsp. almonds, and remaining 1 tbsp. parsley. Serve.

178. Carrot-Almond-Bulgur Salad

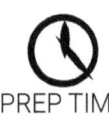
PREP TIME
10 mins

COOK TIME
20 mins

SERVINGS
4 people

NUTRITION

Calories: 287
Protein: 8 g
Fat: 7 g
Carbs: 13 g

INGREDIENTS

- 1/8 tsp. cayenne pepper
- 1/3 cup chopped fresh cilantro
- 1/3 cup chopped fresh mint
- 1/3 cup extra-virgin olive oil
- ½ cup sliced almonds, toasted
- ½ tsp. ground cumin
- 1 cup water
- 1½ cups medium-grind bulgur, rinsed
- 3 scallions, sliced thin
- 4 carrots, peeled and shredded
- 6 tbsp. lemon juice (2 lemons)
- Salt and pepper

DIRECTIONS

1. Mix bulgur, water, ¼ cup lemon juice, and ¼ tsp. salt in a container. Cover and allow to sit at room temperature until grains are softened and liquid is fully absorbed, about 1½ hours.
2. Beat remaining 2 tbsp. lemon juice, oil, cumin, cayenne, and ½ tsp. salt together in a big container.
3. Put in bulgur, carrots, scallions, almonds, mint, and cilantro and gently toss to combine. Sprinkle with salt and pepper to taste. Serve.

179. Chickpea-Spinach Bulgur

PREP TIME: 5 mins
COOK TIME: 20 mins
SERVINGS: 6 people

NUTRITION
Calories: 234
Protein: 18 g
Fat: 14 g
Carbs: 10 g

INGREDIENTS

- ¾ cup chicken or vegetable broth
- ¾ cup water
- 1 (15-oz.) can chickpeas, rinsed
- 1 cup medium-grind bulgur, rinsed
- 1 onion, chopped fine
- 1 tbsp. lemon juice
- 2 tbsp. za'atar
- 3 garlic cloves, minced
- 3 oz. (3 cups) baby spinach, chopped
- 3 tbsp. extra-virgin olive oil
- Salt and pepper

DIRECTIONS

1. Heat 2 tbsp. oil in a big saucepan on moderate heat until it starts to shimmer. Put in onion and ½ tsp. salt and cook till they become tender, approximately five minutes. Mix in garlic and 1 tbsp. za'atar and cook until aromatic, approximately half a minute.
2. Mix in bulgur, chickpeas, broth, and water and bring to simmer. Decrease heat to low, cover, and simmer gently until bulgur is tender, 16 to 18 minutes.
3. Remove from the heat, lay clean dish towel underneath lid and let bulgur sit for about ten minutes. Put in spinach, lemon juice, remaining 1 tbsp. za'atar, and residual 1 tbsp. oil and fluff gently with fork to combine. Sprinkle with salt and pepper to taste. Serve.

180. Classic Baked Brown Rice

PREP TIME: 10 mins
COOK TIME: 20 mins
SERVINGS: 6 people

NUTRITION
Calories: 222
Protein: 18 g
Fat: 10 g
Carbs: 12 g

INGREDIENTS

- 1½ cups long-grain brown rice, rinsed
- 2 tsp. extra-virgin olive oil
- 2 1/3 cups boiling water
- Salt and pepper

DIRECTIONS

1. Place the oven rack in the centre of the oven and pre-heat your oven to 375°F. Mix boiling water, rice, oil, and ½ tsp. salt in 8-inch square baking dish.
2. Cover dish tightly using double layer of aluminium foil. Bake until rice becomes soft and water is absorbed, about 1 hour. Remove dish from oven, uncover, and gently fluff rice with fork, scraping up any rice that has stuck to bottom.
3. Cover dish with clean dish towel and let rice sit for about five minutes. Uncover and let rice sit for about five minutes longer.
4. Sprinkle with salt and pepper to taste. Serve.

181. Classic Italian Seafood Risotto

PREP TIME
10 mins

COOK TIME
20 mins

SERVINGS
4 people

NUTRITION

Calories: 343
Protein: 18 g
Fat: 14 g
Carbs: 33 g

INGREDIENTS

- 1/8 tsp. saffron threads, crumbled
- 1 (14.5-oz.) can diced tomatoes, drained
- 1 cup dry white wine
- 1 onion, chopped fine
- 1 tbsp. lemon juice
- 1 tsp. minced fresh thyme or ¼ tsp. dried
- 12 oz. large shrimp (26 to 30 per lb.), peeled and deveined, shells reserved
- 12 oz. small bay scallops
- 2 bay leaves
- 2 cups Arborio rice
- 2 cups chicken broth
- 2 tbsp. minced fresh parsley
- 2½ cups water
- 4 (8-oz.) bottles clam juice
- 5 garlic cloves, minced
- 5 tbsp. extra-virgin olive oil
- Salt and pepper

DIRECTIONS

1. Bring shrimp shells, broth, water, clam juice, tomatoes, and bay leaves to boil in a big saucepan on moderate to high heat.
2. Decrease the heat to a simmer and cook for 20 minutes. Strain mixture through fine-mesh strainer into big container, pressing on solids to extract as much liquid as possible; discard solids. Return broth to now-empty saucepan, cover, and keep warm on low heat.
3. Heat 2 tbsp. oil in a Dutch oven on moderate heat until it starts to shimmer. Put in onion and cook till they become tender, approximately five minutes.
4. Put in rice, garlic, thyme, and saffron and cook, stirring often, until grain edges begin to turn translucent, approximately three minutes.
5. Put in wine and cook, stirring often, until fully absorbed, approximately three minutes. Mix in 3½ cups warm broth, bring to simmer, and cook, stirring intermittently, until almost fully absorbed, about fifteen minutes.
6. Carry on cooking rice, stirring often and adding warm broth, 1 cup at a time, every few minutes as liquid is absorbed, until rice is creamy and cooked through but still somewhat firm in center, about fifteen minutes.
7. Mix in shrimp and scallops and cook, stirring often, until opaque throughout, approximately three minutes. Remove pot from heat, cover, and allow to sit for about five minutes.
8. Adjust consistency with remaining warm broth as required (you may have broth left over). Mix in remaining 3 tbsp. oil, parsley, and lemon juice and sprinkle with salt and pepper to taste. Serve.

182. Classic Stovetop White Rice

PREP TIME
10 mins

COOK TIME
10 mins

SERVINGS
6 people

NUTRITION

Calories: 252
Protein: 18 g
Fat: 10 g
Carbs: 33 g

INGREDIENTS

- 1 tbsp. extra-virgin olive oil
- 2 cups long-grain white rice, rinsed
- 3 cups water
- Basmati, jasmine, or Texmati rice can be substituted for the long-grain rice.
- Salt and pepper

DIRECTIONS

1. Heat oil in a big saucepan on moderate heat until it starts to shimmer. Put in rice and cook, stirring frequently, until grain edges begin to turn translucent, approximately two minutes.
2. Put in water and 1 tsp. salt and bring to simmer. Cover, decrease the heat to low, and simmer gently until rice becomes soft and water is absorbed, approximately twenty minutes.
3. Remove from the heat, lay clean dish towel underneath lid and let rice sit for about ten minutes. Gently fluff rice with fork. Sprinkle with salt and pepper to taste. Serve.

SOUPS AND STEWS

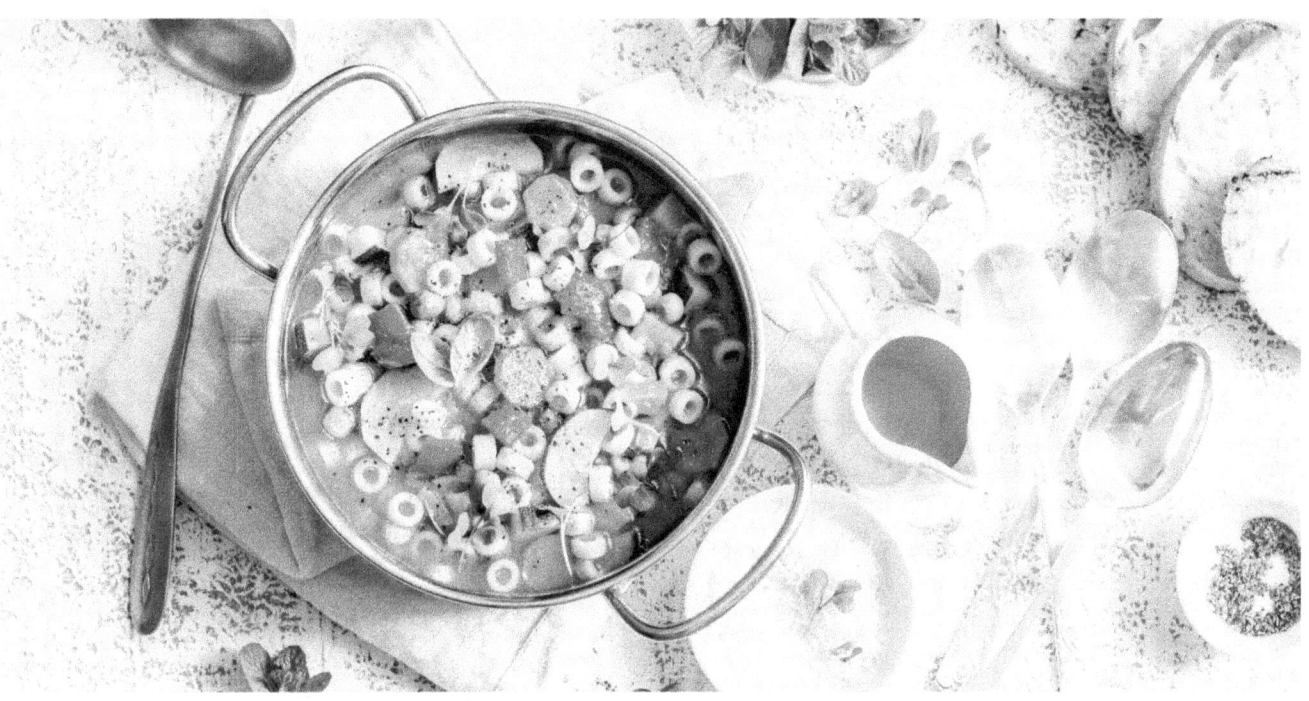

183. Moroccan Lentil Soup

PREP TIME
10 mins

COOK TIME
60 mins

SERVINGS
6 people

NUTRITION

Calories: 551;
Protein: 36.3g;
Carbs: 33.4g;
Fat: 30.3g

INGREDIENTS

- 2 tbsp. extra virgin olive oil
- 1 large yellow onion, finely chopped
- 2 stalks celery, finely chopped
- 1 carrot, peeled and finely chopped
- 1/3 cup chopped parsley, leaves and tender stems
- 1/2 cup chopped cilantro, leaves and tender stems
- 5 large garlic cloves, minced
- 2" piece ginger, minced
- 1 tsp. ground turmeric
- 1 tsp. ground cinnamon
- 2 tsp. sweet paprika
- 1/2 tsp. Aleppo pepper (or substitute freshly ground black pepper)
- 1 1/4 cups dry red lentils, rinsed and picked over
- 1 x 15 oz. can garbanzo beans, drained
- 1 x 28 oz. can sieved tomatoes
- 7-8 cups chicken broth or vegetable broth
- Coarse salt

To Servings:
- Dates
- Lemon wedges

DIRECTIONS

1. Grab a large saucepan, add the olive oil and place over a medium heat.
2. Add the onion, celery, carrots, garlic, and ginger and cook for 5 minutes until soft.
3. Throw in the turmeric, cinnamon, paprika and pepper and continue to cook for another 5 minutes.
4. Add the tomatoes and broth, stir well then bring to a simmer.
5. Add the lentils, garbanzo beans, cilantro and parsley.
6. Cook uncovered for 35 minutes until the lentils become very soft.
7. Season well then serve and enjoy.

184. Roasted Red Pepper and Tomato Soup

PREP TIME
10 mins

COOK TIME
45 mins

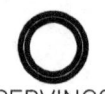
SERVINGS
4 people

NUTRITION

Calories: 531;
Protein: 26.3g;
Carbs: 33.4g;
Fat: 30.3g

INGREDIENTS

- 2 red bell peppers, seeded and halved
- 3 tomatoes, cored and halved
- 1/2 medium onion, quartered
- 2 cloves garlic, peeled and halved
- 1-2 tbsp. olive oil
- 1/4 tsp. salt
- 1/4 tsp. ground black pepper
- 2 cups vegetable broth
- 2 tbsp. tomato paste
- 1/4 cup fresh parsley, chopped
- 1/4 tsp. Italian seasoning blend
- 1/4 tsp. ground paprika
- 1/8 teaspoon. ground cayenne pepper, or more to taste

DIRECTIONS

1. Preheat your oven to 375°F.
2. Grab a medium bowl and add the red peppers, tomatoes, onion, garlic, olive oil and salt and pepper. Toss well to coat.
3. Place onto a baking sheet and pop into the oven for 45 minutes until soft.
4. Next place the veggie broth over a medium heat and add the roasted veggies, tomato paste, parsley, paprika and cayenne.
5. Stir to combine then simmer for 10 minutes.
6. Use an immersion blender to puree the soup then return back to the pan.
7. Reheat if required, add extra seasoning then serve and enjoy.

185. Greek Spring Soup

PREP TIME
10 mins

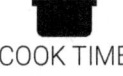
COOK TIME
35 mins

SERVINGS
4 people

NUTRITION

Calories: 551;
Protein: 16.3g;
Carbs: 23.4g;
Fat: 10.3g

INGREDIENTS

- 6 cups chicken broth
- 1 1/2 cups diced or shredded cooked chicken
- 2 tbsp. olive oil
- 1 small onion, diced
- 1 bay leaf
- 1/3 cup arborio rice
- 1 large free-range egg
- 2 tbsp. water
- Juice of half of a lemon
- 1 cup chopped asparagus
- 1 cup diced carrots
- 1/2 cup fresh chopped dill, divided
- Salt and pepper, to taste

DIRECTIONS

1. Find a large pan, add the oil and place over a medium heat.
2. Add the onions and cook for five minutes until soft.
3. Next add ¼ cup dill, plus the chicken broth and bay leaf. Bring to a boil.
4. Add the rice and reduce the heat to low. Simmer for 10 minutes.
5. Add the carrots and asparagus and cook for 10 more minutes until the rice and veggies are tender.
6. Add the chicken and simmer.
7. Meanwhile find a medium bowl and add the egg, lemon and water. Whisk well.
8. Add ½ cup of the stock to the egg mixture, stirring constantly then pour it all back into the pot.
9. Heat through and allow the soup to thicken.
10. Add remaining dill, season well then serve and enjoy.

186. Fast Seafood Gumbo

PREP TIME: 10 mins
COOK TIME: 40 mins
SERVINGS: 4 people

NUTRITION
Calories: 551;
Protein: 36.3g;
Carbs: 33.4g;
Fat: 30.3g

INGREDIENTS

- 1/4 cup olive oil
- 1/4 cup flour
- 1 medium white onion, chopped
- 1 cup celery, chopped
- 1 red or green bell pepper, chopped and deseeded
- 1 red chili, chopped
- 2 cups okra, chopped
- 1 cup canned crushed tomatoes
- 2 large cloves garlic, crushed
- 1 tsp. dried thyme
- 2 cups fish stock
- 1 bay leaf
- 1 tsp. cayenne powder
- 2 x 8 oz. can crab meat with brine
- 1 lb. shrimp, peeled and deveined
- Salt & pepper, to taste
- 1/4 cup fresh parsley, finely chopped

DIRECTIONS

1. Find a large pan, add the oil and place over a medium heat.
2. Add the flour and stir well until it forms a thick paste.
3. Add the onions, celery, peppers and okra and stir well, cooking for 5 minutes.
4. Add the garlic, tomatoes, thyme, stock, bay leaf and cayenne and stir again.
5. Bring to a boil then reduce the heat and simmer for 15 minutes.
6. Add the shrimp and crab and cook for 8 minutes more.

187. Minestrone Soup

PREP TIME: 10 mins
COOK TIME: 60 mins
SERVINGS: 4 people

NUTRITION
Calories 34;
Protein: 26.3g;
Carbs: 33.4g;
Fat: 30.3g

INGREDIENTS

- 1 small white onion, minced
- 4 cloves garlic, minced
- 1/2 cup sliced carrots
- 1 medium zucchini sliced, then cut slices in half
- 1 medium yellow squash sliced, then cut slices in half
- 2 tbsp. minced fresh parsley
- 1/4 cup celery sliced
- 3 tbsp. olive oil
- 2 x 15 oz. cans cannellini beans, rinsed & drained
- 2 x 15 oz. cans red kidney beans, rinsed & drained
- 1 x 14.5 oz. can fire-roasted diced tomatoes, drained
- 4 cups vegetable stock
- 2 cups water
- 1 1/2 tsp. oregano
- 1/2 tsp. basil
- 1/4 tsp. thyme
- 1 tsp. salt
- 1/2 tsp. pepper
- 3/4 cup small pasta shells
- 4 cups fresh baby spinach
- 1/4 cup Parmesan or Romano cheese

DIRECTIONS

1. Grab a stock pot and place over a medium heat.
2. Add the oil then the onions, garlic, carrots, zucchini, squash, parsley and celery.
3. Cook for five minutes until the veggies are getting soft.
4. Pour in the stock, water, beans, tomatoes, herbs and salt and pepper. Stir well.
5. Reduce the heat, cover and simmer for 30 minutes.
6. Add the pasta and spinach, stir well then cover and cook for a further 20 minutes until the pasta is cooked through.
7. Stir through the cheese then serve and enjoy.

188. Lemon Chicken Soup

PREP TIME
10 mins

COOK TIME
20 mins

SERVINGS
6 people

NUTRITION

Calories: 251;
Protein: 16.3g;
Carbs: 23.4g;
Fat: 30.3g

INGREDIENTS

- 10 cups chicken broth
- 3 tbsp. olive oil
- 8 cloves garlic, minced
- 1 sweet onion, sliced
- 1 large lemon, zested
- 2 boneless skinless chicken breasts
- 1 cup Israeli couscous
- 1/2 tsp. crushed red pepper
- 2 oz. crumbled feta
- 1/3 cup chopped chive
- Salt and pepper, to taste

DIRECTIONS

1. Grab a stock pot, add the oil and place over a medium heat.
2. Add the onion and garlic and cook for five minutes until soft.
3. Add the broth, chicken breasts, lemon zest and crushed pepper.
4. Raise the heat, cover and bring to a boil.
5. Reduce the heat then simmer for 5 minutes.
6. Turn off the heat, remove the lid and remove the chicken from the pot.
7. Pop onto a place and use two forks to shred.
8. Pop back into the pot, add the feta, chives and salt and pepper.
9. Stir well then serve and enjoy.

189. Tuscan Vegetable Pasta Soup

PREP TIME
10 mins

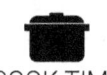
COOK TIME
30 mins

SERVINGS
6 people

NUTRITION

Calories: 151;
Protein: 26.3g;
Carbs: 14.4g;
Fat: 30.3g

INGREDIENTS

- 2 tbsp. extra virgin olive oil
- 4 cloves garlic, minced
- 1 medium yellow onion, diced
- 1/2 cup carrot, chopped
- 1/2 cup celery, chopped
- 1 medium zucchini, sliced and quartered
- 1 x 15 oz. can diced tomatoes
- 6 cups vegetable stock
- 2 tbsp. tomato paste
- 6-8 oz. whole wheat pasta
- 1 x 15 oz. can white beans
- 2 large handfuls baby spinach
- 6 basil cubes
- Salt and pepper, to taste
- Fresh chopped parsley, for garnish

DIRECTIONS

1. Grab a stock pot, add the oil and pop over a medium heat.
2. Add the onion and garlic and cook for five minutes until soft.
3. Throw in the carrots, celery and zucchini and cook for an extra 5 minutes, stirring occasionally.
4. Add the tomato and salt and pepper and cook for 1-2 minutes.
5. Add the veggies broth and tomato paste, stir well then bring to the boil.
6. Throw in the pasta, cook for 10 minutes then add the spinach, white beans, basil cubes and seasoning.
7. Stir well then remove from the heat.
8. Divide between large bowls and serve and enjoy.

190. Dairy Free Zucchini Soup

PREP TIME 10 mins
COOK TIME 25 mins
SERVINGS 8 people

INGREDIENTS
- 2½ lb. zucchini
- 1 medium onion, diced
- 2 tbsp. olive oil
- 4 garlic cloves, chopped
- 4 cups chicken stock
- Sea salt and pepper, to taste
- 1/3 cup fresh basil leaves

DIRECTIONS
1. Grab a pan, add the oil and pop over a medium heat.
2. Add the onion, garlic and zucchini and cook for five minutes until soft.
3. Add the stock and simmer for 15 minutes.
4. Remove from the heat, stir through the basil, add the seasoning and use an immersion blender to whizz until smooth.
5. Serve and enjoy.

NUTRITION
Calories: 551; Protein: 36.3g; Carbs: 33.4g; Fat: 30.3g

191. Farro Stew with Kale & Cannellini Beans

PREP TIME 10 mins
COOK TIME 60 mins
SERVINGS 4 people

INGREDIENTS
- 2 tbsp. olive oil
- 2 medium carrots, diced
- 1 medium onion, chopped
- 2 sticks celery, chopped
- 4 cloves garlic, minced
- 5 cups low-sodium vegetable broth
- 1 x 14.5 oz. can diced tomatoes
- 1 cup farro, rinsed
- 1 tsp. dried oregano
- 1 bay leaf
- Salt, to taste
- 1/2 cup parsley
- 4 cups chopped kale, thick ribs removed
- 1 x 15 oz. can cannellini beans, drained and rinsed
- 1 tbsp. fresh lemon juice
- 1/2 cup feta cheese, crumbled

DIRECTIONS
1. Grab a stock pot, add the oil and place over a medium heat.
2. Add the onion, carrots and celery and cook for five minutes until becoming soft.
3. Add the garlic and cook for another 30 seconds.
4. Stir through the broth, tomatoes, farro, oregano, bay leaf, parsley and salt.
5. Cover with the lid and bring to the boil. Reduce the heat then simmer for 20 minutes.
6. Remove the lid, add the kale and cook for a further 10-15 minutes.
7. Remove the bay leaf, add the beans, stir through the lemon juice and any additional liquid then stir well to combine.
8. Serve and enjoy.

NUTRITION
Calories: 21; Protein: 16.3g; Carbs: 3.4g; Fat: 6.3g

192. Italian Meatball Soup

PREP TIME
10 mins

COOK TIME
45 mins

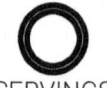
SERVINGS
6 people

NUTRITION

Calories: 331;
Protein: 14.3g;
Carbs: 14.4g;
Fat: 30.3g

INGREDIENTS

- 1/4 - 1/2 cup freshly grated parmesan cheese (optional)
- 1 free-range egg
- 1 cup breadcrumbs, optional
- 2 tbsp. fresh parsley, minced
- 1 tsp. dried oregano
- 1/2 tsp. sea salt
- ½ tsp. black pepper
- 3 tbsp. olive oil
- For the soup…
- 2 quarts chicken broth or beef broth
- 3 tbsp. tomato paste
- 1 onion, diced
- 2 bay leaves
- 4-5 sprigs fresh thyme
- ½ tsp. whole black peppercorns
- To serve…
- Fresh parmesan cheese, grated
- 1-2 tbsp. fresh basil leaves, torn
- 1-2 tbsp. fresh parsley, chopped
- Salt and pepper, to taste

DIRECTIONS

1. Place all the meatball ingredients except the oil into a medium bowl.
2. Using your hands, mix well and form into meatballs.
3. Place the oil into a stock pot, place over a medium heat and add the meatballs, browning on all sides.
4. Remove the meatballs from the pan.
5. Add more oil to the pan if needed and then add the onion. Cook for five minutes until soft.
6. Add the remaining soup ingredients, stir well then cook for 10 minutes.
7. Return the meatballs to the pan and simmer for a few minutes to warm through.
8. Serve and enjoy.

193. Tuscan White Bean Soup with Sausage and Kale

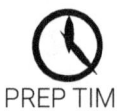
PREP TIME
10 mins

COOK TIME
40 mins

SERVINGS
6 people

NUTRITION

Calories: 551;
Protein: 36.3g;
Carbs: 33.4g;
Fat: 30.3g

INGREDIENTS

- ¼ cup extra virgin olive oil
- 1 lb. hot sausage,
- 1 onion, chopped
- 1 carrot, chopped
- 1 stalk celery, chopped
- 2 cloves garlic, chopped
- ½ lb. kale, stems removed and chopped
- 4 cups chicken broth
- 1 x 28 oz. can cannelloni beans, rinsed and drained
- 1 tsp. rosemary, dried
- 1 bay leaf
- ¼ tsp. pepper
- Salt, to taste
- ½ cup shredded parmesan

DIRECTIONS

1. Find a stock pot, pop over a medium heat and add the oil.
2. Cook the sausage until browned on all sides.
3. Throw in the onion, carrot, celery and garlic then cook for a further five minutes.
4. Add the kale and stir through.
5. Next add the broth, beans, rosemary and bay leaf.
6. Stir well, bring to the boil then cover with the lid.
7. Turn down the heat then simmer for 30 minutes.
8. Serve and enjoy.

194. Vegetable Soup

PREP TIME: 10 mins
COOK TIME: 45 mins
SERVINGS: 4 people

NUTRITION
Calories: 123;
Protein: 12.3g;
Carbs: 33.4g;
Fat: 19.3g

INGREDIENTS

- Extra virgin olive oil, to taste
- 8 oz. sliced baby Bella mushrooms
- 2 medium-size zucchinis, sliced
- 1 bunch flat leaf parsley, chopped
- 1 red onion, chopped
- 2 garlic cloves, chopped
- 2 celery ribs, chopped
- 2 carrots, peeled, chopped
- 2 golden potatoes, peeled, diced
- 1 tsp. ground coriander
- 1/2 tsp. turmeric powder
- 1/2 tsp. sweet paprika
- 1/2 tsp. thyme
- Salt and pepper
- 1 x 32 oz. can whole peeled tomatoes
- 2 bay leaves
- 6 cups turkey or vegetable broth
- 1 x 15 oz. can garbanzo beans, rinsed and drained
- Juice and zest of 1 lime
- 1/3 cup toasted pine nuts, optional

DIRECTIONS

1. Grab a large stockpot, add a tbsp. of olive oil and pop over a medium heat.
2. Add the mushrooms and cook for five minutes, stirring often.
3. Remove from the pan and pop to one side.
4. Add the sliced zucchini and cook for another five minutes. Remove from the pan.
5. Add more oil and add the parsley, onions, garlic, celery, carrots and potatoes. Stir through the spices, salt and pepper.
6. Cook for five minutes until the veggies are softening.
7. Add the tomatoes, bay leaves and broth then bring to a boil.
8. Cover and cook on medium low for 15 minutes.
9. Remove the lid and add the garbanzo beans, mushrooms and zucchini.
10. Heat then serve and enjoy.

195. Sweet Yogurt Bulgur Bowl

PREP TIME: 10 mins
COOK TIME: 0 mins
SERVINGS: 4 people

NUTRITION
Calories: 123;
Protein: 12.3g;
Carbs: 33.4g;
Fat: 19.3g

INGREDIENTS

- 1 cup grapes, halved
- ½ cup bulgur, cooked
- ¼ cup celery stalk, chopped
- 2 oz walnuts, chopped
- ¼ cup plain yogurt
- ½ tsp. ground cinnamon

DIRECTIONS

1. Mix grapes with bulgur, celery stalk, and walnut
2. Then add plain yogurt and ground cinnamon.
3. Stir the mixture with the help of the spoon and transfer in the serving bowls.

196. Spring Farro Plate

PREP TIME
15 mins

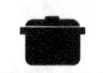
COOK TIME
0 mins

SERVINGS
6 people

INGREDIENTS

- 1 cup farro, cooked
- 2 cups baby spinach
- 2 grapefruits, roughly chopped
- 2 tbsp. balsamic vinegar
- ¼ tsp. white pepper
- 1 tbsp. olive oil

DIRECTIONS

1. Mix baby spinach and farro in the big bowl.
2. Then add grapefruit and shake the ingredients well.
3. Transfer the mixture in the serving plates and sprinkle with white pepper, olive oil, and balsamic vinegar.

NUTRITION

Calories: 113;
Protein: 12.3g;
Carbs: 33.4g;
Fat: 19.3g

197. Sorghum Taboule

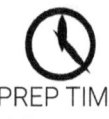
PREP TIME
10 mins

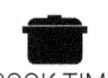
COOK TIME
0 mins

SERVINGS
2 people

INGREDIENTS

- 2 oz sorghum, cooked
- 3 oz pumpkin, diced, boiled
- ½ white onion, diced
- 1 date, pitted, chopped
- 1 tbsp. avocado oil
- ½ tsp. liquid honey
- 2 oz Feta, crumbled

DIRECTIONS

1. Put sorghum, pumpkin, onion, and date in the big bowl.
2. Then sprinkle the ingredients with avocado oil and liquid honey. Stir well.
3. Transfer the cooked taboule in the serving plates and top with crumbled feta.

NUTRITION

Calories: 123;
Protein: 12.3g;
Carbs: 33.4g;
Fat: 19.3g

198. Roasted Sorghum

PREP TIME
10 mins

COOK TIME
15 mins

SERVINGS
4 people

NUTRITION

Calories: 123;
Protein: 2.3g;
Carbs: 3.4g;
Fat: 9.3g

INGREDIENTS

- 1 tbsp. avocado oil
- ½ cup sorghum, cooked
- 1 carrot, diced
- 2 tbsp. dried parsley
- ½ tsp. dried oregano
- 2 tbsp. cream cheese

DIRECTIONS

1. Heat avocado oil and add the carrot.
2. Roast it for 5 minutes.
3. Then add cooked sorghum, parsley, oregano, and cream cheese.
4. Roast the meal for 10 minutes on low heat. Stir it from time to time to avoid burning.

199. Sorghum Stew

PREP TIME
10 mins

COOK TIME
25 mins

SERVINGS
5 people

NUTRITION

Calories: 127;
Protein: 12.3g;
Carbs: 13.4g;
Fat: 19.3g

INGREDIENTS

- 1 cup sorghum
- ½ cup ground sausages
- ½ cup tomatoes
- 1 jalapeno pepper, chopped
- ½ cup bell pepper, chopped
- 4 cups chicken stock

DIRECTIONS

1. Roast the sausages for 5 minutes in the saucepan.
2. Then add tomatoes, jalapeno, and bell pepper.
3. Cook the ingredients for 10 minutes.
4. After this, add sorghum and chicken stock and boil the stew for 10 minutes more.

200. Sorghum Salad

PREP TIME
10 mins

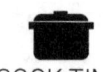
COOK TIME
10 mins

SERVINGS
3 people

INGREDIENTS

- 3 oz butternut squash, chopped
- ¼ cup sorghum
- ¼ cup fresh cilantro, chopped
- 1 tsp. ground cumin
- cups water
- 2 tbsp. organic canola oil
- 2 tbsp. apple cider vinegar

DIRECTIONS

1. Put sorghum and butternut squash in the saucepan.
2. Add water and cook for 10 minutes.
3. Then cool the ingredients and transfer in the salad bowl.
4. Add cilantro, ground cumin, organic canola oil, and apple cider vinegar.
5. Stir the meal well.

NUTRITION

Calories: 123;
Protein: 12.3g;
Carbs: 16.4g;
Fat: 19.3g

201. Sorghum Bake

PREP TIME
10 mins

COOK TIME
25 mins

SERVINGS
4 people

INGREDIENTS

- ½ cup sorghum
- 1 apple, chopped
- 1 oz raisins
- 1.5cup of water

DIRECTIONS

1. Put sorghum in the pan. Flatten it.
2. Then top it with raisins, apple, and water.
3. Cover the meal with baking paper and transfer in the preheated to 375F oven.
4. Bake the meal for 25 minutes.

NUTRITION

Calories: 179;
Protein: 18.3g;
Carbs: 3.4g;
Fat: 19.3g

202. Lamb and Chickpeas Stew

PREP TIME 10 mins
COOK TIME 80 mins
SERVINGS 6 people

NUTRITION
Calories 340, Fat 16gg, Fiber 3g, Carbs 21g, Protein 19g

INGREDIENTS
- 1 and ½ lb. lamb shoulder, cubed
- 3 tbsp. olive oil
- 1 cup yellow onion, chopped
- 1 cup carrots, cubed
- 1 cup celery, chopped
- 3 garlic cloves, minced
- 4 rosemary springs, chopped
- 2 cups chicken stock
- 1 cup tomato puree
- 15 oz. canned chickpeas, drained and rinsed
- 10 oz. baby spinach
- 2 tbsp. black olives, pitted and sliced
- A pinch of salt and black pepper

DIRECTIONS
1. Heat up a pot with the oil over medium-high heat, add the meat, salt and pepper and brown for 5 minutes.
2. Add carrots, celery, onion and garlic, stir and sauté for 5 minutes more.
3. Add the rosemary, stock, chickpeas and the other ingredients except the spinach and olives, stir and cook for 1 hour.
4. Add the rest of the ingredients, cook the stew over medium heat for 10 minutes more, divide into bowls and serve.

203. Chorizo and Lentils Stew

PREP TIME 10 mins
COOK TIME 35 mins
SERVINGS 4 people

NUTRITION
Calories 400, Fat 16gg, Fiber 13g, Carbs 58g, Protein 24g

INGREDIENTS
- 4 cups water
- 1 cup carrots, sliced
- 1 yellow onion, chopped
- 1 tbsp. extra-virgin olive oil
- ¾ cup celery, chopped
- 1 and ½ tsp. garlic, minced
- 1 and ½ lb. gold potatoes, roughly chopped
- 7 oz. chorizo, cut in half lengthwise and thinly sliced
- 1 and ½ cup lentils
- ½ tsp. smoked paprika
- ½ tsp. oregano
- Salt and black pepper to taste
- 14 oz. canned tomatoes, chopped
- ½ cup cilantro, chopped

DIRECTIONS
1. Heat a saucepan with oil over medium high heat, add onion, garlic, celery and carrots, stir and cook for 4 minutes.
2. Add the chorizo, stir and cook for 1 minute more.
3. Add the rest of the ingredients except the cilantro, stir, bring to a boil, reduce heat to medium-low and simmer for 25 minutes.
4. Divide the stew into bowls and serve with the cilantro sprinkled on top. Enjoy!

204. Lamb and Potato Stew

PREP TIME
10 mins

COOK TIME
2 hours

SERVINGS
4 people

NUTRITION

Calories 450,
Fat 12gg,
Fiber 4g,
Carbs 33g,
Protein 39g

INGREDIENTS

- 2 and ½ lb. lamb shoulder, boneless and cut in small pieces
- Salt and black pepper to taste
- 1 yellow onion, chopped
- 3 tbsp. extra virgin olive oil
- 3 tomatoes, grated
- 1 and ½ cups chicken stock
- ½ cup dry white wine
- 1 bay leaf
- 2 and ½ lb. gold potatoes, cut into medium cubes
- ¾ cup green olives

DIRECTIONS

1. Heat a saucepan with the oil over medium high heat, add the lamb, brown for 10 minutes, transfer to a platter and keep warm for now.
2. Heat the pan again, add onion, stir and cook for 4 minutes.
3. Add tomatoes, stir, reduce heat to low and cook for 15 minutes.
4. Return lamb meat to pan, add wine and the rest of the ingredients except the potatoes and olives, stir, increase heat to medium high, bring to a boil, reduce heat again, cover pan and simmer for 30 minutes.
5. Add potatoes and olives, stir, cook for 1 more hour., divide into bowls and serve.

205. Meatball and Pasta Soup

PREP TIME
10 mins

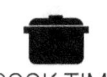
COOK TIME
40 mins

SERVINGS
4 people

NUTRITION

Calories 380,
Fat 17gg,
Fiber 2g,
Carbs 28g,
Protein 26g

INGREDIENTS

- 12 oz. pork meat, ground
- 12 oz. veal, ground
- Salt and black pepper to taste
- 1 garlic clove, minced
- 2 garlic cloves, sliced
- 2 tsp. thyme, chopped
- 1 egg, whisked
- 3 oz. Manchego, grated
- 2 tbsp. extra virgin olive oil
- 1/3 cup panko
- 4 cups chicken stock
- A pinch of saffron
- 15 oz. canned tomatoes, crushed
- 1 tbsp. parsley, chopped
- 8 oz. pasta

DIRECTIONS

1. In a bowl, mix veal with pork, 1 garlic clove, 1 tsp. thyme, ¼ tsp. paprika, salt, pepper to taste, egg, manchego, panko, stir very well and shape medium meatballs out of this mix.
2. Heat a pan with 1 ½ tbsp. oil over medium high heat, add half of the meatballs, cook for 2 minutes on each side, transfer to paper towels, drain grease and put on a plate.
3. Repeat this with the rest of the meatballs.
4. Heat a saucepan with the rest of the oil, add sliced garlic, stir and cook for 1 minute.
5. Add the remaining ingredients and the meatballs, stir, reduce heat to medium low, cook for 25 minutes and season with salt and pepper.
6. Cook pasta according to instructions, drain, put in a bowl and mix with ½ cup soup.
7. Divide pasta into soup bowls, add soup and meatballs on top, sprinkle parsley all over and serve.

206. Peas Soup

PREP TIME
10 mins

COOK TIME
10 mins

SERVINGS
4 people

NUTRITION

Calories 180,
Fat 39gg,
Fiber 4g,
Carbs 10g,
Protein 14g

INGREDIENTS

- 1 tsp. shallot, chopped
- 1 tbsp. butter
- 1-quart chicken stock
- 2 eggs
- 3 tbsp. lemon juice
- 2 cups peas
- 2 tbsp. parmesan, grated
- Salt and black pepper to taste

DIRECTIONS

1. Heat a saucepan with the butter over medium high heat, add shallot, stir and cook for 2 minutes.
2. Add stock, lemon juice, some salt and pepper and the whisked eggs.
3. Add more salt and pepper to taste, peas and parmesan cheese, stir, cook for 3 minutes, divide into bowls and serve.

207. Minty Lamb Stew

PREP TIME
10 mins

COOK TIME
105 mins

SERVINGS
4 people

NUTRITION

Calories 560,
Fat 24gg, Fiber
11g, Carbs 35g,
Protein 33g

INGREDIENTS

- 3 cups orange juice
- ½ cup mint tea
- Salt and black pepper to taste
- 2 lb. lamb shoulder chops
- 1 tbsp. mustard, dry
- 3 tbsp. canola oil
- 1 tbsp. ras el hanout
- 1 carrot, chopped
- 1 yellow onion, chopped
- 1 celery rib, chopped
- 1 tbsp. ginger, grated
- 28 oz. canned tomatoes, crushed
- 1 tbsp. garlic, minced
- 2-star anise
- 1 cup apricots, dried and cut in halves
- 1 cinnamon stick
- ½ cup mint, chopped
- 15 oz. canned chickpeas, drained
- 6 tbsp. yogurt

DIRECTIONS

1. Put orange juice in a saucepan, bring to a boil over medium heat, take off heat, add tea leaves, cover and leave aside for 3 minutes, strain this and leave aside.
2. Heat a saucepan with 2 tbsp. oil over medium high heat, add lamb chops seasoned with salt, pepper, mustard and rasel hanout, toss, brown for 3 minutes on each side and transfer to a plate.
3. Add remaining oil to the saucepan, heat over medium heat, add ginger, onion, carrot, garlic and celery, stir and cook for 5 minutes.
4. Add orange juice, star anise, tomatoes, cinnamon stick, lamb, apricots, stir and cook for 1 hour and 30 minutes.
5. Transfer lamb chops to a cutting board, discard bones and chop.
6. Bring sauce from the pan to a boil, add chickpeas and mint, stir and cook for 10 minutes.
7. Discard cinnamon and star anise, divide into bowls and serve with yogurt on top.

208. Spinach and Orzo Soup

PREP TIME 10 mins

COOK TIME 10 mins

SERVINGS 4 people

INGREDIENTS
- ½ cup orzo
- 6 cups chicken soup
- 1 and ½ cups parmesan, grated
- Salt and black pepper to taste
- 1 and ½ tsp. oregano, dried
- ¼ cup yellow onion, finely chopped
- 3 cups baby spinach
- 2 tbsp. lemon juice
- ½ cup peas, frozen

DIRECTIONS
1. Heat a saucepan with the stock over high heat, add oregano, orzo, onion, salt and pepper, stir, bring to a boil, cover and cook for 10 minutes.
2. Take soup off the heat, add salt and pepper to taste and the rest of the ingredients, stir well and divide into soup bowls. Serve right away.

NUTRITION
Calories 201,
Fat 5g,
Fiber 3g,
Carbs 28g,
Protein 17g

209. Minty Lentil and Spinach Soup

PREP TIME 10 mins

COOK TIME 30 mins

SERVINGS 6 people

INGREDIENTS
- 2 tbsp. olive oil
- 1 yellow onion, chopped
- A pinch of salt and black pepper
- 2 garlic cloves, minced
- 1 tsp. coriander, ground
- 1 tsp. cumin, ground
- 1 tsp. sumac
- 1 tsp. red pepper, crushed
- 2 tsp. mint, dried
- 1 tbsp. flour
- 6 cups veggie stock
- 3 cups water
- 12 oz. spinach, torn
- 1 and ½ cups brown lentils, rinsed
- 2 cups parsley, chopped
- Juice of 1 lime

DIRECTIONS
1. Heat up a pot with the oil over medium heat, add the onions, stir and sauté for 5 minutes.
2. Add garlic, salt, pepper, coriander, cumin, sumac, red pepper, mint and flour, stir and cook for another minute.
3. Add the stock, water and the other ingredients except the parsley and lime juice, stir, bring to a simmer and cook for 20 minutes.
4. Add the parsley and lime juice, cook the soup for 5 minutes more, ladle into bowls and serve.

NUTRITION
Calories 170,
Fat 7g,
Fiber 6g,
Carbs 22g,
Protein 8g

210. Chicken and Apricots Stew

PREP TIME: 10 mins
COOK TIME: 130 mins
SERVINGS: 4 people

NUTRITION
Calories 560,
Fat 10g,
Fiber 4g,
Carbs 34g,
Protein 44g

INGREDIENTS

- 3 garlic cloves, minced
- 1 tbsp. parsley, chopped
- 20 saffron threads
- 3 tbsp. cilantro, chopped
- Salt and black pepper to taste
- 1 tsp. ginger, ground
- 2 tbsp. olive oil
- 3 red onions, thinly sliced
- 4 chicken drumsticks
- 5 oz. apricots, dried
- 2 tbsp. butter
- ¼ cup honey
- 2/3 cup walnuts, chopped
- ½ cinnamon stick

DIRECTIONS

1. Heat a pan over medium high heat, add saffron threads, toast them for 2 minutes, transfer to a bowl, cool down and crush.
2. Add the chicken pieces, 1 tbsp. cilantro, parsley, garlic, ginger, salt, pepper, oil and 2 tbsp. water, toss really well and keep in the fridge for 30 minutes.
3. Arrange onion on the bottom of a saucepan.
4. Add chicken and marinade, add 1 tbsp. butter, place on stove over medium high heat and cook for 15 minutes.
5. Add ¼ cup water, stir, cover pan, reduce heat to medium-low and simmer for 45 minutes.
6. Heat a pan over medium heat, add 2 tbsp. honey, cinnamon stick, apricots and ¾ cup water, stir, bring to a boil, reduce to low and simmer for 15 minutes.
7. Take off heat, discard cinnamon and leave to cool down.
8. Heat a pan with remaining butter over medium heat, add remaining honey and walnuts, stir, cook for 5 minutes and transfer to a plate.
9. Add chicken to apricot sauce, also season with salt, pepper and the rest of the cilantro stir, cook for 10 minutes and serve on top of walnuts.

211. Fish and Veggie Stew

PREP TIME: 10 mins
COOK TIME: 90 mins
SERVINGS: 4 people

NUTRITION
Calories 440,
Fat 18g,
Fiber 8g,
Carbs 43g,
Protein 30g

INGREDIENTS

- 6 lemon wedges, pulp separated and chopped and some of the peel reserved
- 2 tbsp. parsley, chopped
- 2 tomatoes, cut in halves, peeled and grated
- 2 tbsp. cilantro, chopped
- 2 garlic cloves, minced
- ½ tsp. paprika
- 2 tbsp. water
- ½ cup water
- ½ tsp. cumin, ground
- Salt and black pepper to taste
- 4 bass fillets
- ¼ cup olive oil
- 3 carrots, sliced
- 1 red bell pepper, sliced lengthwise and thinly cut in strips
- 1 and ¼ lb. potatoes, peeled and sliced
- ½ cup olives
- 1 red onion, thinly sliced

DIRECTIONS

1. In a bowl, mix tomatoes with lemon pulp, cilantro, parsley, cumin, garlic, paprika, salt, pepper, 2 tbsp. water, 2 tsp. oil and the fish, toss to coat and keep in the fridge for 30 minutes.
2. Heat a saucepan with the water and some salt over medium high heat, add potatoes and carrots, stir, cook for 10 minutes and drain.
3. Heat a pan over medium heat, add bell pepper and ¼ cup water, cover, cook for 5 minutes and take off heat.
4. Coat a saucepan with remaining oil, add potatoes and carrots, ¼ cup water, onion slices, fish and its marinade, bell pepper strips, olives, salt and pepper, toss gently, cook for 45 minutes, divide into bowls and serve.

212. Tomato Soup

PREP TIME
60 mins

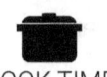
COOK TIME
2 mins

SERVINGS
4 people

NUTRITION

Calories 260
Fat 23g
Fiber 2g
Carbs 11g
Protein 2g

INGREDIENTS

- ½ green bell pepper, chopped
- ½ red bell pepper, chopped
- 1 and ¾ lb. tomatoes, chopped
- ¼ cup bread, torn
- 9 tbsp. extra virgin olive oil
- 1 garlic clove, minced
- 2 tsp. sherry vinegar
- Salt and black pepper to taste
- 1 tbsp. cilantro, chopped
- A pinch of cumin, ground

DIRECTIONS

1. In a blender, mix green and red bell peppers with tomatoes, salt, pepper, 6 tbsp. oil, and the other ingredients except the bread and cilantro, and pulse well. Keep in the fridge for 1 hour.
2. Heat up a pan with remaining oil over medium high heat, add bread pieces, and toast them for 1 minute.
3. Divide cold soup into bowls, top with bread cubes and cilantro then serve.

213. Chickpeas Soup

PREP TIME
10 mins

COOK TIME
35 mins

SERVINGS
4 people

NUTRITION

Calories 360
Fat 14g
Fiber 11g
Carbs 53g
Protein 14g

INGREDIENTS

- 1 bunch kale, leaves torn
- Salt and black pepper to taste
- 3 tbsp. olive oil
- 1 celery stalk, chopped
- 1 yellow onion, chopped
- 1 carrot, chopped
- 30 oz. canned chickpeas, drained
- 14 oz. canned tomatoes, chopped
- 1 bay leaf
- 3 rosemary sprigs
- 4 cups veggie stock

DIRECTIONS

1. In a bowl, mix kale with half of the oil, salt and pepper, toss to coat., spread on a lined baking sheet, cook at 425°F for 12 minutes and leave aside to cool down.
2. Heat a saucepan with remaining oil over medium high heat, add carrot, celery, onion, some salt and pepper, stir and cook for 5 minutes.
3. Add the rest of the ingredients, toss and simmer for 20 minutes.
4. Discard rosemary and bay leaf, puree using a blender and divide into soup bowls. Top with roasted kale and serve.

214. Fish Soup

PREP TIME: 10 mins
COOK TIME: 35 mins
SERVINGS: 6 people

NUTRITION
Calories 340
Fat 20g
Fiber 3g
Carbs 23g
Protein 45g

INGREDIENTS

- 2 garlic cloves, minced
- 2 tbsp. olive oil
- 1 fennel bulb, sliced
- 1 yellow onion, chopped
- 1 pinch saffron, soaked in some orange juice for 10 minutes and drained
- 14 oz. canned tomatoes, peeled
- 1 strip orange zest
- 6 cups seafood stock
- 10 halibut fillet, cut into big pieces
- 20 shrimp, peeled and deveined
- 1 bunch parsley, chopped
- Salt and white pepper to taste

DIRECTIONS

1. Heat a saucepan with oil over medium high heat, add onion, garlic and fennel, stir and cook for 10 minutes.
2. Add saffron, tomatoes, orange zest and stock, stir, bring to a boil and simmer for 20 minutes.
3. Add fish and shrimp, stir and cook for 6 minutes..
4. Sprinkle parsley, salt and pepper, divide into bowls and serve.

215. Chili Watermelon Soup

PREP TIME: 4 mins
COOK TIME: 5 mins
SERVINGS: 4 people

NUTRITION
Calories 115
Fat 0g
Fiber 2g
Carbs 18g,
Protein 2g

INGREDIENTS

- 3 lb. watermelon, sliced
- ½ tsp. chipotle chili powder
- 2 tbsp. olive oil
- Salt to taste
- 1 tomato, chopped
- 1 tbsp. shallot, chopped
- ¼ cup cilantro, chopped
- 1 small cucumber, chopped
- 1 small Serrano chili pepper, chopped
- 3 and ½ tbsp. lime juice
- ¼ cup crème Fraiche
- ½ tbsp. red wine vinegar

DIRECTIONS

1. In a bowl, mix 1 tbsp. oil with chipotle powder, stir and brush the watermelon with this mix.
2. Put the watermelon slices preheated grill pan over medium high heat, grill for 1 minute on each side, cool down, chop and put in a blender.
3. Add cucumber and the rest of the ingredients except the vinegar and the lime juice and pulse well.
4. Transfer to bowls, top with lime juice and vinegar, keep in the fridge for 4 hours and then serve.

216. Shrimp Soup

PREP TIME
30 mins

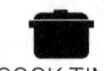
COOK TIME
5 mins

SERVINGS
6 people

NUTRITION

Calories 230
Fat 7g
Fiber 10g
Carbs 24g
Protein 13g

INGREDIENTS

- 1 English cucumber, chopped
- 3 cups tomato juice
- 3 jarred roasted red peppers, chopped
- ½ cup olive oil
- 2 tbsp. sherry vinegar
- 1 tsp. sherry vinegar
- 1 garlic clove, mashed
- 2 baguette slices, cut into cubes and toasted
- Salt and black pepper to taste
- ½ tsp. cumin, ground
- ¾ lb. shrimp, peeled and deveined
- 1 tsp. thyme, chopped

DIRECTIONS

1. In a blender, mix cucumber with tomato juice, red peppers and pulse well, bread, 6 tbsp. oil, 2 tbsp. vinegar, cumin, salt, pepper and garlic, pulse again, transfer to a bowl and keep in the fridge for 30 minutes.
2. Heat a saucepan with 1 tbsp. oil over high heat, add shrimp, stir and cook for 2 minutes.
3. Add thyme, and the rest of the ingredients, cook for 1 minute and transfer to a plate. .
4. Divide cold soup into bowls, top with shrimp and serve. Enjoy!

217. Halibut and Veggies Stew

PREP TIME
10 mins

COOK TIME
50 mins

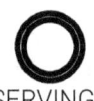
SERVINGS
4 people

NUTRITION

Calories 450,
Fat 12g,
Fiber 13g,
Carbs 47g,
Protein 34g

INGREDIENTS

- 1 yellow onion, chopped
- 2 tbsp. oil
- 1 fennel bulb, stalks removed, sliced and roughly chopped
- 1 carrot, thinly sliced crosswise
- 1 red bell pepper, chopped
- 2 garlic cloves, minced
- 3 tbsp. tomato paste
- 16 oz. canned chickpeas, drained
- ½ cup dry white wine
- 1 tsp. thyme, chopped
- A pinch of smoked paprika
- Salt and black pepper to taste
- 1 bay leaf
- 2 pinches saffron
- 4 baguette slices, toasted
- 3 and ½ cups water
- 13 mussels, debearded
- 11 oz. halibut fillets, skinless and cut into chunks

DIRECTIONS

1. Heat a saucepan with the oil over medium high heat, add fennel, onion, bell pepper, garlic, tomato paste and carrot, stir and cook for 5 minutes. .
2. Add wine, stir and cook for 2 minutes. Add the rest of the ingredients except the halibut and mussels, stir, bring to a boil, cover and boil for 25 minutes.
3. Add, halibut and mussels, cover and simmer for 6 minutes more.
4. Discard unopened mussels, ladle into bowls and serve with toasted bread on the side.

218. Cucumber Soup

PREP TIME 10 mins
COOK TIME 6 mins
SERVINGS 4 people

NUTRITION
Calories 200,
Fat 12g
Fiber 3g
Carbs 20g,
Protein 6g

INGREDIENTS

- 3 bread slices
- ¼ cup almonds
- 4 tsp. almonds
- 3 cucumbers, peeled and chopped
- 3 garlic cloves, minced
- ½ cup warm water
- 6 scallions, thinly sliced
- ¼ cup white wine vinegar
- 3 tbsp. olive oil
- Salt to taste
- 1 tsp. lemon juice
- ½ cup green grapes, cut in halves

DIRECTIONS

1. Heat a pan over medium high heat, add almonds, stir, toast for 5 minutes, transfer to a plate and leave aside.
2. Soak bread in warm water for 2 minutes, transfer to a blender, add almost all the cucumber, salt, the oil, garlic, 5 scallions, lemon juice, vinegar and half of the almonds and pulse well.
3. Ladle soup into bowls, top with reserved ingredients and 2 tbsp. grapes and serve.

219. Chickpeas, Tomato and Kale Stew

PREP TIME 10 mins
COOK TIME 30 mins
SERVINGS 4 people

NUTRITION
Calories 280
Fat 6g
Fiber 9g
Carbs 53g
Protein 10g

INGREDIENTS

- 1 yellow onion, chopped
- 1 tbsp. extra-virgin olive oil
- 2 cups sweet potatoes, peeled and chopped
- 1 ½ tsp. cumin, ground
- 4-inch cinnamon stick
- 14 oz. canned tomatoes, chopped
- 14 oz. canned chickpeas, drained
- 1 ½ tsp. honey
- 6 tbsp. orange juice
- 1 cup water
- Salt and black pepper to taste
- ½ cup green olives, pitted
- 2 cups kale leaves, chopped

DIRECTIONS

1. Heat a saucepan with the oil over medium high heat, add onion, cumin and cinnamon stir and cook for 5 minutes.
2. Add potatoes and the rest of the ingredients except the kale, stir, cover, reduce heat to medium-low and cook for 15 minutes.
3. Add kale, stir, cover again and cook for 10 minutes more. Divide into bowls and serve.

220. Veggie Stew

PREP TIME
10 mins

COOK TIME
50 mins

SERVINGS
4 people

NUTRITION

Calories 80
Fat 2g
Fiber 4g
Carbs 12g
Protein 3g

INGREDIENTS

- 3 eggplants, chopped
- Salt and black pepper to taste
- 6 zucchinis, chopped
- 2 yellow onions, chopped
- 3 red bell peppers, chopped
- 56 oz. canned tomatoes, chopped
- A handful black olives, pitted and chopped
- A pinch of allspice, ground
- A pinch of cinnamon, ground
- 1 tsp. oregano, dried
- A drizzle of honey
- 1 tbsp. garbanzo bean flour mixed with 1 tbsp. water
- A drizzle of olive oil
- A pinch of red chili flakes
- 3 tbsp. Greek yogurt

DIRECTIONS

1. Heat a saucepan with the oil over medium high heat, add bell peppers, onions, some salt and pepper, stir and sauté for 4 minutes.
2. Add eggplant and the rest of the ingredients except the flour, olives, chili flakes and the yogurt, stir, bring to a boil, cover, reduce heat to medium-low and cook for 45 minutes.
3. Add the remaining ingredients except the yogurt, stir, cook for 1 minute, divide into bowls and serve with some Greek yogurt on top.

221. Beef and Eggplant Soup

PREP TIME
10 mins

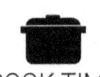
COOK TIME
30 mins

SERVINGS
8 people

NUTRITION

Calories 241
Fat 3g
Fiber 5g
Carbs 7g
Protein 10g

INGREDIENTS

- 1 yellow onion, chopped
- 1 tbsp. olive oil
- 1 garlic clove, minced
- 1 lb. beef, ground
- 1 lb. eggplant, chopped
- ¾ cup celery, chopped
- ¾ cup carrots, chopped
- Salt and black pepper to taste
- 29 oz. canned tomatoes, drained and chopped
- 28 oz. beef stock
- ½ tsp. nutmeg, ground
- ½ cup macaroni
- 2 tsp. parsley, chopped
- ½ cup parmesan cheese, grated

DIRECTIONS

1. Heat a large saucepan with the oil over medium heat, add onion, garlic and meat, stir and brown for 5 minutes..
2. Add celery, carrots and the other ingredients except the macaroni and the cheese, stir, bring to a simmer and cook for 20 minutes.
3. Add macaroni, stir and cook for 12 minutes.
4. Ladle into soup bowls, top with grated cheese and serve.

SALAD AND SIDE DISHES

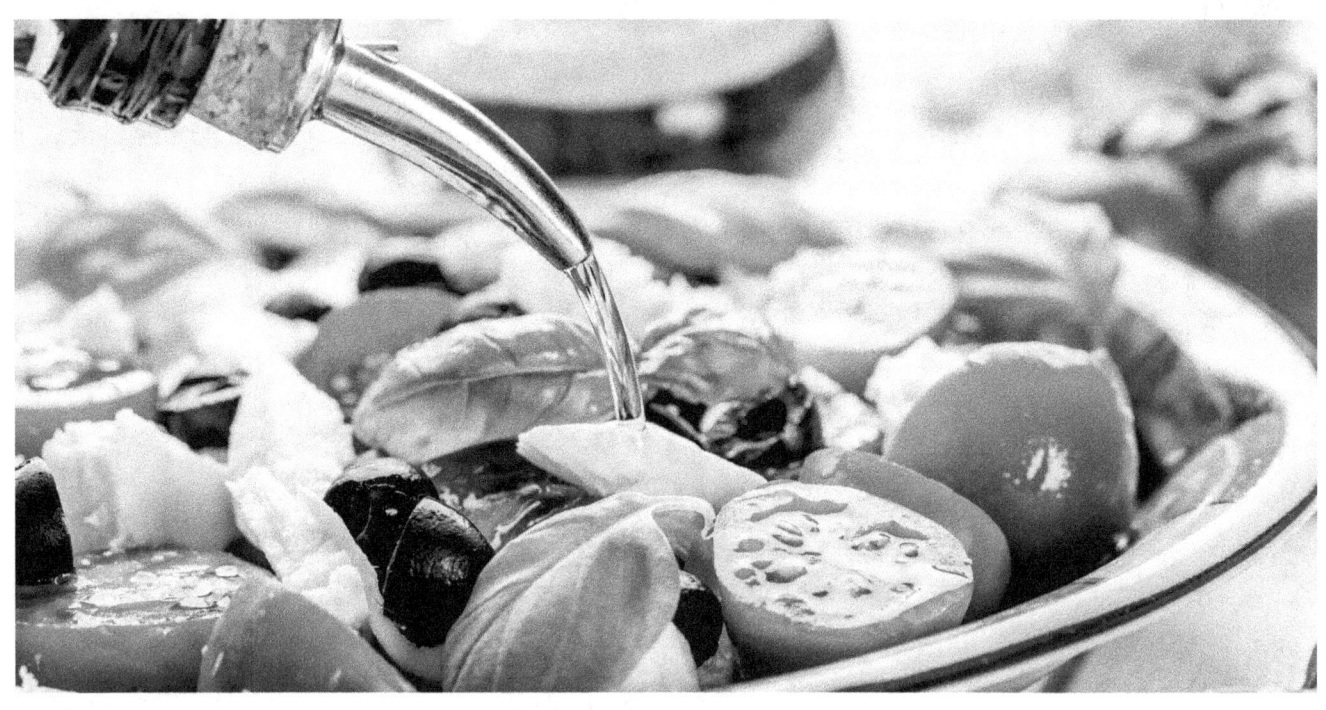

222. Melon Salad

PREP TIME: 10 mins
COOK TIME: 20 mins
SERVINGS: 6 people

NUTRITION
Calories: 218
Protein: 10 g
Fat: 13 g
Carbs: 17 g

INGREDIENTS

- ¼ tsp. Sea Salt
- ¼ tsp. Black Pepper
- 1 tbsp. Balsamic Vinegar
- 1 Cantaloupe, Quartered & Seeded
- 12 Watermelon, Small & Seedless
- 2 Cups Mozzarella Balls, Fresh
- 1/3 Cup Basil, Fresh & Torn
- 2 tbsp. Olive Oil

DIRECTIONS

1. Get out a melon baller and scoop out balls of cantaloupe, and the put them in a colander over a serving bowl.
2. Use your melon baller to cut the watermelon as well, and then put them in with your cantaloupe.
3. Allow your fruit to drain for ten minutes, and then refrigerate the juice for another recipe. It can even be added to smoothies.
4. Wipe the bowl dry, and then place your fruit in it.
5. Add in your basil, oil, vinegar, mozzarella and tomatoes before seasoning with salt and pepper.
6. Gently mix and serve immediately or chilled.

223. Orange Celery Salad

PREP TIME
5 mins

COOK TIME
15 mins

SERVINGS
6 people

NUTRITION

Calories: 65
Protein: 2 g
Fat: 0 g
Carbs: 9 g

INGREDIENTS

- 1 tbsp. Lemon Juice, Fresh
- ¼ tsp. Sea Salt, Fine
- ¼ tsp. Black Pepper
- 1 tbsp. Olive Brine
- 1 tbsp. Olive Oil
- ¼ Cup Red Onion, Sliced
- ½ Cup Green Olives
- 2 Oranges, Peeled & Sliced
- 3 Celery Stalks, Sliced Diagonally in ½ Inch Slices

DIRECTIONS

1. Put your oranges, olives, onion and celery in a shallow bowl.
2. In a different bowl whisk your oil, olive brine and lemon juice, pour this over your salad.
3. Season with salt and pepper before serving.

224. Roasted Broccoli Salad

PREP TIME
30 mins

COOK TIME
30 mins

SERVINGS
4 people

NUTRITION

Calories: 226
Protein: 7 g
Fat: 12 g
Carbs: 26 g

INGREDIENTS

- 1 lb. Broccoli, Cut into Florets & Stem Sliced
- 3 tbsp. Olive Oil, Divided
- 1 Pint Cherry Tomatoes
- 1 ½ Teaspoons Honey, Raw & Divided
- 3 Cups Cubed Bread, Whole Grain
- 1 tbsp. Balsamic Vinegar
- ½ tsp. Black Pepper
- ¼ tsp. Sea Salt, Fine
- Grated Parmesan for Serving

DIRECTIONS

1. Start by heating your oven to 450, and then get out a rimmed baking sheet. Place it in the oven to heat up.
2. Drizzle your broccoli with a tbsp. of oil, and toss to coat.
3. Remove the baking sheet form the oven, and spoon the broccoli on it. Leave oil it eh bottom of the bowl and add in your tomatoes, toss to coat, and then toss your tomatoes with a tbsp. of honey. Pour them on the same baking sheet as your broccoli.
4. Roast for fifteen minutes, and stir halfway through your cooking time.
5. Add in your bread, and then roast for three more minutes.
6. Whisk two tbsp. of oil, vinegar, and remaining honey. Season with salt and pepper. Pour this over your broccoli mix to serve.

225. Tomato Salad

PREP TIME 5 mins
COOK TIME 20 mins
SERVINGS 4 people

INGREDIENTS

- 1 Cucumber, Sliced
- ¼ Cup Sun Dried Tomatoes, Chopped
- 1 lb. Tomatoes, Cubed
- ½ Cup Black Olives
- 1 Red Onion, Sliced
- 1 tbsp. Balsamic Vinegar
- ¼ Cup Parsley, Fresh & Chopped
- 2 tbsp. Olive Oil
- Sea Salt & Black Pepper to Taste

DIRECTIONS

1. Get out a bowl and combine all of your vegetables together. To make your dressing mix all your seasoning, olive oil and vinegar.
2. Toss with your salad and serve fresh.

NUTRITION

Calories: 126
Protein: 2.1 g
Fat: 9.2 g
Carbs: 11.5 g

---

226. Feta Beet Salad

PREP TIME 5 mins
COOK TIME 5 mins
SERVINGS 4 people

INGREDIENTS

- 6 Red Beets, Cooked & Peeled
- 3 Oz. Feta Cheese, Cubed
- 2 tbsp. Olive Oil
- 2 tbsp. Balsamic Vinegar

DIRECTIONS

1. Combine everything together, and then serve.

NUTRITION

Calories: 230
Protein: 7.3 g
Fat: 12 g
Carbs: 26.3 g

227. Cauliflower & Tomato Salad

PREP TIME
5 mins

COOK TIME
15 mins

SERVINGS
4 people

INGREDIENTS

- 1 Head Cauliflower, Chopped
- 2 tbsp. Parsley, Fresh & chopped
- 2 Cups Cherry Tomatoes, Halved
- 2 tbsp. Lemon Juice, Fresh
- 2 tbsp. Pine Nuts
- Sea Salt & Black Pepper to Taste

DIRECTIONS

1. Mix your lemon juice, cherry tomatoes, cauliflower and parsley together, and then season. Top with pine nuts, and mix well before serving.

NUTRITION

Calories: 64
Protein: 2.8 g
Fat: 3.3 g
Carbs: 7.9 g

228. Tuna Salad

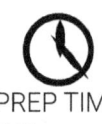

PREP TIME
10 mins

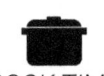

COOK TIME
0 mins

SERVINGS
2 people

INGREDIENTS

- 12 oz. canned tuna in water, drained and flaked
- ¼ cup roasted red peppers, chopped
- 2 tbsp. capers, drained
- 8 kalamata olives, pitted and sliced
- 2 tbsp. olive oil
- 1 tbsp. parsley, chopped
- 1 tbsp. lemon juice
- A pinch of salt and black pepper

DIRECTIONS

1. In a bowl, combine the tuna with roasted peppers and the rest of the ingredients, toss, divide between plates and serve for breakfast.

NUTRITION

Calories 250,
Fat 17.5 g,
Fiber 0.6 g,
Carbs 2.6 g,
Protein 10.4 g

229. Corn and Shrimp Salad

PREP TIME: 10 mins
COOK TIME: 10 mins
SERVINGS: 4 people

INGREDIENTS

- 4 ears of sweet corn, husked
- 1 avocado, peeled, pitted and chopped
- ½ cup basil, chopped
- A pinch of salt and black pepper
- 1 lb. shrimp, peeled and deveined
- 1 and ½ cups cherry tomatoes, halved
- ¼ cup olive oil

DIRECTIONS

1. Put the corn in a pot, add water to cover, bring to a boil over medium heat, cook for 6 minutes, drain, cool down, cut corn from the cob and put it in a bowl.
2. Thread the shrimp onto skewers and brush with some of the oil.
3. Place the skewers on the preheated grill, cook over medium heat for 2 minutes on each side, remove from skewers and add over the corn.
4. Add the rest of the ingredients to the bowl, toss, divide between plates and serve for breakfast.

NUTRITION
Calories 316, Fat 22.5 g, Fiber 5.6 g, Carbs 23.6 g, Protein 15.4 g

---

230. Tahini Spinach

PREP TIME: 5 mins
COOK TIME: 5 mins
SERVINGS: 4 people

INGREDIENTS

- 10 Spinach, Chopped
- ½ Cup Water
- 1 tbsp. Tahini
- 2 Cloves Garlic, Minced
- ¼ tsp. Cumin
- ¼ tsp. Paprika
- ¼ tsp. Cayenne Pepper
- 1/3 Cup Red Wine Vinegar
- Sea Salt & Black Pepper to Taste

DIRECTIONS

1. Add your spinach and water to the saucepan, and then boil it on high heat. Once boiling reduce to low, and cover. Allow it to cook on simmer for five minutes.
2. Add in your garlic, cumin, cayenne, red wine vinegar, paprika and tahini. Whisk well, and season with salt and pepper.
3. Drain your spinach and top with tahini sauce to serve.

NUTRITION
Calories: 69
Protein: 5 g
Fat: 3 g
Carbs: 8 g

231. Asparagus Couscous

PREP TIME
15 mins

COOK TIME
30 mins

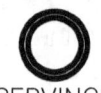
SERVINGS
6 people

NUTRITION

Calories: 263
Protein: 11 g
Fat: 9 g
Carbs: 36 g

INGREDIENTS

- 1 Cup Goat Cheese, Garlic & Herb Flavored
- 1 ½ lbs. Asparagus, Trimmed & Chopped into 1 Inch Pieces
- 1 tbsp. Olive Oil
- 1 Clove Garlic, Minced
- ¼ tsp. Black Pepper
- 1 ¾ Cup Water
- 8 Oz. Whole Wheat Couscous, Uncooked
- ¼ tsp. Sea Salt, Fine

DIRECTIONS

1. Start by heating your oven to 425°F, and then put your goat cheese on the counter. It needs to come to room temperature.
2. Get out a bowl and mix your oil, pepper, garlic and asparagus. Spread the asparagus on a baking sheet and roast for ten minutes. Make sure to stir at least once.
3. Remove it from the pan, and place your asparagus in a serving bowl.
4. Get out a medium saucepan, and bring your water to a boil. Add in your salt and couscous. Reduce the heat to medium-low, and then cover your saucepan. Cook for twelve minutes. All your water should be absorbed.
5. Pour the couscous in a bowl with asparagus, and ad din your goat cheese. Stir until melted, and serve warm.

232. Easy Spaghetti Squash

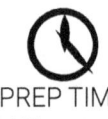
PREP TIME
15 mins

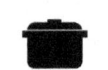
COOK TIME
25 mins

SERVINGS
4 people

NUTRITION

Calories: 423
Protein: 18 g
Fat: 30 g
Carbs: 22 g

INGREDIENTS

- 2 Spring Onions, Chopped Fine
- 3 Cloves Garlic, Minced
- 1 Zucchini, Diced 1 Red Bell Pepper, Diced
- 1 tbsp. Italian Seasoning
- 1 Tomato, Small & Chopped Fine
- 1 tbsp. Parsley, Fresh & Chopped
- Pinch Lemon Pepper
- Dash Sea Salt, Fine
- 4 Oz. Feta Cheese, Crumbled
- 3 Italian Sausage Links, Casing Removed
- 2 tbsp. Olive Oil
- 1 Spaghetti Sauce, Halved Lengthwise

DIRECTIONS

1. Start by heating your oven to 350°F, and get out a large baking sheet. Coat it with cooking spray, and then put your squash on it with the cut side down.
2. Bake at 350°F for forty-five minutes. It should be tender.
3. Turn the squash over, and bake for five more minutes. Scrape the strands into a larger bowl.
4. Heat up a tbsp. of olive oil in a skillet, and then add in your Italian sausage. Cook at eight minutes before removing it and placing it in a bowl.
5. Add another tbsp. of olive oil to the skillet and cook your garlic and onions until softened. This will take five minutes.
6. Throw in your Italian seasoning, red peppers and zucchini. Cook for another five minutes. Your vegetables should be softened.
7. Mix in your feta cheese and squash, cooking until the cheese has melted.
8. Stir in your sausage, and then season with lemon pepper and salt. Serve with parsley and tomato.

233. Garbanzo Bean Salad

PREP TIME: 10 mins
COOK TIME: 0 mins
SERVINGS: 4 people

NUTRITION
Calories 268, Fat 16.5 g, Fiber 7.6 g, Carbs 36.6 g, Protein 9.4 g

INGREDIENTS

- 1 and ½ cups cucumber, cubed
- 15 oz. canned garbanzo beans, drained and rinsed
- 3 oz. black olives, pitted and sliced
- 1 tomato, chopped
- ¼ cup red onion, chopped
- 5 cups salad greens
- A pinch of salt and black pepper
- ½ cup feta cheese, crumbled
- 3 tbsp. olive oil
- 1 tbsp. lemon juice
- ¼ cup parsley, chopped

DIRECTIONS

1. In a salad bowl, combine the garbanzo beans with the cucumber, tomato and the rest of the ingredients except the cheese and toss.
2. Divide the mix into small bowls, sprinkle the cheese on top and serve for breakfast.

234. Spiced Chickpeas Bowls

PREP TIME: 10 mins
COOK TIME: 30 mins
SERVINGS: 4 people

NUTRITION
Calories 519, Fat 34.5 g, Fiber 13.6 g, Carbs 36.6 g, Protein 11.4 g

INGREDIENTS

- 15 oz. canned chickpeas, drained and rinsed
- ¼ tsp. cardamom, ground
- ½ tsp. cinnamon powder
- 1 and ½ tsp. turmeric powder
- 1 tsp. coriander, ground
- 1 tbsp. olive oil
- A pinch of salt and black pepper
- ¾ cup Greek yogurt
- ½ cup green olives, pitted and halved
- ½ cup cherry tomatoes, halved
- 1 cucumber, sliced

DIRECTIONS

1. Spread the chickpeas on a lined baking sheet, add the cardamom, cinnamon, turmeric, coriander, the oil, salt and pepper, toss and bake at 375°F for 30 minutes.
2. In a bowl, combine the roasted chickpeas with the rest of the ingredients, toss and serve for breakfast.

235. Tomato and Lentils Salad

PREP TIME
10 mins

COOK TIME
35 mins

SERVINGS
4 people

NUTRITION

Calories 294,
Fat 3.5 g,
Fiber 9.6 g,
Carbs 26.6 g,
Protein 15.4 g

INGREDIENTS

- 2 yellow onions, chopped
- 4 garlic cloves, minced
- 2 cups brown lentils
- 1 tbsp. olive oil
- A pinch of salt and black pepper
- ½ tsp. sweet paprika
- ½ tsp. ginger, grated
- 3 cups water
- ¼ cup lemon juice
- ¾ cup Greek yogurt
- 3 tbsp. tomato paste

DIRECTIONS

1. Heat up a pot with the oil over medium-high heat, add the onions and sauté for 2 minutes.
2. Add the garlic and the lentils, stir and cook for 1 minute more.
3. Add the water, bring to a simmer and cook covered for 30 minutes.
4. Add the lemon juice and the remaining ingredients except the yogurt. Toss, divide the mix into bowls, top with the yogurt and serve.

236. Egg and Arugula Salad

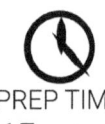
PREP TIME
15 mins

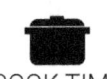
COOK TIME
20 mins

SERVINGS
4 people

NUTRITION

Calories 169,
Fat 6.5 g,
Fiber 2.6 g,
Carbs 10.6 g,
Protein 9.4 g

INGREDIENTS

- 3 tomatoes
- 1 cucumber
- 4 eggs, boiled, peeled
- ½ cup black olives, pitted
- ¼ red onion, peeled
- ½ cup arugula
- 1/3 cup Plain yogurt
- 1 tsp. lemon juice
- ¼ tsp. paprika
- 1/3 tsp. Sea salt
- ½ tsp. dried oregano

DIRECTIONS

1. Chop tomatoes and cucumber into the medium cubes and transfer in the salad bowl.
2. Then tear arugula and add it in the salad bowl.
3. In the shallow bowl whisk together Plain yogurt, lemon juice, paprika, sea salt, and dried oregano.
4. Chop the boiled eggs roughly and add in the salad.
5. Add black olives (slice them if desired).
6. Then add red onion.
7. Shake the salad well.
8. Pour Plain yogurt dressing over the salad and stir it only before serving.

237. Roasted Veggies

PREP TIME: 5 mins
COOK TIME: 20 mins
SERVINGS: 12 people

NUTRITION
Calories: 675
Protein: 13 g
Fat: 21 g
Carbs: 112 g

INGREDIENTS

- 6 Cloves Garlic
- 6 tbsp. Olive Oil
- 1 Fennel Bulb, Diced
- 1 Zucchini, Diced
- 2 Red Bell Peppers, Diced
- 6 Potatoes, Large & Diced
- 2 Teaspoons Sea Salt
- ½ Cup Balsamic Vinegar
- ¼ Cup Rosemary, Chopped & Fresh
- 2 Teaspoons Vegetable Bouillon Powder

DIRECTIONS

1. Start by heating your oven to 400°F.
2. Get out a baking dish and place your potatoes, fennel, zucchini, garlic and fennel on a baking dish, drizzling with olive oil.
3. Sprinkle with salt, bouillon powder, and rosemary. Mix well, and then bake at 450 for thirty to forty minutes. Mix your vinegar into the vegetables before serving.

238. Roasted Eggplant Salad

PREP TIME: 15 mins
COOK TIME: 40 mins
SERVINGS: 6 people

NUTRITION
Calories: 148
Protein: 3.5 g
Fat: 7.7 g
Carbs: 20.5 g

INGREDIENTS

- 1 Red Onion, Sliced
- 2 tbsp. Parsley, Fresh & Chopped
- 1 tsp. Thyme
- 2 Cups Cherry Tomatoes, Halved
- Sea Salt & Black Pepper to Taste
- 1 tsp. Oregano
- 3 tbsp. Olive Oil
- 1 tsp. Basil
- 3 Eggplants, Peeled & Cubed

DIRECTIONS

1. Start by heating your oven to 350°F.
2. Season your eggplant with basil, salt, pepper, oregano, thyme and olive oil.
3. Spread it on a baking tray, and bake for a half hour.
4. Toss with your remaining ingredients before serving.

239. Penne with Tahini Sauce

PREP TIME
10 mins

COOK TIME
20 mins

SERVINGS
8 people

NUTRITION

Calories: 332
Proteins: 11 g
Fat: 12 g
Carbs: 48 g

INGREDIENTS

- 1/3 Cup Water
- 1 Cup Yogurt, Plain
- 1/8 Cup Lemon Juice
- 3 tbsp. Tahini
- 3 Cloves Garlic
- 1 Onion, Chopped
- ¼ Cup Olive Oil
- 2 Portobello Mushrooms, Large & Sliced
- ½ Red Bell Pepper, Diced
- 16 Oz. Penne Pasta
- ½ Cup Parsley, Fresh & Chopped
- Black Pepper to Taste

DIRECTIONS

1. Start by getting out a pot and bring a pot of salted water to a boil. Cook your pasta al dente per package instructions.
2. Mix your lemon juice and tahini together, and then place it tin a food processor. Process with garlic, water and yogurt. It should be smooth.
3. Get out a saucepan, and place it over medium heat. Heat up your oil, and cook your onions until soft.
4. Add in your mushroom and continue to cook until softened.
5. Add in your bell pepper, and cook until crispy.
6. Drain your pasta, and then toss with your tahini sauce, top with parsley and pepper and serve with vegetables.

240. Parmesan Barley Risotto

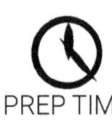
PREP TIME
15 mins

COOK TIME
30 mins

SERVINGS
6 people

NUTRITION

Calories; 346
Protein: 14 g
Fat: 7 g
Carbs: 56 g

INGREDIENTS

- 1 Cup yellow Onion, Chopped
- 1 tbsp. Olive Oil
- 4 Cups Vegetable Broth, Low Sodium
- 2 Cups Pearl Barley, Uncooked
- ½ Cup Dry White Wine
- 1 Cup Parmesan Cheese, Grated Fine & Divided
- Sea Salt & Black Pepper to Taste
- Fresh Chives, Chopped for Serving
- Lemon Wedges for Serving

DIRECTIONS

1. Add your broth into a saucepan and bring it to a simmer over medium-high heat.
2. Get out a stock pot and put it over medium-high heat as well. Heat up your oil before adding in your onion.
3. Cook for eight minutes and stir occasionally. Add in your barley and cook for two minutes more. Stir in your barley, cooking until it's toasted.
4. Pour in the wine, cooking for a minute more. Most of the liquid should have evaporated before adding in a cup of warm broth.
5. Cook and stir for two minutes. Your liquid should be absorbed. Add in the remaining broth by the cup, and cook until ach cup is absorbed fore adding more. It should take about two minutes each time. It will take a little longer for the last cup to be absorbed.
6. Remove from heat, and stir in a half a cup of cheese, and top with remaining cheese chives and lemon wedges.

241. Zucchini Pasta

PREP TIME: 15 mins
COOK TIME: 30 mins
SERVINGS: 4 people

NUTRITION
Calories: 410
Protein: 15 g
Fat: 17 g
Carbs: 45 g

INGREDIENTS
- 3 tbsp. Olive Oil
- 2 Cloves Garlic, Minced
- 3 Zucchini, Large & Diced
- Sea Salt & Black Pepper to Taste
- ½ Cup Milk, 2%
- ¼ tsp. Nutmeg
- 1 tbsp. Lemon Juice, Fresh
- ½ Cup Parmesan, Grated
- 8 Oz. Uncooked Farfalle Pasta

DIRECTIONS
1. Get out a skillet and place it over medium heat, and then heat up the oil. Add in your garlic and cook for a minute. Stir often so that it doesn't burn. Add in your salt, pepper and zucchini. Stir well, and cook covered for fifteen minutes. During this time, you'll want to stir the mixture twice.
2. Get out a microwave safe bowl, and heat the milk for thirty seconds. Stir in your nutmeg, and then pour it into the skillet. Cook uncovered for five minutes. Stir occasionally to keep from burning.
3. Get out a stockpot and cook your pasta per package instructions. Drain the pasta, and then save two tbsp. of pasta water.
4. Stir everything together, and add in the cheese and lemon juice and pasta water.

242. Quinoa and Eggs Salad

PREP TIME: 5 mins
COOK TIME: 0 mins
SERVINGS: 4 people

NUTRITION
Calories 519,
Fat 32.5 g,
Fiber 11.6 g,
Carbs 43.6 g,
Protein 19.4 g

INGREDIENTS
- 4 eggs, soft boiled, peeled and cut into wedges
- 2 cups baby arugula
- 2 cups cherry tomatoes, halved
- 1 cucumber, sliced
- 1 cup quinoa, cooked
- 1 cup almonds, chopped
- 1 avocado, peeled, pitted and sliced
- 1 tbsp. olive oil
- ½ cup mixed dill and mint, chopped
- A pinch of salt and black pepper
- Juice of 1 lemon

DIRECTIONS
1. In a large salad bowl, combine the eggs with the arugula and the rest of the ingredients, toss, divide between plates and serve for breakfast.

243. Feta & Spinach Pita Bake

PREP TIME
10 mins

COOK TIME
20 mins

SERVINGS
6 people

INGREDIENTS

- 2 Roma Tomatoes, Chopped
- 6 Whole Wheat Pita Bread
- 1 Jar Sun Dried Tomato Pesto
- 4 Mushrooms, Fresh & Sliced
- 1 Bunch Spinach, Rinsed & Chopped
- 2 tbsp. Parmesan Cheese, Grated
- 3 tbsp. Olive Oil
- ½ Cup Feta Cheese, Crumbled
- Dash Black Pepper

DIRECTIONS

1. Start by heating the oven to 350°F, and get to your pita bread. Spread the tomato pesto on the side of each one. Put them in a baking pan with the tomato side up.
2. Top with tomatoes, spinach, mushrooms, parmesan and feta. Drizzle with olive oil and season with pepper.
3. Bake for twelve minutes, and then serve cut into quarters.

NUTRITION

Calories; 350
Protein: 12 g
Fat: 17 g
Carbs: 42 g

244. Pistachio Arugula Salad

PREP TIME
10 mins

COOK TIME
20 mins

SERVINGS
6 people

INGREDIENTS

- 6 Cups Kale, Chopped
- ¼ Cup Olive Oil
- 2 tbsp. Lemon Juice, Fresh
- ½ tsp. Smoked Paprika
- 2 Cups Arugula
- 1/3 Cup Pistachios, Unsalted & Shelled
- 6 tbsp. Parmesan Cheese, Grated

DIRECTIONS

1. Get out a salad bowl and combine your oil, lemon, smoked paprika and kale. Gently massage the leaves for half a minute. Your kale should be coated well.
2. Gently mix your arugula and pistachios when ready to serve.

NUTRITION

Calories: 150
Protein: 5 g
Fat: 12 g
Carbs: 8 g

245. Easy Salad Wraps

PREP TIME
10 mins

COOK TIME
20 mins

SERVINGS
4 people

NUTRITION

Calories: 262
Protein: 7 g
Fat: 15 g
Carbs: 23 g

INGREDIENTS

- 1 ½ Cups Cucumber, Seedless, Peeled & Chopped
- 1 Cup Tomato, Chopped
- ½ Cup Mint, Fresh & Chopped Fine
- Ounce Can Black Olives, Sliced & Drained
- ¼ Cup Red Onion, Diced
- 2 tbsp. olive Oil
- Sea Salt & Black Pepper to Taste
- 1 tbsp. Red Wine Vinegar
- ½ Cup Goat Cheese, Crumbled
- 4 Flatbread Wraps, Whole Wheat

DIRECTIONS

1. Get out a bowl and mix your tomato, mint, cucumber, onion and olives together.
2. Get out another bowl and whisk your vinegar, oil, pepper and salt. Drizzle this over your salad, and mix well.
3. Spread your goat cheese over the four wraps, and then spoon your salad filling in each one. Fold up to serve.

246. Margherita Slices

PREP TIME
5 mins

COOK TIME
15 mins

SERVINGS
4 people

NUTRITION

Calories: 297
Protein: 12 g
Fat: 11 g
Carbs: 38 g

INGREDIENTS

- 1 Tomato, Cut into 8 Slices
- 1 Clove Garlic, Halved
- 1 tbsp. Olive Oil
- ¼ tsp. Oregano
- 1 Cup Mozzarella, Fresh & Sliced
- ¼ Cup Basil Leaves, Fresh, Tron & Lightly Packed
- Sea Salt & Black Pepper to Taste
- 2 Hoagie Rolls, 6 Inches Each

DIRECTIONS

1. Start by heating your oven broiler to high. Your rack should be four inches under the heating element.
2. Place the sliced bread on a rimmed baking sheet. Broil for a minute. Your bread should be toasted lightly. Brush each one down with oil and rub your garlic over each half.
3. Place the bread back on your baking sheet. Distribute the tomato slices on each one, and then sprinkle with oregano and cheese.
4. Bake for one to two minutes, but check it after a minute. Your cheese should be melted.
5. Top with basil and pepper before serving.

247. Vegetable Panini

PREP TIME
15 mins

COOK TIME
25 mins

SERVINGS
4 people

NUTRITION

Calories: 352
Protein: 16 g
Fat: 15 g
Carbs: 45 g

INGREDIENTS

- 2 tbsp. Olive Oil, Divided
- ¼ Cup Onion, Diced
- 1 Cup Zucchini, Diced
- 1 ½ Cups Broccoli, Diced
- ¼ tsp. Oregano
- Sea Salt & Black Pepper to Taste
- 12 Oz. Jar Roasted Red Peppers, Drained & Chopped Fine
- 2 tbsp. Parmesan Cheese, Grated
- 1 Cup Mozzarella, Fresh & Sliced
- 2-Foot-Long Whole Grain Italian Loaf, Cut into 4 Pieces

DIRECTIONS

1. Heat your oven to 450°F, and then get out a baking sheet. Heat the oven with your baking sheet inside.
2. Get out a bowl and mix your broccoli, zucchini, oregano, pepper, onion and salt with a tbsp. of olive oil.
3. Remove your baking sheet from the oven and coat it in a nonstick cooking spray. Spread the vegetable mixture over it to roast for five minutes. Stir halfway through.
4. Remove it from the oven, and add your red pepper, and sprinkle with parmesan cheese. Mix everything together.
5. Get out a panini maker or grill pan, placing it over medium-high heat. Heat up a tbsp. of oil.
6. Spread the bread horizontally on it, but don't cut it all the way through. Fill with the vegetable mix, and then a slice of mozzarella cheese on top.
7. Close the sandwich and cook like you would a normal panini. With a press it should grill for five minutes. For a grill pan cook for two and a half minutes per side. Repeat for the remaining sandwiches.

248. Baked Tomato

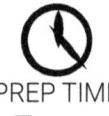

PREP TIME
7 mins

COOK TIME
25 mins

SERVINGS
4 people

NUTRITION

Calories: 342
Protein: 16 g
Fat: 10 g
Carbs: 45 g

INGREDIENTS

- Whole grain bread
- Salt and pepper to taste
- 1 tbsp. of finely chopped basil
- 2 cloves of garlic. Finely chopped
- Extra virgin oil
- 2 large tomatoes

DIRECTIONS

1. Preheat your oven to 400°F.
2. Use the olive oil to brush the bottom of a baking dish. Set aside.
3. Slice the tomatoes into a thickness of a ½ inch. Lay the tomato pieces into the baking dish that you had prepared earlier. Sprinkle some basil and garlic on top of the tomatoes, season with pepper and salt to taste.
4. Then drizzle the slices of tomatoes with olive oil and then place the baking dish into the oven. Bake for about 20-25 minutes.
5. Remove from the oven, give it a few seconds to cool down and then serve and enjoy.
6. Tip: The tomato juice and olive oil at the bottom of the pan can be used as a dipping sauce. So if you want, you can put it into a small bowl and enjoy it with warm whole grain bread.

249. Mediterranean Humus Filled Roasted Veggies

PREP TIME: 7 mins
COOK TIME: 25 mins
SERVINGS: 12 people

NUTRITION
Calories: 342
Protein: 10 g
Fat: 15 g
Carbs: 35 g

INGREDIENTS

- 6 pitted kalamata olives quartered
- ½ cup (2oz.) of feta cheese
- 1 cup of hummus
- 2 tbsp. of olive oil
- 1 medium red bell pepper
- 1 small zucchini (6 inch)

DIRECTIONS

1. Heat a closed medium sized contact grill at 375°F for about 5 minutes.
2. Cut the summer squash and zucchini into half lengthwise. Use a spoon to scoop out the seeds from the two vegetables and discard the seeds.
3. Cut the red bell pepper around the stem and remove the stem and the seeds; cut them into quarters and set aside.
4. Use olive oil to brush the bell pepper, squash and zucchini pieces. Once done, place them on the grill. Do not close the grill.
5. Cook them for 4-6 minutes and turn only once. The vegetables should be tender by the end of the sixth minute. Remove from the grill and let them cool for 2 minutes. Cut the vegetables into 1-inch pieces.
6. Use a spoon to scoop 2 tbsp. of humus onto each piece of vegetable. Light drizzle the vegetables with cheese and top it with one piece of olive. Serve cold or warm.

250. Cucumber and Nuts Salad

PREP TIME: 20 mins
COOK TIME: 3 hours
SERVINGS: 10 people

NUTRITION
Calories: 252
Protein: 16 g
Fat: 10 g
Carbs: 35 g

INGREDIENTS

- ½ cup (2 oz.) of crumbled feta cheese
- 1/3 cup of chopped walnuts, toasted
- 1 chopped orange, peeled and sectioned
- ½ tsp. of salt
- 1 tbsp. of grated orange peel
- 1/3 cup of chopped fresh mint leaves that are loosely packed
- 1/3 cup of loosely packed flat-leafed chopped parsley
- ½ cup of sweetened dried cranberries
- ½ cup of chopped red onion
- ½ medium cucumber, unpeeled, seeded and chopped
- 2 tbsp. of olive oil
- ¼ cup of orange juice
- 1 cup of boiling water
- cup of uncooked bulgur

DIRECTIONS

1. Start by placing the bulgur in a large heatproof bowl. Pour in some hot boiling water into the heatproof bowl and give the mixture a stir. Let the bulgur sit for about 1 hour or until the water has been absorbed.
2. Add in orange peel, mint, parsley, cranberries, onion, cucumber, salt, oil and orange juice and toss well. Cover the large bowl and refrigerate it for 2-3 hours or until the mixture is chilled.
3. Remove the mixture from the fridge and stir in some chopped oranges. Lightly sprinkle the mixture with cheese and walnuts. Serve and enjoy.

251. Courgette, Fennel, and Orange Salad

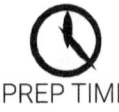
PREP TIME
15 mins

COOK TIME
0 mins

SERVINGS
4 people

NUTRITION

Calories: 170
Protein: 3 g
Fat: 12 g
Carbs: 10 g

INGREDIENTS

- 1 orange
- 2 small courgettes (green or yellow)
- 2 small fennel bulbs
- 2 tsp. sherry vinegar
- 4 tbsp. olive oil
- 1 Baby Gem lettuce, washed and leaves separated
- Juice ½ lemon

DIRECTIONS

1. Cut the peel off the orange. Remove any pith. Slice the orange and halve each slice. Ideally, you should be cutting the orange on a plate or the chopping board since we are going to collect the juice left over from the cutting.
2. Take the fennel and remove any outer leaves that are tough. Cut the cores into halves and then slice them as thinly as you can.
3. Remove the ends of the courgettes and shave thin and long slices using a vegetable peeler. You can toss away the watery and seedy centers.
4. Take a small bowl and mix together olive oil, vinegar, and the orange juice left over on the plate or chopping board.
5. Take out another bowl and mix the courgette, fennel, orange slices, and lettuce leaves.
6. Serve the fennel mixture and top it with the orange juice dressing.

252. Potato Salad

PREP TIME
10 mins

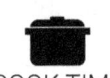
COOK TIME
6 mins

SERVINGS
4 people

NUTRITION

Calories: 111
Protein: 3 g
Fat: 4 g
Carbs: 16 g

INGREDIENTS

- 1 small onion, thinly sliced
- 1 tbsp. olive oil
- 1 garlic clove, crushed
- 3.5 oz. roasted red pepper sliced
- 25 g black olive, sliced
- 1 tsp. fresh oregano
- 7 oz. canned cherry tomatoes
- 10 oz. new potato, halved if large
- Handful basil leaves, torn

DIRECTIONS

1. Take out a saucepan and place it over medium heat. Pour the olive oil into it and allow it to heat. Add the onions and cook for about 10 minutes, or until the onions have become soft.
2. Add oregano and garlic. Cook for another 1 minute.
3. Add the peppers and tomato. Let the mixture simmer for about 10 minutes.
4. Use a pan and place it over medium-high heat. Bring it to a boil and then add the potatoes into the water. Cook the potatoes for about 15 minutes, or until they turn tender. Drain the potatoes.
5. Take out a small bowl and add the pepper and tomato sauce into it. Toss in the potatoes and mix well.
6. Serve your salad with a sprinkle of basil and olives.

253. Tomato, Cucumber, and Feta Salad

PREP TIME
10 mins

COOK TIME
0 mins

SERVINGS
4 people

NUTRITION

Calories: 153 Calories
Protein: 3 g
Fat: 13.1 g
Carbs: 6.1 g

INGREDIENTS

- 3 tbsp. extra-virgin olive oil
- ½ tsp. Dijon mustard
- 4 medium Persian cucumbers, thinly sliced crosswise
- 1 tsp. chopped fresh oregano, plus extra for garnish
- 1 1/2 tbsp. red-wine vinegar
- 1 cup (8 oz.) tomatoes, cut into wedges
- 1/4 tsp. salt
- 1 1/2 oz. feta cheese, crumbled

DIRECTIONS

1. Take out a medium bowl and combine oregano, vinegar, mustard, and salt.
2. Drizzle the oil on top. Add tomatoes, cucumbers, and feta.
3. Mix them well and serve with oregano leaves toppings, if you prefer.
4. Refrigerate if you are planning to serve later.

254. Goat Cheese Stuffed Tomatoes

PREP TIME
10 mins

COOK TIME
6 mins

SERVINGS
4 people

NUTRITION

Calories: 142
Protein: 7 g
Fat: 13.1 g
Carbs: 7 g

INGREDIENTS

- 6-8 arugula leaves
- 3 oz. crumbled feta cheese
- 2 medium ripe tomatoes
- Extra-virgin olive oil to drizzle
- Balsamic vinegar to drizzle
- 1 red onion, very thinly sliced for garnish
- Fresh chopped parsley for garnish
- Salt and freshly ground pepper to taste

DIRECTIONS

1. Arrange the arugula leaves in the center of a plate.
2. Remove the tops and the core of the tomatoes. Ideally, you should remove the top first and scoop out the core.
3. Fill the tomatoes with feta cheese. Add salt and pepper, to taste
4. Drizzle with olive oil and balsamic vinegar.
5. Garnish with chopped parsley and red onion.
6. Serve at room temperature.

255. Classic Tabbouleh

PREP TIME
10 mins

COOK TIME
10 mins

SERVINGS
4 people

NUTRITION

Calories: 177
Protein: 12 g
Fat: 11 g
Carbs: 28 g

INGREDIENTS

- ¾ cup bulgur
- 2 cups freshly chopped parsley
- 1½ cups water
- ½ cup fresh lemon juice
- ½ cup extra-virgin olive oil
- ½ red bell pepper, diced
- 3 ripe plum tomatoes, peeled, seeded, and diced
- 1 large cucumber, peeled, seeded, and diced
- ¾ cup chopped scallions, white and green parts
- ½ green bell pepper, diced
- ½ cup finely chopped fresh mint
- Handful of greens for serving
- Seasoned pita wedges
- Sea salt and freshly ground pepper to taste

DIRECTIONS

1. Preheat the oven to around 375°F.
2. Take a medium-sized bowl and add the asparagus with 2 tbsp. of salt and olive oil.
3. Take out a baking dish and add the asparagus. Place the tray in the oven and roast for about 10 minutes, or until the asparagus becomes tender.
4. Take out the asparagus and set aside.
5. Use another medium-sized bowl and add garlic, lime juice, orange juice, and remaining 2 tbsp. of olive oil. Whisk all the ingredients together. Add salt and pepper to taste.
6. Take the lettuce and split it into 6 plates. Take out the asparagus and place it on top of the lettuce.
7. Pour the dressing over the asparagus and lettuce salad. Top the salad with basil and pine nuts. Add a small amount of Romano cheese for garnish, if you prefer.
8. You can also toast the pine nuts in the oven. Use the method below:
9. Take out a baking tray and line it with a non-stick baking sheet. Add the pine nuts on top.
10. Bake at 375°F for about 5-10 minutes, or until the nuts are lightly browned.
11. Remove from the oven and set aside to cool.
12. Add the nuts to the salad as a topping.

256. Mediterranean Greens

PREP TIME
10 mins

COOK TIME
0 mins

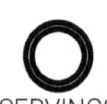
SERVINGS
4 people

NUTRITION

Calories: 140
Protein: 2 g
Fat: 12 g
Carbs: 6 g

INGREDIENTS

- 6 cups assorted fresh mixed greens (such as radicchio, arugula, watercress, baby spinach, and romaine)
- 1 small red onion, thinly sliced
- 20 cherry tomatoes, halved
- ¼ cup dried cranberries
- ¼ cup chopped walnuts
- Crumbled feta cheese
- Freshly ground pepper to taste
- 2 tbsp. balsamic vinegar
- 2 cloves fresh garlic, finely minced
- 4 tbsp. extra-virgin olive oil
- 1 tbsp. water
- ½ tsp. crushed dried oregano

DIRECTIONS

1. Take out a large salad bowl, combine walnuts, greens, tomatoes, onion, and cranberries. Gently toss.
2. For the dressing, combine water, vinegar, oregano, olive oil, and garlic. Mix the ingredients well. Pour over the salad and lightly toss.
3. Add feta cheese as garnish, if preferred.
4. Add pepper to taste.

257. Classic Greek Salad

PREP TIME: 15 mins
COOK TIME: 0 mins
SERVINGS: 6 people

NUTRITION
Calories: 268
Protein: 23 g
Fat: 17 g
Carbs: 44 g

INGREDIENTS

- 6 large firm tomatoes, quartered
- 20 Greek black olives
- ½ lb. Greek feta cheese, cut into small cubes
- ½ head of escarole, shredded
- 3 tbsp. red wine vinegar
- ¼ cup extra-virgin olive oil
- 1 tbsp. dried oregano
- ½ English cucumber, peeled, seeded, and thinly sliced
- 2 cloves fresh garlic, finely minced
- ½ red onion, sliced
- 1 medium red bell pepper, seeded and sliced
- ¼ cup freshly chopped Italian parsley
- Salt and freshly ground pepper to taste

DIRECTIONS

1. Take out a large bowl and add vinegar, oregano, olive oil, and garlic. Add salt and pepper to taste. Set aside the bowl.
2. In another large bowl, add onion, tomatoes, escarole, cucumber, bell pepper, and cheese and mix them well.
3. Take the vinegar mixture and pour it over the salad in the second bowl.
4. Top the salad with olives and parsley.

258. North African Zucchini Salad

PREP TIME: 10 mins
COOK TIME: 0 mins
SERVINGS: 4 people

NUTRITION
Calories: 140
Protein: 2 g
Fat: 12 g
Carbs: 6 g

INGREDIENTS

- 1 lb. firm green zucchini, thinly sliced
- ½ tsp. ground cumin
- 2 cloves fresh garlic, finely minced
- Juice from 1 large lemon
- 1 tbsp. extra-virgin olive oil
- 1½ tbsp. plain low-fat yogurt
- Crumbled feta cheese
- Finely chopped parsley for garnish
- Salt and freshly ground pepper to taste

DIRECTIONS

1. Add the zucchini into a large saucepan and steam it for about 2-5 minutes, or until it becomes tender and crispy. Place the zucchini under cold water and drain well.
2. Take out a large bowl and mix cumin, olive oil, lemon juice, garlic, and yogurt. Add salt and pepper to taste.
3. Add the zucchini into the mixture in the bowl and toss gently.
4. Serve with feta cheese and parsley as garnish.

259. Tunisian Style Carrot Salad

PREP TIME
15 mins

COOK TIME
0 mins

SERVINGS
6 people

NUTRITION

Calories: 138
Protein: 7 g
Fat: 5 g
Carbs: 13 g

INGREDIENTS

- 10 medium carrots, peeled and sliced
- 1 cup crumbled feta cheese, divided
- 2 tsp. caraway seed
- ¼ cup extra-virgin olive oil
- 6 tbsp. apple cider vinegar
- 5 tsp. freshly minced garlic
- 1 tbsp. Harissa paste (choose the level of heat based on your preference)
- 20 pitted Kalamata olives, reserving some for garnish
- Salt to taste

DIRECTIONS

1. Take out a medium saucepan and place it on medium heat. Fill it with water and add the carrots. Cook carrots until tender. Drain and cool the carrots under cold water. Drain again to remove any excess water.
2. Take out a large bowl and place the carrots in them.
3. Take out a mortar and combine salt, garlic, and caraway seeds. Grind them until they form a paste. Otherwise, you can also use a small bowl, preferably one not made out of glass for grind. The final option would be to toss the ingredients into a blender and pulse them.
4. Add vinegar and Harissa into the bowl with the carrots and mix them well.
5. Use a large spoon and mash the carrots. Add the garlic mixture into the carrot and mix again until they have all blended well. Add the olive oil and mix again.
6. Finally, add about ½ the feta cheese and all the olives and mix well again.
7. Take out a large bowl and add the salad to it. Top it with the remaining feta cheese.

260. Caesar Salad

PREP TIME
5 mins

COOK TIME
0 mins

SERVINGS
6 people

NUTRITION

Calories: 49
Protein: 4 g
Fat: 1 g
Carbs: 4 g

INGREDIENTS

- 10 small pitted black olives, chopped
- 1-2 bunches romaine lettuce, cleaned and torn in pieces
- 2 tsp. lemon juice
- 2½ tsp. balsamic vinegar
- ½ cup grated parmesan cheese
- ½ cup nonfat plain yogurt
- 1 tsp. worcestershire sauce
- ½ tsp. anchovy paste
- 2 cloves freshly minced garlic

DIRECTIONS

1. Take out a large bowl and place romaine lettuce in it.
2. Take out your blended and add mix lemon juice, yogurt, garlic, anchovy paste, vinegar, worcestershire sauce, and ¼ cup parmesan cheese. Mix all the ingredients well until they are smooth.
3. Pour the yogurt mixture over the lettuce and toss lightly.
4. Top the salad with the remaining parmesan cheese.

261 Avocado Salad

PREP TIME: 10 mins
COOK TIME: 0 mins
SERVINGS: 3 people

INGREDIENTS

- 1 small onion, finely chopped
- 1 large ripe avocado, pitted and peeled
- 2 tbsp. chopped fresh parsley
- 2 tsp. fresh lime juice
- ½ small hot pepper, finely chopped (optional)
- 1 cup halved cherry tomatoes
- Salt and freshly ground pepper to taste

DIRECTIONS

1. Start with the avocado and cut it into bite-sized pieces.
2. Add parsley, lime juice, tomatoes, onion, and hot pepper. Mix all the ingredients well. Add salt and pepper to taste.
3. Finally, add the avocado into the mixture and mix them well.

NUTRITION

Calories: 130
Protein: 2 g
Fat: 10 g
Carbs: 10 g

262. Spanish Salad

PREP TIME: 10 mins
COOK TIME: 0 mins
SERVINGS: 6 people

INGREDIENTS

- 2 bunches romaine lettuce, cleaned and trimmed
- 1 large sweet onion, thinly sliced
- 3 medium ripe tomatoes, chopped
- 3 tbsp. balsamic vinegar
- ¼ cup extra-virgin olive oil
- 1 red bell pepper, seeded and thinly sliced
- 1 green bell pepper, seeded and thinly sliced
- ¼ cup chopped and pitted black olives
- ¼ cup chopped and pitted marinated green olives
- Salt and freshly ground pepper to taste

DIRECTIONS

1. Take out 6 plates and place romaine lettuce on them to form a base.
2. Add peppers, tomatoes, onion, and olives on top of each of the lettuce bases.
3. In a small bowl, combine olive oil and vinegar together. Add the dressing over the salad.
4. Add salt and pepper to taste, if preferred.

NUTRITION

Calories: 107
Protein: 2 g
Fat: 9 g
Carbs: 6 g

263. Parsley Couscous Salad

PREP TIME
2 hours

COOK TIME
0 mins

SERVINGS
4 people

NUTRITION

Calories: 120
Protein: 5 g
Fat: 2 g
Carbs: 18 g

INGREDIENTS

- ¼ cup couscous
- 2 tsp. extra-virgin olive oil
- ¼ cup water
- 2 tsp. lemon zest
- 1 medium ripe tomato, peeled, seeded, and diced
- 2 tbsp. pine nuts
- 2 tbsp. fresh lemon juice
- ¼ cup finely chopped fresh flat parsley leaves
- 2 tbsp. finely chopped fresh mint leaves
- 2 heads Belgian endive, leaves for scooping
- Whole wheat pita rounds, cut into wedges and toasted until crispy
- Salt and freshly ground pepper to taste

DIRECTIONS

1. Take out a medium bowl and then combine lemon juice and water. All the mixture to stand for about 1 hour.
2. After the hour, add mint, parsley, lemon zest, olive oil, and pine nuts. Mix the ingredients well.
3. Add in the couscous to the mixture. Allow it to stand for about 1 hour. After 1 hour, add salt and pepper to taste.
4. Place couscous mixture in the center of a plate and top it with tomato. You can surround the couscous salad with toasted pita wedges and endive leaves, which makes for a wonderful presentation.
5. Refrigerator overnight so that you can have it the next day.

264. Cress and Tangerine Salad

PREP TIME
15 mins

COOK TIME
0 mins

SERVINGS
4 people

NUTRITION

Calories: 195
Protein: 3 g
Fat: 16 g
Carbs: 14 g

INGREDIENTS

- 4 large sweet tangerines
- ¼ cup extra-virgin olive oil
- 2 large bunches watercress, washed and stems removed
- Juice from 1 fresh lemon
- 10 cherry tomatoes, halved
- 16 pitted Kalamata olives
- Sea salt and freshly ground pepper to taste

DIRECTIONS

1. Take the tangerines and peel them into a medium-sized bowl. Make sure that you remove any pits and squeeze the sections. You should have around ¼ cup of tangerine juice. Set sections aside.
2. Take a large bowl and add lemon juice, tangerine juice, and olive oil. Mix them together and add salt and pepper for flavor, if you prefer.
3. Use paper towels to pat the cress dry. Add watercress, tomatoes, and olives to the bowl containing the tangerine sections (not to be confused with the bowl containing tangerine juice). Toss them lightly.
4. Pour the tangerine juice mixture on top. Mix well and serve.

265. Prosciutto and Figs Salad

PREP TIME 10 mins
COOK TIME 0 mins
SERVINGS 4 people

NUTRITION
Calories: 190
Protein: 26 g
Fat: 9 g
Carbs: 17 g

INGREDIENTS

- One 10-12-oz. package fresh baby spinach
- 1 small hot red chili pepper, finely diced
- 1 carton figs, stems removed and quartered
- ½ cup walnuts, coarsely chopped
- 1 tbsp. fresh orange juice
- 1 tbsp. honey
- 4 slices prosciutto, cut into strips
- Shaved parmesan cheese for garnish

DIRECTIONS

1. Take your spinach and divide them into 4 equal portions. Each portion should be on a separate plate and will act as a base. Add quartered prosciutto, figs, and walnuts on each spinach as toppings.
2. For the dressing, take a small bowl and add honey, orange juice, and diced pepper. Add the mixture over the salad.
3. Finally, toss the salad lightly and use parmesan cheese for the garnish.

266. Garden Vegetables and Chickpeas Salad

PREP TIME 10 mins
COOK TIME 0 mins
SERVINGS 4 people

NUTRITION
Calories: 195
Protein: 16 g
Fat: 7 g
Carbs: 24 g

INGREDIENTS

- 2 tbsp. freshly squeezed lemon juice
- 1/8 tsp. freshly ground pepper
- 1 cup cubed part-skim mozzarella cheese
- 1 tbsp. fresh basil leaf, snipped
- 1 (15-oz.) can chickpeas, rinsed and well drained
- 2 cups coarsely chopped fresh broccoli
- 2 cloves fresh garlic, finely minced
- ½ cup sliced fresh carrots
- 1 7½-oz. can diced tomatoes, undrained

DIRECTIONS

1. Use a large bowl and add garlic, basil, lemon juice, and ground pepper. Mix them well.
2. Add the chickpeas, carrots, tomatoes with juice, broccoli, and mozzarella cheese. Toos all the ingredients well.
3. You can serve immediately, or you can keep it refrigerated overnight.

267. Peppered Watercress Salad

PREP TIME: 5 mins
COOK TIME: 0 mins
SERVINGS: 4 people

INGREDIENTS

- 2 tsp. champagne vinegar
- 2 bunches (about 8 cups) watercress, rinsed and rough stems removed
- 2 tbsp. extra-virgin olive oil
- Salt and freshly ground pepper to taste

DIRECTIONS

1. Drain the watercress properly.
2. Take out a small bowl and then add salt, pepper, vinegar, and olive oil. Mix them well together.
3. Transfer the watercress to a bowl. Add the vinegar mixture into it and toss well.
4. Serve immediately.

NUTRITION

Calories: 67
Protein: 4 g
Fat: 7 g
Carbs: 1 g

VEGETARIAN DISHES

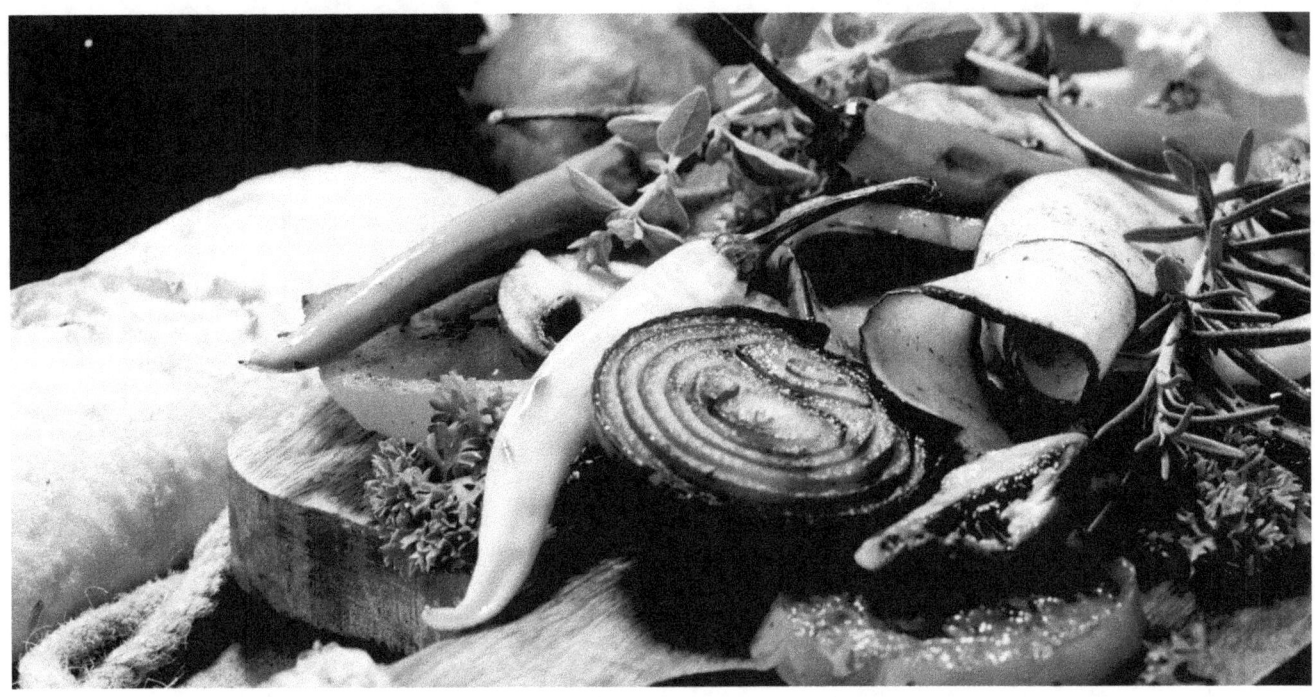

268. Rustic Vegetable and Brown Rice Bowl

PREP TIME: 15 mins
COOK TIME: 10 mins
SERVINGS: 4 people

NUTRITION
Calories: 192;
Carbs: 12.7g;
Protein: 3.8g;
Fat: 15.5g

INGREDIENTS

- Nonstick cooking spray
- 2 cups broccoli florets
- 2 cups cauliflower florets
- 1 (15-oz.) can chickpeas, drained and rinsed
- 1 cup carrots sliced 1 inch thick
- 2 to 3 tbsp. extra-virgin olive oil, divided
- Salt and freshly ground black pepper
- 2 to 3 tbsp. sesame seeds, for garnish
- 2 cups cooked brown rice
- For the dressing
- 3 to 4 tbsp. tahini
- 2 tbsp. honey
- 1 lemon, juiced
- 1 garlic clove, minced
- Salt
- Freshly ground black pepper

DIRECTIONS

1. Preheat the oven to 400°F. Spray two baking sheets with cooking spray.
2. Cover the first baking sheet with the broccoli and cauliflower and the second with the chickpeas and carrots. Toss each sheet with half of the oil and season with salt and pepper before placing in oven.
3. Cook the carrots and chickpeas for 10 minutes, leaving the carrots still just crisp, and the broccoli and cauliflower for 20 minutes, until tender. Stir each halfway through cooking.
4. To make the dressing, in a small bowl, mix the tahini, honey, lemon juice, and garlic. Season with salt and pepper and set aside.
5. Divide the rice into individual bowls, then layer with vegetables and drizzle dressing over the dish.

269. Roasted Brussels sprouts And Pecans

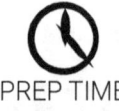
PREP TIME
10 mins

COOK TIME
15 mins

SERVINGS
4 people

INGREDIENTS

- 1 ½ lb. fresh Brussels sprouts
- 4 tbsp. olive oil
- 4 cloves of garlic, minced
- 3 tbsp. water
- Salt and pepper to taste
- ½ cup chopped pecans

DIRECTIONS

1. Place all ingredients in the Instant Pot.
2. Combine all ingredients until well combined.
3. Close the lid and make sure that the steam release vent is set to "Venting."
4. Press the "Slow Cook" button and adjust the cooking time to 3 hours.
5. Sprinkle with a dash of lemon juice if desired.

NUTRITION

Calories: 161;
Carbs: 10.2g;
Protein: 4.1g;
Fat: 13.1g

270. Eggs with Zucchini Noodles

PREP TIME
10 mins

COOK TIME
11 mins

SERVINGS
2 people

INGREDIENTS

- 2 tbsp. extra-virgin olive oil
- 3 zucchinis, cut with a spiralizer
- 4 eggs
- Salt and black pepper to the taste
- A pinch of red pepper flakes
- Cooking spray
- 1 tbsp. basil, chopped

DIRECTIONS

1. In a bowl, combine the zucchini noodles with salt, pepper and the olive oil and toss well.
2. Grease a baking sheet with cooking spray and divide the zucchini noodles into 4 nests on it.
3. Crack an egg on top of each nest, sprinkle salt, pepper and the pepper flakes on top and bake at 350°F for 11 minutes.
4. Divide the mix between plates, sprinkle the basil on top and serve.

NUTRITION

Calories 296,
Fat 23.6,
Fiber 3.3,
Carbs 10.6,
Protein 14.7

271. Roasted Root Veggies

PREP TIME: 20 mins
COOK TIME: 90 mins
SERVINGS: 6 people

NUTRITION
Calories: 298;
Carbs: 61.1g;
Protein: 7.4g;
Fat: 5.0g

INGREDIENTS

- 2 tbsp. olive oil
- 1 head garlic, cloves separated and peeled
- 1 large turnip, peeled and cut into ½-inch pieces
- 1 medium sized red onion, cut into ½-inch pieces
- 1 ½ lbs. beets, trimmed but not peeled, scrubbed and cut into ½-inch pieces
- 1 ½ lbs. Yukon gold potatoes, unpeeled, cut into ½-inch pieces
- 2 ½ lbs. butternut squash, peeled, seeded, cut into ½-inch pieces

DIRECTIONS

1. Grease 2 rimmed and large baking sheets. Preheat oven to 425oF.
2. In a large bowl, mix all ingredients thoroughly.
3. Into the two baking sheets, evenly divide the root vegetables, spread in one layer.
4. Season generously with pepper and salt.
5. Pop into the oven and roast for 1 hour and 15 minute or until golden brown and tender.
6. Remove from oven and let it cool for at least 15 minutes before serving.

272. Roasted Vegetables and Zucchini Pasta

PREP TIME: 10 mins
COOK TIME: 7 mins
SERVINGS: 2 people

NUTRITION
Calories: 288;
Carbs: 23.6g;
Protein: 8.2g;
Fat: 19.2g

INGREDIENTS

- ¼ cup raw pine nuts
- 4 cups leftover vegetables
- 2 garlic cloves, minced
- 1 tbsp. extra virgin olive oil
- 4 medium zucchinis, cut into long strips resembling noodles

DIRECTIONS

1. Heat oil in a large skillet over medium heat and sauté the garlic for 2 minutes.
2. Add the leftover vegetables and place the zucchini noodles on top. Let it cook for five minutes. Garnish with pine nuts.

273. Sautéed Collard Greens

PREP TIME
10 mins

COOK TIME
0 mins

○
SERVINGS
4 people

INGREDIENTS

- 1-lb. fresh collard greens, cut into 2-inch pieces
- 1 pinch red pepper flakes
- 3 cups chicken broth
- 1 tsp. pepper
- 1 tsp. salt
- 2 cloves garlic, minced
- 1 large onion, chopped
- 3 slices bacon
- 1 tbsp. olive oil

DIRECTIONS

1. Using a large skillet, heat oil on medium-high heat. Sauté bacon until crisp. Remove it from the pan and crumble it once cooled. Set it aside.
2. Using the same pan, sauté onion and cook until tender. Add garlic until fragrant. Add the collard greens and cook until they start to wilt.
3. Pour in the chicken broth and season with pepper, salt and red pepper flakes. Reduce the heat to low and simmer for 45 minutes.

NUTRITION

Calories: 20;
Carbs: 3.0g;
Protein: 1.0g;
Fat: 1.0g

274. Savoy Cabbage with Coconut Cream Sauce

PREP TIME
5 mins

COOK TIME
20 mins

SERVINGS
4 people

INGREDIENTS

- 3 tbsp. olive oil
- 1 onion, chopped
- 4 cloves of garlic, minced
- 1 head savoy cabbage, chopped finely
- 2 cups bone broth
- 1 cup coconut milk, freshly squeezed
- 1 bay leaf
- Salt and pepper to taste
- 2 tbsp. chopped parsley

DIRECTIONS

1. Heat oil in a pot for 2 minutes.
2. Stir in the onions, bay leaf, and garlic until fragrant, around 3 minutes.
3. Add the rest of the ingredients, except for the parsley and mix well.
4. Cover pot, bring to a boil, and let it simmer for 5 minutes or until cabbage is tender to taste.
5. Stir in parsley and serve.

NUTRITION

Calories: 195;
Carbs: 12.3g;
Protein: 2.7g;
Fat: 19.7g

275. Slow Cooked Buttery Mushrooms

PREP TIME: 10 mins
COOK TIME: 10 mins
SERVINGS: 2 people

INGREDIENTS

- 2 tbsp. butter
- 2 tbsp. olive oil
- 3 cloves of garlic, minced
- 16 oz. fresh brown mushrooms, sliced
- 7 oz. fresh shiitake mushrooms, sliced
- A dash of thyme
- Salt and pepper to taste

DIRECTIONS

1. Heat the butter and oil in a pot.
2. Sauté the garlic until fragrant, around 1 minute.
3. Stir in the rest of the ingredients and cook until soft, around 9 minutes.

NUTRITION
Calories: 192; Carbs: 12.7g; Protein: 3.8g; Fat: 15.5g

---

276. Steamed Squash Chowder

PREP TIME: 20 mins
COOK TIME: 40 mins
SERVINGS: 4 people

INGREDIENTS

- 3 cups chicken broth
- 2 tbsp. ghee
- 1 tsp. chili powder
- ½ tsp. cumin
- 1 ½ tsp. salt
- 2 tsp. cinnamon
- 3 tbsp. olive oil
- 2 carrots, chopped
- 1 small yellow onion, chopped
- 1 green apple, sliced and cored
- 1 large butternut squash, peeled, seeded, and chopped to ½-inch cubes

DIRECTIONS

1. In a large pot on medium high fire, melt ghee.
2. Once ghee is hot, sauté onions for 5 minutes or until soft and translucent.
3. Add olive oil, chili powder, cumin, salt, and cinnamon. Sauté for half a minute.
4. Add chopped squash and apples.
5. Sauté for 10 minutes while stirring once in a while.
6. Add broth, cover and cook on medium fire for twenty minutes or until apples and squash are tender.
7. With an immersion blender, puree chowder. Adjust consistency by adding more water.
8. Add more salt or pepper depending on desire.
9. Serve and enjoy.

NUTRITION
Calories: 228; Carbs: 17.9g; Protein: 2.2g; Fat: 18.0g

277. Steamed Zucchini-Paprika

PREP TIME
15 mins

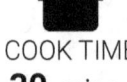
COOK TIME
30 mins

SERVINGS
2 people

NUTRITION
Calories: 93;
Carbs: 3.1g;
Protein: 0.6g;
Fat: 10.2g

INGREDIENTS
- 4 tbsp. olive oil
- 3 cloves of garlic, minced
- 1 onion, chopped
- 3 medium-sized zucchinis, sliced thinly
- A dash of paprika
- Salt and pepper to taste

DIRECTIONS
1. Place all ingredients in the Instant Pot.
2. Give a good stir to combine all ingredients.
3. Close the lid and make sure that the steam release valve is set to "Venting."
4. Press the "Slow Cook" button and adjust the cooking time to 4 hours.
5. Halfway through the cooking time, open the lid and give a good stir to brown the other side.

278. Stir Fried Brussels sprouts and Carrots

PREP TIME
10 mins

COOK TIME
15 mins

SERVINGS
6 people

NUTRITION
Calories: 98;
Carbs: 13.9g;
Protein: 3.5g;
Fat: 4.2g

INGREDIENTS
- 1 tbsp. cider vinegar
- 1/3 cup water
- 1 lb. Brussels sprouts, halved lengthwise
- 1 lb. carrots cut diagonally into ½-inch thick lengths
- 3 tbsp. unsalted butter, divided
- 2 tbsp. chopped shallot
- ½ tsp. pepper
- ¾ tsp. salt

DIRECTIONS
1. On medium high fire, place a nonstick medium fry pan and heat 2 tbsp. butter.
2. Add shallots and cook until softened, around one to two minutes while occasionally stirring.
3. Add pepper salt, Brussels sprouts and carrots. Stir fry until vegetables starts to brown on the edges, around 3 to 4 minutes.
4. Add water, cook and cover.
5. After 5 to 8 minutes, or when veggies are already soft, add remaining butter.
6. If needed season with more pepper and salt to taste.
7. Turn off fire, transfer to a platter, serve and enjoy.

279. Stir Fried Eggplant

PREP TIME: 10 mins
COOK TIME: 30 mins
SERVINGS: 2 people

NUTRITION
Calories: 369;
Carbs: 28.4g;
Protein: 11.4g;
Fat: 25.3g

INGREDIENTS
- 1 tsp. cornstarch + 2 tbsp. water, mixed
- 1 tsp. brown sugar
- 2 tbsp. oyster sauce
- 1 tbsp. fish sauce
- 2 tbsp. soy sauce
- ½ cup fresh basil
- 2 tbsp. oil
- ¼ cup water
- 2 cups Chinese eggplant, spiral
- 1 red chili
- 6 cloves garlic, minced
- ½ purple onion, sliced thinly
- 1 3-oz package medium firm tofu, cut into slivers

DIRECTIONS
1. Prepare sauce by mixing cornstarch and water in a small bowl. In another bowl mix brown sugar, oyster sauce and fish sauce and set aside.
2. On medium high fire, place a large nonstick saucepan and heat 2 tbsp. oil. Sauté chili, garlic and onion for 4 minutes. Add tofu, stir fry for 4 minutes.
3. Add eggplant noodles and stir fry for 10 minutes. If pan dries up, add water in small amounts to moisten pan and cook noodles.
4. Pour in sauce and mix well. Once simmering, slowly add cornstarch mixer while continuing to mix vigorously. Once sauce thickens add fresh basil and cook for a minute.
5. Remove from fire, transfer to a serving plate and enjoy.

280. Summer Vegetables

PREP TIME: 20 mins
COOK TIME: 100 mins
SERVINGS: 6 people

NUTRITION
Calories: 150;
Carbs: 11.8g;
Protein: 3.3g;
Fat: 10.8g

INGREDIENTS
- 1 tsp. dried marjoram
- 1/3 cup Parmesan cheese
- 1 small eggplant, sliced into ¼-inch thick circles
- 1 small summer squash, peeled and sliced diagonally into ¼-inch thickness
- 3 large tomatoes, sliced into ¼-inch thick circles
- ½ cup dry white wine
- ½ tsp. freshly ground pepper, divided
- ½ tsp. salt, divided
- 5 cloves garlic, sliced thinly
- 2 cups leeks, sliced thinly
- 4 tbsp. extra virgin olive oil, divided

DIRECTIONS
1. On medium fire, place a large nonstick saucepan and heat 2 tbsp. oil.
2. Sauté garlic and leeks for 6 minutes or until garlic is starting to brown. Season with pepper and salt, ¼ tsp. each.
3. Pour in wine and cook for another minute. Transfer to a 2-quart baking dish.
4. In baking dish, layer in alternating pattern the eggplant, summer squash, and tomatoes. Do this until dish is covered with vegetables. If there are excess vegetables, store for future use.
5. Season with remaining pepper and salt. Drizzle with remaining olive oil and pop in a preheated 425oF oven.
6. Bake for 75 minutes. Remove from oven and top with marjoram and cheese.
7. Return to oven and bake for 15 minutes more or until veggies are soft and edges are browned.
8. Allow to cool for at least 5 minutes before serving.

281. Stir Fried Bok Choy

PREP TIME
5 mins

COOK TIME
13 mins

SERVINGS
4 people

INGREDIENTS

- 3 tbsp. coconut oil
- 4 cloves of garlic, minced
- 1 onion, chopped
- 2 heads bok choy, rinsed and chopped
- 2 tsp. coconut aminos
- Salt and pepper to taste
- 2 tbsp. sesame oil
- 2 tbsp. sesame seeds, toasted

DIRECTIONS

1. Heat the oil in a pot for 2 minutes.
2. Sauté the garlic and onions until fragrant, around 3 minutes.
3. Stir in the bok choy, coconut aminos, salt and pepper.
4. Cover pan and cook for 5 minutes.
5. Stir and continue cooking for another 3 minutes.
6. Drizzle with sesame oil and sesame seeds on top before serving.

NUTRITION

Calories: 358;
Carbs: 5.2g;
Protein: 21.5g;
Fat: 28.4g

282. Summer Veggies in Instant Pot

PREP TIME
10 mins

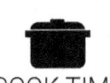
COOK TIME
7 mins

SERVINGS
6 people

INGREDIENTS

- 2 cups okra, sliced
- 1 cup grape tomatoes
- 1 cup mushroom, sliced
- 1 ½ cups onion, sliced
- 2 cups bell pepper, sliced
- 2 ½ cups zucchini, sliced
- 2 tbsp. basil, chopped
- 1 tbsp. thyme, chopped
- ½ cups balsamic vinegar
- ½ cups olive oil
- Salt and pepper

DIRECTIONS

1. Place all ingredients in the Instant Pot.
2. Stir the contents and close the lid.
3. Close the lid and press the Manual button.
4. Adjust the cooking time to 7 minutes.
5. Do quick pressure release.
6. Once cooled, evenly divide into serving size, keep in your preferred container, and refrigerate until ready to eat.

NUTRITION

Calories 233;
Carbs: 7g;
Protein: 3g;
Fat: 18g

283. Sumptuous Tomato Soup

PREP TIME
10 mins

COOK TIME
30 mins

SERVINGS
2 people

NUTRITION

Calories: 179;
Carbs: 26.7g;
Protein: 5.2g;
Fat: 7.7g

INGREDIENTS

- Pepper and salt to taste
- 2 tbsp. tomato paste
- 1 ½ cups vegetable broth
- 1 tbsp. chopped parsley
- 1 tbsp. olive oil
- 5 garlic cloves
- ½ medium yellow onion
- 4 large ripe tomatoes

DIRECTIONS

1. Preheat oven to 350°F.
2. Chop onion and tomatoes into thin wedges. Place on a rimmed baking sheet. Season with parsley, pepper, salt, and olive oil. Toss to combine well. Hide the garlic cloves inside tomatoes to keep it from burning.
3. Pop in the oven and bake for 30 minutes.
4. On medium pot, bring vegetable stock to a simmer. Add tomato paste.
5. Pour baked tomato mixture into pot. Continue simmering for another 10 minutes.
6. With an immersion blender, puree soup.
7. Adjust salt and pepper to taste before serving.

284. Superfast Cajun Asparagus

PREP TIME
10 mins

COOK TIME
8 mins

SERVINGS
2 people

NUTRITION

Calories: 81;
Carbs: 0g;
Protein: 0g;
Fat: 9g

INGREDIENTS

- 1 tsp. Cajun seasoning
- 1-lb. asparagus
- 1 tsp. Olive oil

DIRECTIONS

1. Snap the asparagus and make sure that you use the tender part of the vegetable.
2. Place a large skillet on stovetop and heat on high for a minute.
3. Then grease skillet with cooking spray and spread asparagus in one layer.
4. Cover skillet and continue cooking on high for 5 to eight minutes.
5. Halfway through cooking time, stir skillet and then cover and continue to cook.
6. Once done cooking, transfer to plates, serve, and enjoy!

285. Sweet and Nutritious Pumpkin Soup

PREP TIME
20 mins

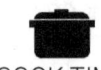
COOK TIME
40 mins

SERVINGS
8 people

NUTRITION

Calories: 58;
Carbs: 6.6g;
Protein: 5.1g;
Fat: 1.7g

INGREDIENTS

- 1 tsp. chopped fresh parsley
- ½ cup half and half
- ½ tsp. chopped fresh thyme
- 1 tsp. salt
- 4 cups pumpkin puree
- 6 cups vegetable stock, divided
- 1 clove garlic, minced
- 1 1-inch piece gingerroot, peeled and minced
- 1 cup chopped onion

DIRECTIONS

1. On medium high fire, place a heavy bottomed pot and for 5 minutes heat ½ cup vegetable stock, ginger, garlic and onions or until veggies are tender.
2. Add remaining stock and cook for 30 minutes.
3. Season with thyme and salt.
4. With an immersion blender, puree soup until smooth.
5. Turn off fire and mix in half and half.
6. Transfer pumpkin soup into 8 bowls, garnish with parsley, serve and enjoy.

286. Sweet Potato Puree

PREP TIME
10 mins

COOK TIME
15 mins

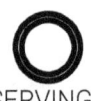
SERVINGS
6 people

NUTRITION

Calories: 619;
Carbs: 97.8g;
Protein: 4.8g;
Fat: 24.3g;

INGREDIENTS

- 2 lb. sweet potatoes, peeled
- 1 ½ cups water
- 5 Medjool dates, pitted and chopped

DIRECTIONS

1. Place all ingredients in a pot.
2. Close the lid and allow to boil for 15 minutes until the potatoes are soft.
3. Drain the potatoes and place in a food processor together with the dates.
4. Pulse until smooth.
5. Place in individual containers.
6. Put a label and store in the fridge.
7. Allow to thaw at room temperature before heating in the microwave oven.

287. Sweet Potato Soup

PREP TIME 10 mins
COOK TIME 30 mins
SERVINGS 4 people

NUTRITION
Calories: 112;
Carbs: 17.5g;
Protein: 3.5g;
Fat: 4.6g

INGREDIENTS

- Pepper and salt to taste
- 2 tbsp. thyme leaves
- Juice of half a lemon
- 1 tsp. ground cumin
- 2 cups mashed sweet potato
- 4 cups chicken stock
- 4 bell pepper, diced
- 1 onion, diced
- 1 tbsp. coconut oil

DIRECTIONS

1. On medium low fire, place a heavy bottomed pot and heat coconut oil.
2. Sauté peppers and onions for 5 minutes or until slightly soft.
3. Meanwhile, in a blender puree mashed sweet potatoes with 2 cups chicken stock. Pour into pot.
4. Add cumin and remaining chicken stock. Cover and bring to a boil.
5. Lower fire to a simmer and cook for 20 minutes or until peppers are tender.
6. Season with pepper, salt, thyme and lemon juice.
7. Serve while hot.

288. Sweet Potatoes Oven Fried

PREP TIME 10 mins
COOK TIME 30 mins
SERVINGS 7 people

NUTRITION
Calories: 176;
Carbs: 36.6g;
Protein: 2.5g;
Fat: 2.5g

INGREDIENTS

- 1 small garlic clove, minced
- 1 tsp. grated orange rind
- 1 tbsp. fresh parsley, chopped finely
- ¼ tsp. pepper
- ¼ tsp. salt
- 1 tbsp. olive oil
- 4 medium sweet potatoes, peeled and sliced to ¼-inch thickness

DIRECTIONS

1. In a large bowl mix well pepper, salt, olive oil and sweet potatoes.
2. In a greased baking sheet, in a single layer arrange sweet potatoes.
3. Pop in a preheated 400oF oven and bake for 15 minutes, turnover potato slices and return to oven. Bake for another 15 minutes or until tender.
4. Meanwhile, mix well in a small bowl garlic, orange rind and parsley, sprinkle over cooked potato slices and serve.
5. You can store baked sweet potatoes in a lidded container and just microwave whenever you want to eat it. Do consume within 3 days.

289. Tasty Avocado Sauce over Zoodles

PREP TIME
10 mins

COOK TIME
10 mins

SERVINGS
2 people

INGREDIENTS

- 1 zucchini peeled and spiralized into noodles
- 4 tbsp. pine nuts
- 2 tbsp. lemon juice
- 1 avocado peeled and pitted
- 12 sliced cherry tomatoes
- 1/3 cup water
- 1 1/4 cup basil
- Pepper and salt to taste

DIRECTIONS

1. Make the sauce in a blender by adding pine nuts, lemon juice, avocado, water, and basil. Pulse until smooth and creamy. Season with pepper and salt to taste. Mix well.
2. Place zoodles in salad bowl. Pour over avocado sauce and toss well to coat.
3. Add cherry tomatoes, serve, and enjoy.

NUTRITION

Calories: 313;
Protein: 6.8g;
Carbs: 18.7g;
Fat: 26.8g

290. Tomato Basil Cauliflower Rice

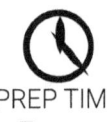
PREP TIME
5 mins

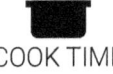
COOK TIME
10 mins

SERVINGS
4 people

INGREDIENTS

- Salt and pepper to taste
- Dried parsley for garnish
- ¼ cup tomato paste
- ½ tsp. garlic, minced
- ½ tsp. onion powder
- ½ tsp. marjoram
- 1 ½ tsp. dried basil
- 1 tsp. dried oregano
- 1 large head of cauliflower
- 1 tsp. oil

DIRECTIONS

1. Cut the cauliflower into florets and place in the food processor.
2. Pulse until it has a coarse consistency similar with rice. Set aside.
3. In a skillet, heat the oil and sauté the garlic and onion for three minutes. Add the rest of the ingredients. Cook for 8 minutes.

NUTRITION

Calories: 106;
Carbs: 15.1g;
Protein: 3.3g;
Fat: 5.0g

291. Vegan Sesame Tofu and Eggplants

PREP TIME: 10 mins
COOK TIME: 20 mins
SERVINGS: 4 people

INGREDIENTS
- 5 tbsp. olive oil
- 1-lb. firm tofu, sliced
- 3 tbsp. rice vinegar
- 2 tsp. Swerve sweetener
- 2 whole eggplants, sliced
- ¼ cup soy sauce
- Salt and pepper to taste
- 4 tbsp. toasted sesame oil
- ¼ cup sesame seeds
- 1 cup fresh cilantro, chopped

DIRECTIONS
1. Heat the oil in a pan for 2 minutes.
2. Pan fry the tofu for 3 minutes on each side.
3. Stir in the rice vinegar, sweetener, eggplants, and soy sauce. Season with salt and pepper to taste.
4. Cover and cook for 5 minutes on medium fire. Stir and continue cooking for another 5 minutes.
5. Toss in the sesame oil, sesame seeds, and cilantro.
6. Serve and enjoy.

NUTRITION
Calories: 616;
Carbs: 27.4g;
Protein: 23.9g;
Fat: 49.2g

---

292. Vegetarian Coconut Curry

PREP TIME: 10 mins
COOK TIME: 30 mins
SERVINGS: 4 people

INGREDIENTS
- 4 tbsp. coconut oil
- 1 medium onion, chopped
- 1 tsp. minced garlic
- 1 tsp. minced ginger
- 1 cup broccoli florets
- 2 cups fresh spinach leaves
- 2 tsp. fish sauce
- 1 tbsp. garam masala
- ½ cup coconut milk
- Salt and pepper to taste

DIRECTIONS
1. Heat oil in a pot.
2. Sauté the onion and garlic until fragrant, around 3 minutes.
3. Stir in the rest of the ingredients, except for spinach leaves.
4. Season with salt and pepper to taste.
5. Cover and cook on medium fire for 5 minutes.
6. Stir and add spinach leaves. Cover and cook for another 2 minutes.
7. Turn off fire and let it sit for two more minutes before serving.

NUTRITION
Calories: 210;
Carbs: 6.5g;
Protein: 2.1g;
Fat: 20.9g

293. Veggie Lo Mein

PREP TIME
10 mins

COOK TIME
4 mins

SERVINGS
6 people

NUTRITION

Calories 288;
Carbs: 48.7g;
Protein: 7.6g;
Fat: 11g;

INGREDIENTS

- 2 tbsp. olive oil
- 5 cloves of garlic, minced
- 2-inch knob of ginger, grated
- 8 oz. mushrooms, sliced
- ½ lb. zucchini, spiralized
- 1 carrot, julienned
- 1 spring green onions, chopped
- 3 tbsp. coconut aminos
- Salt and pepper to taste
- 1 tbsp. sesame oil

DIRECTIONS

1. Heat the oil in a skillet and sauté the garlic and ginger until fragrant.
2. Stir in the mushrooms, zucchini, carrot, and green onions.
3. Season with coconut aminos, salt and pepper.
4. Close the lid and allow to simmer for 5 minutes.
5. Drizzle with sesame oil last.
6. Place in individual containers.
7. Put a label and store in the fridge.
8. Allow to thaw at room temperature before heating in the microwave oven.

294. Veggie Jamaican Stew

PREP TIME
15 mins

COOK TIME
30 mins

SERVINGS
4 people

NUTRITION

Calories: 531;
Carbs: 59.7g;
Protein: 8.3g;
Fat: 32.7g

INGREDIENTS

- 1 tbsp. cilantro, chopped
- 1 tsp. salt
- 1 tsp. pepper
- 1 tbsp. lime juice
- 2 cups collard greens, sliced
- 3 cups carrots, cut into bite-sized chunks
- ½ yellow plantain, cut into bite-sized pieces
- 1 cup okra, cut into ½" pieces
- 2 cups potatoes, cut into bite-sized cubes
- 2 cups taro, cut into bite sized cubes
- 2 cups pumpkin, cut into bite sized cubes
- 2 cups water
- 2 cups coconut milk
- 2 bay leaves
- 3 green onions, white bottom removed
- ½ tsp. dried thyme
- ½ tsp. ground allspice
- 4 garlic cloves, minced
- 1 onion, chopped
- 1 tbsp. olive oil

DIRECTIONS

1. On medium fire, place a stockpot and heat oil. Sauté onions for 4 minutes or until translucent and soft. Add thyme, all spice and garlic. Sauté for a minute.
2. Pour in water and coconut milk and bring to a simmer. Add bay leaves and green onions.
3. Once simmering, slow fire to keep broth at a simmer and add taro and pumpkin. Cook for 5 minutes.
4. Add potatoes and cook for three minutes.
5. Add carrots, plantain and okra. Mix and cook for five minutes.
6. Then remove and fish for thyme sprigs, bay leaves and green onions and discard.
7. Add collard greens and cook for four minutes or until bright green and darker in color.
8. Turn off fire, add pepper, salt and lime juice to taste. Once it tastes good, mix well, transfer to a serving bowl, serve and enjoy.

295. Vegetable Soup Moroccan Style

PREP TIME: 10 mins
COOK TIME: 10 mins
SERVINGS: 6 people

NUTRITION
Calories: 268;
Carbs: 12.9g;
Protein: 28.1g;
Fat: 11.7g

INGREDIENTS

- ½ tsp. pepper
- 1 tsp. salt
- 2 oz whole wheat orzo
- 1 large zucchini, peeled and cut into ¼-insh cubes
- 8 sprigs fresh cilantro, plus more leaves for garnish
- 12 sprigs flat leaf parsley, plus more for garnish
- A pinch of saffron threads
- 2 stalks celery leaves included, sliced thinly
- 2 carrots, diced
- 2 small turnips, peeled and diced
- 1 14-oz can diced tomatoes
- 6 cups water
- 1 lb. lamb stew meat, trimmed and cut into ½-inch cubes
- 2 tsp. ground turmeric
- 1 medium onion, diced finely
- 2 tbsp. extra virgin olive oil

DIRECTIONS

1. On medium high fire, place a large Dutch oven and heat oil.
2. Add turmeric and onion, stir fry for two minutes.
3. Add meat and sauté for 5 minutes.
4. Add saffron, celery, carrots, turnips, tomatoes and juice, and water.
5. With a kitchen string, tie cilantro and parsley sprigs together and into pot.
6. Cover and bring to a boil. Once boiling reduce fire to a simmer and continue to cook for 45 to 50 minutes or until meat is tender.
7. Once meat is tender, stir in zucchini. Cover and cook for 8 minutes.
8. Add orzo; cook for 10 minutes or until soft.
9. Remove and discard cilantro and parsley sprigs.
10. 1 Season with pepper and salt.
11. 1 Transfer to a serving bowl and garnish with cilantro and parsley leaves before serving.

296. Veggie Ramen Miso Soup

PREP TIME: 5 mins
COOK TIME: 20 mins
SERVINGS: 1 people

NUTRITION
Calories: 335;
Carbs: 19.0g;
Protein: 30.6g;
Fat: 17.6g

INGREDIENTS

- 2 tsp. thinly sliced green onion
- A pinch of salt
- ½ tsp. shoyu
- 2 tbsp. mellow white miso
- 1 cup zucchini, cut into angel hair spirals
- ½ cup thinly sliced cremini mushrooms
- ½ medium carrot, cut into angel hair spirals
- 1/2 cup baby spinach leaves – optional
- 2 ¼ cups water
- ½ box of medium firm tofu, cut into ¼-inch cubes
- 1 hardboiled egg

DIRECTIONS

1. In a small bowl, mix ¼ cup of water and miso. Set aside.
2. In a small saucepan on medium high fire, bring to a boil 2 cups water, mushrooms, tofu and carrots. Add salt, shoyu and miso mixture. Allow to boil for 5 minutes. Remove from fire and add green onion, zucchini and baby spinach leaves if using.
3. Let soup stand for 5 minutes before transferring to individual bowls. Garnish with ½ of hardboiled egg per bowl, serve and enjoy.

297. Yummy Cauliflower Fritters

PREP TIME
10 mins

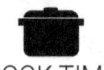
COOK TIME
15 mins

SERVINGS
6 people

NUTRITION

Calories 157;
Carbs: 2.8g;
Protein: 3.9g;
Fat: 15.3g;
Fiber: 0.9g

INGREDIENTS

- 1 large cauliflower head, cut into florets
- 2 eggs, beaten
- ½ tsp. turmeric
- ½ tsp. salt
- ¼ tsp. black pepper
- 6 tbsp. coconut oil

DIRECTIONS

1. Place the cauliflower florets in a pot with water.
2. Bring to a boil and drain once cooked.
3. Place the cauliflower, eggs, turmeric, salt, and pepper into the food processor.
4. Pulse until the mixture becomes coarse.
5. Transfer into a bowl. Using your hands, form six small flattened balls and place in the fridge for at least 1 hour until the mixture hardens.
6. Heat the oil in a skillet and fry the cauliflower patties for 3 minutes on each side
7. Place in individual containers.
8. Put a label and store in the fridge.
9. Allow to thaw at room temperature before heating in the microwave oven.

298. Zucchini Garlic Fries

PREP TIME
15 mins

COOK TIME
20 mins

SERVINGS
6 people

NUTRITION

Calories: 11;
Carbs: 1.1g;
Protein: 1.5g;
Fat: 0.1g

INGREDIENTS

- ¼ tsp. garlic powder
- ½ cup almond flour
- 2 large egg whites, beaten
- 3 medium zucchinis, sliced into fry sticks
- Salt and pepper to taste

DIRECTIONS

1. Preheat oven to 400°F.
2. Mix all ingredients in a bowl until the zucchini fries are well coated.
3. Place fries on cookie sheet and spread evenly.
4. Put in oven and cook for 20 minutes.
5. Halfway through cooking time, stir fries.

299. Zucchini Pasta with Mango-Kiwi Sauce

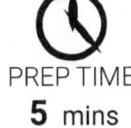
PREP TIME
5 mins

COOK TIME
20 mins

SERVINGS
2 people

INGREDIENTS

- 1 tsp. dried herbs – optional
- ½ Cup Raw Kale leaves, shredded
- 2 small dried figs
- 3 medjool dates
- 4 medium kiwis
- 2 big mangos, seed discarded
- 2 cup zucchini, spiralized
- ¼ cup roasted cashew

DIRECTIONS

1. On a salad bowl, place kale then topped with zucchini noodles and sprinkle with dried herbs. Set aside.
2. In a food processor, grind to a powder the cashews. Add figs, dates, kiwis and mangoes then puree to a smooth consistency.
3. Pour over zucchini pasta, serve and enjoy.

NUTRITION

Calories: 530;
Carbs: 95.4g;
Protein: 8.0g;
Fat: 18.5g

300. Quinoa with Almonds and Cranberries

PREP TIME
10 mins

COOK TIME
15 mins

SERVINGS
4 people

INGREDIENTS

- 2 cups cooked quinoa
- 1/3 tsp. cranberries or currants
- ¼ cup sliced almonds
- 2 garlic cloves, minced
- 1 ¼ tsp. salt
- ½ tsp. ground cumin
- ½ tsp. turmeric
- ¼ tsp. ground cinnamon
- ¼ tsp. freshly ground black pepper

DIRECTIONS

1. In a large bowl, toss the quinoa, cranberries, almonds, garlic, salt, cumin, turmeric, cinnamon, and pepper and stir to combine. Enjoy alone or with roasted cauliflower.

NUTRITION

Calories: 430;
Carbs: 65.4g;
Protein: 8.0g;
Fat: 15.5g

301. Mediterranean Baked Chickpeas

PREP TIME 15 mins

COOK TIME 15 mins

SERVINGS 6 people

NUTRITION

Calories: 330;
Carbs: 75.4g;
Protein: 9.0g;
Fat: 18.5g

INGREDIENTS

- 1 tbsp. extra-virgin olive oil
- ½ medium onion, chopped
- 3 garlic cloves, chopped
- 2 tsp. smoked paprika
- ¼ tsp. ground cumin
- 4 cups halved cherry tomatoes
- 2 (15-oz.) cans chickpeas, drained and rinsed
- ½ cup plain, unsweetened, full-fat Greek yogurt, for serving
- 1 cup crumbled feta, for serving

DIRECTIONS

1. Preheat the oven to 425°F.
2. In an oven-safe sauté pan or skillet, heat the oil over medium heat and sauté the onion and garlic. Cook for about 5 minutes, until softened and fragrant. Stir in the paprika and cumin and cook for 2 minutes. Stir in the tomatoes and chickpeas.
3. Bring to a simmer for 5 to 10 minutes before placing in the oven.
4. Roast in oven for 25 to 30 minutes, until bubbling and thickened. To serve, top with Greek yogurt and feta.

302. Falafel Bites

PREP TIME 10 mins

COOK TIME 15 mins

SERVINGS 4 people

NUTRITION

Calories: 530;
Carbs: 95.4g;
Protein: 8.0g;
Fat: 18.5g

INGREDIENTS

- 1 2/3 cups falafel mix
- 1¼ cups water
- Extra-virgin olive oil spray
- 1 tbsp. Pickled Onions (optional)
- 1 tbsp. Pickled Turnips (optional)
- 2 tbsp. Tzatziki Sauce (optional)

DIRECTIONS

1. In a large bowl, carefully stir the falafel mix into the water. Mix well. Let stand 15 minutes to absorb the water. Form mix into 1-inch balls and arrange on a baking sheet.
2. Preheat the broiler to high.
3. Take the balls and flatten slightly with your thumb (so they won't roll around on the baking sheet). Spray with olive oil, and then broil for 2 to 3 minutes on each side, until crispy and brown.
4. To fry the falafel, fill a pot with ½ inch of cooking oil and heat over medium-high heat to 375°F. Fry the balls for about 3 minutes, until brown and crisp. Drain on paper towels and serve with pickled onions, pickled turnips, and tzatziki sauce (if using).

303. Quick Vegetable Kebabs

PREP TIME: 15 mins
COOK TIME: 20 mins
SERVINGS: 6 people

NUTRITION
Calories: 235;
Carbs: 30.4g;
Protein: 8.0g;
Fat: 14.5g

INGREDIENTS

- 4 medium red onions, peeled and sliced into 6 wedges
- 4 medium zucchini, cut into 1-inch-thick slices
- 4 bell peppers, cut into 2-inch squares
- 2 yellow bell peppers, cut into 2-inch squares
- 2 orange bell peppers, cut into 2-inch squares
- 2 beefsteak tomatoes, cut into quarters
- 3 tbsp. Herbed Oil

DIRECTIONS

1. Preheat the oven or grill to medium-high or 350°F.
2. Thread 1 piece red onion, zucchini, different colored bell peppers, and tomatoes onto a skewer. Repeat until the skewer is full of vegetables, up to 2 inches away from the skewer end, and continue until all skewers are complete.
3. Put the skewers on a baking sheet and cook in the oven for 10 minutes or grill for 5 minutes on each side. The vegetables will be done with they reach your desired crunch or softness.
4. Remove the skewers from heat and drizzle with Herbed Oil.

304. Tortellini in Red Pepper Sauce

PREP TIME: 15 mins
COOK TIME: 10 mins
SERVINGS: 4 people

NUTRITION
Calories: 530;
Carbs: 95.4g;
Protein: 8.0g;
Fat: 18.5g

INGREDIENTS

- 1 (16-oz.) container fresh cheese tortellini (usually green and white pasta)
- 1 (16-oz.) jar roasted red peppers, drained
- 1 tsp. garlic powder
- ¼ cup tahini
- 1 tbsp. red pepper oil (optional)

DIRECTIONS

1. Bring a large pot of water to a boil and cook the tortellini according to package directions.
2. In a blender, combine the red peppers with the garlic powder and process until smooth. Once blended, add the tahini until the sauce is thickened. If the sauce gets too thick, add up to 1 tbsp. red pepper oil (if using).
3. Once tortellini are cooked, drain and leave pasta in colander. Add the sauce to the bottom of the empty pot and heat for 2 minutes. Then, add the tortellini back into the pot and cook for 2 more minutes. Serve and enjoy!

305. Freekeh, Chickpea, and Herb Salad

PREP TIME
15 mins

COOK TIME
10 mins

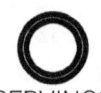
SERVINGS
6 people

NUTRITION

Calories: 230;
Carbs: 25.4g;
Protein: 8.0g;
Fat: 18.5g

INGREDIENTS

- 1 (15-oz.) can chickpeas, rinsed and drained
- 1 cup cooked freekeh
- 1 cup thinly sliced celery
- 1 bunch scallions, both white and green parts, finely chopped
- ½ cup chopped fresh flat-leaf parsley
- ¼ cup chopped fresh mint
- 3 tbsp. chopped celery leaves
- ½ tsp. kosher salt
- 1/3 cup extra-virgin olive oil
- ¼ cup freshly squeezed lemon juice
- ¼ tsp. cumin seeds
- 1 tsp. garlic powder

DIRECTIONS

1. In a large bowl, combine the chickpeas, freekeh, celery, scallions, parsley, mint, celery leaves, and salt and toss lightly.
2. In a small bowl, whisk together the olive oil, lemon juice, cumin seeds, and garlic powder. Once combined, add to freekeh salad.

306. Kate's Warm Mediterranean Farro Bowl

PREP TIME
15 mins

COOK TIME
10 mins

SERVINGS
4 people

NUTRITION

Calories: 530;
Carbs: 95.4g;
Protein: 8.0g;
Fat: 13.5g

INGREDIENTS

- 1/3 cup extra-virgin olive oil
- ½ cup chopped red bell pepper
- 1/3 cup chopped red onions
- 2 garlic cloves, minced
- 1 cup zucchini, cut in ½-inch slices
- ½ cup canned chickpeas, drained and rinsed
- ½ cup coarsely chopped artichokes
- 3 cups cooked farro
- Salt
- Freshly ground black pepper
- ¼ cup sliced olives, for serving (optional)
- ½ cup crumbled feta cheese, for serving (optional)
- 2 tbsp. fresh basil, chiffonade, for serving (optional)
- 3 tbsp. balsamic reduction, for serving (optional)

DIRECTIONS

1. In a large sauté pan or skillet, heat the oil over medium heat and sauté the pepper, onions, and garlic for about 5 minutes, until tender.
2. Add the zucchini, chickpeas, and artichokes, then stir and continue to sauté vegetables, approximately 5 more minutes, until just soft.
3. Stir in the cooked farro, tossing to combine and cooking enough to heat through. Season with salt and pepper and remove from the heat.
4. Transfer the contents of the pan into the serving vessels or bowls.
5. Top with olives, feta, and basil (if using). Drizzle with balsamic reduction (if using) to finish.

307. Creamy Chickpea Sauce with Whole-Wheat Fusilli

PREP TIME
15 mins

COOK TIME
20 mins

SERVINGS
4 people

NUTRITION

Calories: 230;
Carbs: 20.4g;
Protein: 8.0g;
Fat: 18.5g

INGREDIENTS

- ¼ cup extra-virgin olive oil
- ½ large shallot, chopped
- 5 garlic cloves, thinly sliced
- 1 (15-oz.) can chickpeas, drained and rinsed, reserving ½ cup canning liquid
- Pinch red pepper flakes
- 1 cup whole-grain fusilli pasta
- ¼ tsp. salt
- 1/8 tsp. freshly ground black pepper
- ¼ cup shaved fresh Parmesan cheese
- ¼ cup chopped fresh basil
- 2 tsp. dried parsley
- 1 tsp. dried oregano
- Red pepper flakes

DIRECTIONS

1. In a medium pan, heat the oil over medium heat, and sauté the shallot and garlic for 3 to 5 minutes, until the garlic is golden. Add ¾ of the chickpeas plus 2 tbsp. of liquid from the can, and bring to a simmer.
2. Remove from the heat, transfer into a standard blender, and blend until smooth. At this point, add the remaining chickpeas. Add more reserved chickpea liquid if it becomes thick.
3. Bring a large pot of salted water to a boil and cook pasta until al dente, about 8 minutes. Reserve ½ cup of the pasta water, drain the pasta, and return it to the pot.
4. Add the chickpea sauce to the hot pasta and add up to ¼ cup of the pasta water. You may need to add more pasta water to reach your desired consistency.
5. Place the pasta pot over medium heat and mix occasionally until the sauce thickens. Season with salt and pepper.
6. Serve, garnished with Parmesan, basil, parsley, oregano, and red pepper flakes.

308. Linguine and Brussels sprouts

PREP TIME
10 mins

COOK TIME
25 mins

SERVINGS
4 people

NUTRITION

Calories: 530;
Carbs: 95.4g;
Protein: 5.0g;
Fat: 16.5g

INGREDIENTS

- 8 oz. whole-wheat linguine
- 1/3 cup, plus 2 tbsp. extra-virgin olive oil, divided
- 1 medium sweet onion, diced
- 2 to 3 garlic cloves, smashed
- 8 oz. Brussels sprouts, chopped
- ½ cup chicken stock, as needed
- 1/3 cup dry white wine
- ½ cup shredded Parmesan cheese
- 1 lemon, cut in quarters

DIRECTIONS

1. Bring a large pot of water to a boil and cook the pasta according to package directions. Drain, reserving 1 cup of the pasta water. Mix the cooked pasta with 2 tbsp. of olive oil, then set aside.
2. In a large sauté pan or skillet, heat the remaining 1/3 cup of olive oil on medium heat. Add the onion to the pan and cook for about 5 minutes, until softened. Add the smashed garlic cloves and cook for 1 minute, until fragrant.
3. Add the Brussels sprouts and cook covered for 15 minutes. Add chicken stock as needed to prevent burning. Once Brussels sprouts have wilted and are fork-tender, add white wine and cook down for about 7 minutes, until reduced.
4. Add the pasta to the skillet and add the pasta water as needed.
5. Serve with the Parmesan cheese and lemon for squeezing over the dish right before eating.

187

309. Peppers and Lentils Salad

PREP TIME 10 mins

COOK TIME 0 mins

SERVINGS 4 people

INGREDIENTS

- 14 oz. canned lentils, drained and rinsed
- 2 spring onions, chopped
- 1 red bell pepper, chopped
- 1 green bell pepper, chopped
- 1 tbsp. fresh lime juice
- 1/3 cup coriander, chopped
- 2 tsp. balsamic vinegar

DIRECTIONS

1. In a salad bowl, combine the lentils with the onions, bell peppers and the rest of the ingredients, toss and serve.

NUTRITION

Calories 200, Fat 2.45g, Fiber 6.7g, Carbs 10.5g, Protein 5.6g

310. Cashews and Red Cabbage Salad

PREP TIME 10 mins

COOK TIME 0 mins

SERVINGS 4 people

INGREDIENTS

- 1 lb. red cabbage, shredded
- 2 tbsp. coriander, chopped
- ½ cup cashews, halved
- 2 tbsp. olive oil
- 1 tomato, cubed
- A pinch of salt and black pepper
- 1 tbsp. white vinegar

DIRECTIONS

1. In a salad bowl, combine the cabbage with the coriander and the rest of the ingredients, toss and serve cold.

NUTRITION

Calories 210, Fat 6.3g, Fiber 5.2g, Carbs 5.5g, Protein 8g

311. Apples and Pomegranate Salad

PREP TIME: 10 mins
COOK TIME: 0 mins
SERVINGS: 4 people

INGREDIENTS

- 3 big apples, cored and cubed
- 1 cup pomegranate seeds
- 3 cups baby arugula
- 1 cup walnuts, chopped
- 1 tbsp. olive oil
- 1 tsp. white sesame seeds
- 2 tbsp. apple cider vinegar
- Salt and black pepper to the taste

DIRECTIONS

1. In a bowl, mix the apples with the arugula and the rest of the ingredients, toss and serve cold.

NUTRITION
Calories 160, Fat 4.3g, Fiber 5.3g, Carbs 8.7g, Protein 10g

312. Cranberry Bulgur Mix

PREP TIME: 10 mins
COOK TIME: 0 mins
SERVINGS: 4 people

INGREDIENTS

- 1 and ½ cups hot water
- 1 cup bulgur
- Juice of ½ lemon
- 4 tbsp. cilantro, chopped
- ½ cup cranberries, chopped
- 1 and ½ tsp. curry powder
- ¼ cup green onions, chopped
- ½ cup red bell peppers, chopped
- ½ cup carrots, grated
- 1 tbsp. olive oil
- A pinch of salt and black pepper

DIRECTIONS

1. Put bulgur into a bowl, add the water, stir, cover, leave aside for 10 minutes, fluff with a fork and transfer to a bowl.
2. Add the rest of the ingredients, toss, and serve cold.

NUTRITION
Calories 300, Fat 6.4g, Fiber 6.1g, Carbs 7.6g, Protein 13g

313. Chickpeas, Corn and Black Beans Salad

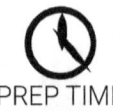
PREP TIME
10 mins

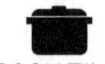
COOK TIME
0 mins

SERVINGS
4 people

NUTRITION

Calories 300,
Fat 13.4g,
Fiber 4.1g,
Carbs 8.6g,
Protein 13g

INGREDIENTS

- 1 and ½ cups canned black beans, drained and rinsed
- ½ tsp. garlic powder
- 2 tsp. chili powder
- A pinch of sea salt and black pepper
- 1 and ½ cups canned chickpeas, drained and rinsed
- 1 cup baby spinach
- 1 avocado, pitted, peeled and chopped
- 1 cup corn kernels, chopped
- 2 tbsp. lemon juice
- 1 tbsp. olive oil
- 1 tbsp. apple cider vinegar
- 1 tsp. chives, chopped

DIRECTIONS

1. In a salad bowl, combine the black beans with the garlic powder, chili powder and the rest of the ingredients, toss and serve cold.

314. Olives and Lentils Salad

PREP TIME
10 mins

COOK TIME
0 mins

SERVINGS
2 people

NUTRITION

Calories 279,
Fat 6.5g,
Fiber 4.5g,
Carbs 9.6g,
Protein 12g

INGREDIENTS

- 1/3 cup canned green lentils, drained and rinsed
- 1 tbsp. olive oil
- 2 cups baby spinach
- 1 cup black olives, pitted and halved
- 2 tbsp. sunflower seeds
- 1 tbsp. Dijon mustard
- 2 tbsp. balsamic vinegar
- 2 tbsp. olive oil

DIRECTIONS

1. In a bowl, mix the lentils with the spinach, olives and the rest of the ingredients, toss and serve cold.

315. Lime Spinach and Chickpeas Salad

INGREDIENTS

- 16 oz. canned chickpeas, drained and rinsed
- 2 cups baby spinach leaves
- ½ tbsp. lime juice
- 2 tbsp. olive oil
- 1 tsp. cumin, ground
- A pinch of sea salt and black pepper
- ½ tsp. chili flakes

DIRECTIONS

1. In a bowl, mix the chickpeas with the spinach and the rest of the ingredients, toss and serve cold.

PREP TIME: 10 mins
COOK TIME: 0 mins
SERVINGS: 4 people

NUTRITION
Calories 240, Fat 8.2g, Fiber 5.3g, Carbs 11.6g, Protein 12g

---

316. Beans and Cucumber Salad

INGREDIENTS

- 15 oz. canned great northern beans, drained and rinsed
- 2 tbsp. olive oil
- ½ cup baby arugula
- 1 cup cucumber, sliced
- 1 tbsp. parsley, chopped
- 2 tomatoes, cubed
- A pinch of sea salt and black pepper
- 2 tbsp. balsamic vinegar

DIRECTIONS

1. In a bowl, mix the beans with the cucumber and the rest of the ingredients, toss and serve cold.

PREP TIME: 10 mins
COOK TIME: 0 mins
SERVINGS: 4 people

NUTRITION
Calories 233, Fat 9g, Fiber 6.5g, Carbs 13g, Protein 8g

317. Minty Olives and Tomatoes Salad

PREP TIME
10 mins

COOK TIME
0 mins

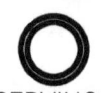
SERVINGS
4 people

NUTRITION

Calories 190,
Fat 8.1g,
Fiber 5.8g,
Carbs 11.6g,
Protein 4.6g

INGREDIENTS

- 1 cup kalamata olives, pitted and sliced
- 1 cup black olives, pitted and halved
- 1 cup cherry tomatoes, halved
- 4 tomatoes, chopped
- 1 red onion, chopped
- 2 tbsp. oregano, chopped
- 1 tbsp. mint, chopped
- 2 tbsp. balsamic vinegar
- ¼ cup olive oil
- 2 tsp. Italian herbs, dried
- A pinch of sea salt and black pepper

DIRECTIONS

1. In a salad bowl, mix the olives with the tomatoes and the rest of the ingredients, toss and serve cold.

318. Tomato And Avocado Salad

PREP TIME
10 mins

COOK TIME
0 mins

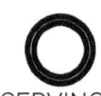
SERVINGS
4 people

NUTRITION

Calories 148,
Fat 7.8g,
Fiber 2.9g,
Carbs 5.4g,
Protein 5.5g

INGREDIENTS

- 1 lb. cherry tomatoes, cubed
- 2 avocados, pitted, peeled and cubed
- 1 sweet onion, chopped
- A pinch of sea salt and black pepper
- 2 tbsp. lemon juice
- 1 and ½ tbsp. olive oil
- A handful basil, chopped

DIRECTIONS

1. In a salad bowl, mix the tomatoes with the avocados and the rest of the ingredients, toss and serve right away.

319. Corn and Tomato Salad

PREP TIME: 10 mins
COOK TIME: 0 mins
SERVINGS: 4 people

INGREDIENTS

- 2 avocados, pitted, peeled and cubed
- 1 pint mixed cherry tomatoes, halved:
- 2 tbsp. avocado oil
- 1 tbsp. lime juice
- ½ tsp. lime zest, grated
- A pinch of salt and black pepper
- ¼ cup dill, chopped

DIRECTIONS

1. In a salad bowl, mix the avocados with the tomatoes and the rest of the ingredients, toss and serve cold.

NUTRITION

Calories 188, Fat 7.3g, Fiber 4.9g, Carbs 6.4g, Protein 6.5g

320. Orange and Cucumber Salad

PREP TIME: 10 mins
COOK TIME: 0 mins
SERVINGS: 4 people

INGREDIENTS

- 2 cucumbers, sliced
- 1 orange, peeled and cut into segments
- 1 cup cherry tomatoes, halved
- 1 small red onion, chopped
- 3 tbsp. olive oil
- 4 and ½ tsp. balsamic vinegar
- Salt and black pepper to the taste
- 1 tbsp. lemon juice

DIRECTIONS

1. In a bowl, mix the cucumbers with the orange and the rest of the ingredients, toss and serve cold.

NUTRITION

Calories 102, Fat 7.5g, Fiber 3g, Carbs 6.1g, Protein 3.4g

321. Parsley and Corn Salad

PREP TIME
10 mins

COOK TIME
0 mins

SERVINGS
4 people

INGREDIENTS

- 1 and ½ tsp. balsamic vinegar
- 2 tbsp. lime juice
- 2 tbsp. olive oil
- A pinch of sea salt and black pepper
- Black pepper to the taste
- 4 cups corn
- ½ cup parsley, chopped
- 2 spring onions, chopped

DIRECTIONS

1. In a salad bowl, combine the corn with the onions and the rest of the ingredients, toss and serve cold.

NUTRITION

Calories 121,
Fat 9.5g,
Fiber 1.8g,
Carbs 4.1g,
Protein 1.9g

322. Radish and Corn Salad

PREP TIME
10 mins

COOK TIME
0 mins

SERVINGS
2 people

INGREDIENTS

- 1 tbsp. lemon juice
- 1 jalapeno, chopped
- 2 tbsp. olive oil
- ¼ tsp. oregano, dried
- A pinch of sea salt and black pepper
- 2 cups fresh corn
- 6 radishes, sliced

DIRECTIONS

1. In a salad bowl, combine the corn with the radishes and the rest of the ingredients, toss and serve cold.

NUTRITION

Calories 134,
Fat 4.5g,
Fiber 1.8g,
Carbs 4.1g,
Protein 1.9g

323. Arugula and Corn Salad

INGREDIENTS

- 1 red bell pepper, thinly sliced
- 2 cups corn
- Juice of 1 lime
- Zest of 1 lime, grated
- 8 cups baby arugula
- A pinch of sea salt and black pepper

DIRECTIONS

1. In a salad bowl, mix the corn with the arugula and the rest of the ingredients, toss and serve cold.

PREP TIME 10 mins
COOK TIME 0 mins
SERVINGS 4 people

NUTRITION
Calories 172, Fat 8.5g, Fiber 1.8g, Carbs 5.1g, Protein 1.4g

324. Balsamic Bulgur Salad

INGREDIENTS

- 1 cup bulgur
- 2 cups hot water
- 1 cucumber, sliced
- A pinch of sea salt and black pepper
- 2 tbsp. lemon juice
- 2 tbsp. balsamic vinegar
- ¼ cup olive oil

DIRECTIONS

1. In a bowl, mix bulgur with the water, cover, leave aside for 30 minutes, fluff with a fork and transfer to a salad bowl.
2. Add the rest of the ingredients, toss and serve.

PREP TIME 30 mins
COOK TIME 0 mins
SERVINGS 4 people

NUTRITION
Calories 171, Fat 5.1g, Fiber 6.1g, Carbs 11.3g, Protein 4.4g

SNACKS

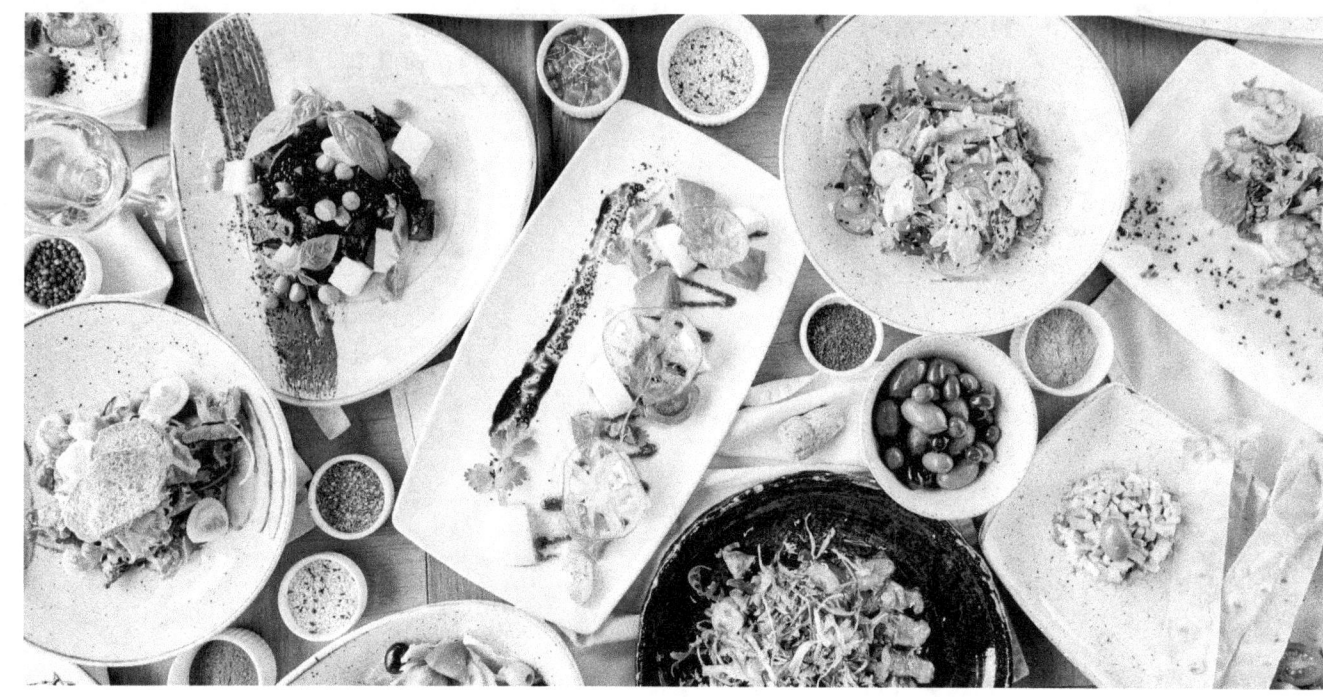

325. Healthy Coconut Blueberry Balls

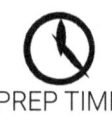
PREP TIME
10 mins

COOK TIME
10 mins

SERVINGS
12 people

NUTRITION

Calories 129,
Fat 7.4g,
Carbs 14.1g,
Sugar 7g,
Protein 4 g,

INGREDIENTS

- ¼ cup flaked coconut
- ¼ cup blueberries
- ½ tsp. vanilla
- ¼ cup honey
- ½ cup creamy almond butter
- ¼ tsp. cinnamon
- 1 ½ tbsp. chia seeds
- ¼ cup flaxseed meal
- 1 cup rolled oats, gluten-free

DIRECTIONS

1. In a large bowl, add oats, cinnamon, chia seeds, and flaxseed meal and mix well.
2. Add almond butter in microwave-safe bowl and microwave for 30 seconds. Stir until smooth.
3. Add vanilla and honey in melted almond butter and stir well.
4. Pour almond butter mixture over oat mixture and stir to combine.
5. Add coconut and blueberries and stir well.
6. Make small balls from oat mixture and place onto the baking tray and place in the refrigerator for 1 hour.
7. Serve and enjoy.

326. Crunchy Roasted Chickpeas

PREP TIME: 10 mins
COOK TIME: 25 mins
SERVINGS: 4 people

INGREDIENTS
- 15 oz can chickpeas, drained, rinsed and pat dry
- ¼ tsp. paprika
- 1 tbsp. olive oil
- ¼ tsp. pepper
- Pinch of salt

DIRECTIONS
1. Preheat the oven to 450°F.
2. Spray a baking tray with cooking spray and set aside.
3. In a large bowl, toss chickpeas with olive oil and spread chickpeas onto the prepared baking tray.
4. Roast chickpeas in preheated oven for 25 minutes. Shake after every 10 minutes.
5. Once chickpeas are done then immediately toss with paprika, pepper, and salt.
6. Serve and enjoy.

NUTRITION
Calories 157, Fat 4.7g, Carbs 24.2g, Protein 5.3g,

---

327. Tasty Zucchini Chips

PREP TIME: 10 mins
COOK TIME: 15 mins
SERVINGS: 8 people

INGREDIENTS
- 2 medium zucchini, sliced 4mm thick
- ½ tsp. paprika
- ¼ tsp. garlic powder
- ¾ cup parmesan cheese, grated
- 4 tbsp. olive oil
- ¼ tsp. pepper
- Pinch of salt

DIRECTIONS
1. Preheat the oven to 375°F.
2. Spray a baking tray with cooking spray and set aside.
3. In a bowl, combine the oil, garlic powder, paprika, pepper, and salt.
4. Add sliced zucchini and toss to coat.
5. Arrange zucchini slices onto the prepared baking tray and sprinkle grated cheese on top.
6. Bake in preheated oven for 15 minutes or until lightly golden brown.
7. Serve and enjoy.

NUTRITION
Calories 110, Fat 9.8g, Carbs 2.2g, Protein 4.4g

328. Roasted Green Beans

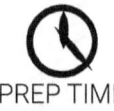
PREP TIME
10 mins

COOK TIME
15 mins

SERVINGS
4 people

INGREDIENTS
- 1 lb green beans
- 4 tbsp. parmesan cheese
- 2 tbsp. olive oil
- ¼ tsp. garlic powder
- Pinch of salt

DIRECTIONS
1. Preheat the oven to 400°F.
2. Add green beans in a large bowl.
3. Add remaining ingredients on top of green beans and toss to coat.
4. Spread green beans onto the baking tray and roast in preheated oven for 15 minutes. Stir halfway through.
5. Serve and enjoy.

NUTRITION
Calories 101,
Fat 7.5g,
Carbs 8.3g,
Sugar 1.6g,
Protein 2.6g,
Cholesterol 1mg

329. Savory Pistachio Balls

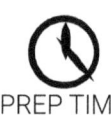
PREP TIME
10 mins

COOK TIME
5 mins

SERVINGS
16 people

INGREDIENTS
- ½ cup pistachios, unsalted
- 1 cup dates, pitted
- ½ tsp. ground fennel seeds
- ½ cup raisins
- Pinch of pepper

DIRECTIONS
1. Add all ingredients into the food processor and process until well combined.
2. Make small balls and place onto the baking tray and place in the refrigerator for 1 hour.
3. Serve and enjoy.

NUTRITION
Calories 55,
Fat 0.9g,
Carbs 12.5g,
Sugar 9.9g,
Protein 0.8g,
Cholesterol 0mg

330. Roasted Almonds

PREP TIME
10 mins

COOK TIME
20 mins

SERVINGS
12 people

NUTRITION
Calories 137,
Fat 11.2g,
Carbs 7.3g,
Protein 4.2g,

INGREDIENTS
- 2 ½ cups almonds
- ¼ tsp. cayenne
- ¼ tsp. ground coriander
- ¼ tsp. cumin
- ¼ tsp. chili powder
- 1 tbsp. fresh rosemary, chopped
- 1 tbsp. olive oil
- 2 ½ tbsp. maple syrup
- Pinch of salt

DIRECTIONS
1. Preheat the oven to 325°F.
2. Spray a baking tray with cooking spray and set aside.
3. In a mixing bowl, whisk together oil, cayenne, coriander, cumin, chili powder, rosemary, maple syrup, and salt.
4. Add almond and stir to coat.
5. Spread almonds onto the prepared baking tray.
6. Roast almonds in preheated oven for 20 minutes. Stir halfway through.
7. Serve and enjoy.

331. Banana Strawberry Popsicles

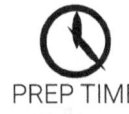
PREP TIME
5 mins

COOK TIME
0 mins

SERVINGS
8 people

NUTRITION
Calories 31,
Fat 0. g,
Carbs 6.2g,
Protein 1.2g.

INGREDIENTS
- ½ cup Greek yogurt
- 1 banana, peeled and sliced
- 1 ¼ cup fresh strawberries
- ¼ cup of water

DIRECTIONS
1. Add all ingredients into the blender and blend until smooth.
2. Pour blended mixture into the popsicles molds and place in the refrigerator for 4 hours or until set.
3. Serve and enjoy.

332. Chocolate Matcha Balls

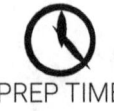
PREP TIME
10 mins

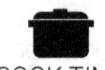
COOK TIME
5 mins

SERVINGS
15 people

INGREDIENTS

- 2 tbsp. unsweetened cocoa powder
- 3 tbsp. oats, gluten-free
- ½ cup pine nuts
- ½ cup almonds
- 1 cup dates, pitted
- 2 tbsp. matcha powder

DIRECTIONS

1. Add oats, pine nuts, almonds, and dates into a food processor and process until well combined.
2. Place matcha powder in a small dish.
3. Make small balls from mixture and coat with matcha powder.
4. Enjoy or store in refrigerator until ready to eat.

NUTRITION

Calories 88
Fat 4.9g
Carbs 11.3g
Protein 1.9g

333. Chia Almond Butter Pudding

PREP TIME
5 mins

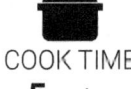
COOK TIME
5 mins

SERVINGS
1 people

INGREDIENTS

- ¼ cup chia seeds
- 1 cup unsweetened almond milk
- 1 ½ tbsp. maple syrup
- 2 ½ tbsp. almond butter

DIRECTIONS

1. Add almond milk, maple syrup, and almond butter in a bowl and stir well.
2. Add chia seeds and stir to mix.
3. Pour pudding mixture into the Mason jar and place in the refrigerator for overnight.
4. Serve and enjoy.

NUTRITION

Calories 354
Fat 21.3g
Carbs 31.1g
Protein 11.2g

334. Refreshing Strawberry Popsicles

PREP TIME 5 mins
COOK TIME 5 mins
SERVINGS 8 people

INGREDIENTS
- ½ cup almond milk
- 2 ½ cup fresh strawberries

DIRECTIONS
1. Add strawberries and almond milk into the blender and blend until smooth.
2. Pour strawberry mixture into popsicles molds and place in the refrigerator for 4 hours or until set.
3. Serve and enjoy.

NUTRITION
Calories 49, Fat 3.7g, Carbs 4.3g, Protein 0.6g,

335. Dark Chocolate Mousse

PREP TIME 10 mins
COOK TIME 10 mins
SERVINGS 4 people

INGREDIENTS
- 3.5oz unsweetened dark chocolate, grated
- ½ tsp. vanilla
- 1 tbsp. honey
- 2 cups Greek yogurt
- ¾ cup unsweetened almond milk

DIRECTIONS
1. Add chocolate and almond milk in a saucepan and heat over medium heat until just chocolate melted. Do not boil.
2. Once the chocolate and almond milk combined then add vanilla and honey and stir well.
3. Add yogurt in a large mixing bowl.
4. Pour chocolate mixture on top of yogurt and mix until well combined.
5. Pour chocolate yogurt mixture into the serving bowls and place in refrigerator for 2 hours.
6. Top with fresh raspberries and serve.

NUTRITION
Calories 278, Fat 15.4g, Carbs 20g, Protein 10.5g,

336. Warm & Soft Baked Pears

PREP TIME
10 mins

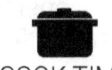
COOK TIME
25 mins

SERVINGS
4 people

INGREDIENTS

- 4 pears, cut in half and core
- ½ tsp. vanilla
- ¼ tsp. cinnamon
- ½ cup maple syrup

DIRECTIONS

1. Preheat the oven to 375°F.
2. Spray a baking tray with cooking spray.
3. Arrange pears, cut side up on a prepared baking tray and sprinkle with cinnamon.
4. In a small bowl, whisk vanilla and maple syrup and drizzle over pears.
5. Bake pears in preheated oven for 25 minutes.
6. Serve and enjoy.

NUTRITION

Calories 226,
Fat 0.4g,
Carbs 58.4g,
Sugar 43.9g,
Protein 0.8g,

337. Healthy & Quick Energy Bites

PREP TIME
10 mins

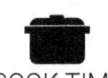
COOK TIME
0 mins

SERVINGS
20 people

INGREDIENTS

- 2 cups cashew nuts
- ¼ tsp. cinnamon
- 1 tsp. lemon zest
- 4 tbsp. dates, chopped
- 1/3 cup unsweetened shredded coconut
- ¾ cup dried apricots

DIRECTIONS

1. Line baking tray with parchment paper and set aside.
2. Add all ingredients in a food processor and process until the mixture is crumbly and well combined.
3. Make small balls from mixture and place on a prepared baking tray.
4. Place in refrigerator for 1 hour.
5. Serve and enjoy.

NUTRITION

Calories 100,
Fat 7.5g,
Carbs 7.2g,
Protein 2.4g,

338. Creamy Yogurt Banana Bowls

PREP TIME 10 mins

COOK TIME 0 mins

SERVINGS 4 people

INGREDIENTS
- 2 bananas, sliced
- ½ tsp. ground nutmeg
- 3 tbsp. flaxseed meal
- ¼ cup creamy peanut butter
- 4 cups Greek yogurt

DIRECTIONS
1. Divide Greek yogurt between 4 serving bowls and top with sliced bananas.
2. Add peanut butter in microwave-safe bowl and microwave for 30 seconds.
3. Drizzle 1 tbsp. of melted peanut butter on each bowl on top of the sliced bananas.
4. Sprinkle cinnamon and flax meal on top and serve.

NUTRITION
Calories 351, Fat 13.1g, Carbs 35.6g, , Protein 19.6g,

---

339. Chicken Wings Platter

PREP TIME 10 mins

COOK TIME 20 mins

SERVINGS 4 people

INGREDIENTS
- 2 lb. chicken wings
- ½ cup tomato sauce
- A pinch of salt and black pepper
- 1 tsp. smoked paprika
- 1 tbsp. cilantro, chopped
- 1 tbsp. chives, chopped

DIRECTIONS
1. In your instant pot, combine the chicken wings with the sauce and the rest of the ingredients, stir, put the lid on and cook on High for 20 minutes.
2. Release the pressure naturally for 10 minutes, arrange the chicken wings on a platter and serve as an appetizer.

NUTRITION
Calories 203, Fat 13g, Fiber 3g, Carbs 5g, Protein 8g

340. Carrot Spread

PREP TIME
10 mins

COOK TIME
10 mins

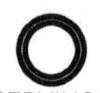
SERVINGS
4 people

NUTRITION

Calories 124,
Fat 1g,
Fiber 2g,
Carbs 5g,
Protein 8g

INGREDIENTS

- ¼ cup veggie stock
- A pinch of salt and black pepper
- 1 tsp. onion powder
- ½ tsp. garlic powder
- ½ tsp. oregano, dried
- 1 lb. carrots, sliced
- ½ cup coconut cream

DIRECTIONS

1. In your instant pot, combine all the ingredients except the cream, put the lid on and cook on High for 10 minutes.
2. Release the pressure naturally for 10 minutes, transfer the carrots mix to food processor, add the cream, pulse well, divide into bowls and serve cold

341. Chocolate Mousse

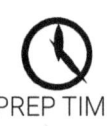
PREP TIME
10 mins

COOK TIME
6 mins

SERVINGS
5 people

NUTRITION

Calories 128,
Fat 11.9g,
Carbs 4g,
Protein 3.6g

INGREDIENTS

- 4 egg yolks
- ½ tsp. vanilla
- ½ cup unsweetened almond milk
- 1 cup whipping cream
- ¼ cup cocoa powder
- ¼ cup water
- ½ cup Swerve
- 1/8 tsp. salt

DIRECTIONS

1. Add egg yolks to a large bowl and whisk until well beaten.
2. In a saucepan, add swerve, cocoa powder, and water and whisk until well combined.
3. Add almond milk and cream to the saucepan and whisk until well mix.
4. Once saucepan mixtures are heated up then turn off the heat.
5. Add vanilla and salt and stir well.
6. Add a tbsp. of chocolate mixture into the eggs and whisk until well combined.
7. Slowly pour remaining chocolate to the eggs and whisk until well combined.
8. Pour batter into the ramekins.
9. Pour 1 ½ cups of water into the instant pot then place a trivet in the pot.
10. Place ramekins on a trivet.
11. Seal pot with lid and select manual and set timer for 6 minutes.
12. Release pressure using quick release method than open the lid.
13. Carefully remove ramekins from the instant pot and let them cool completely.
14. Serve and enjoy.

342. Veggie Fritters

PREP TIME 10 mins
COOK TIME 10 mins
SERVINGS 4 people

NUTRITION
Calories 209;
Fat 11.2 g;
Fiber 3 g;
Carbs 4.4 g;
Protein 4.8 g

INGREDIENTS

- 2 garlic cloves, minced
- 2 yellow onions, chopped
- 4 scallions, chopped
- 2 carrots, grated
- 2 tsp. cumin, ground
- ½ tsp. turmeric powder
- Salt and black pepper to the taste
- ¼ tsp. coriander, ground
- 2 tbsp. parsley, chopped
- ¼ tsp. lemon juice
- ½ cup almond flour
- 2 beets, peeled and grated
- 2 eggs, whisked
- ¼ cup tapioca flour
- 3 tbsp. olive oil

DIRECTIONS

1. In a bowl, combine the garlic with the onions, scallions and the rest of the ingredients except the oil, stir well and shape medium fritters out of this mix.
2. Heat up a pan with the oil over medium-high heat, add the fritters, cook for 5 minutes on each side, arrange on a platter and serve.

343. White Bean Dip

PREP TIME 10 mins
COOK TIME 0 mins
SERVINGS 4 people

NUTRITION
Calories 274;
Fat 11.7 g;
Carbs 18.5 g;
Protein 16.5 g

INGREDIENTS

- 15 oz. canned white beans, drained and rinsed
- 6 oz. canned artichoke hearts, drained and quartered
- 4 garlic cloves, minced
- 1 tbsp. basil, chopped
- 2 tbsp. olive oil
- Juice of ½ lemon
- Zest of ½ lemon, grated
- Salt and black pepper to the taste

DIRECTIONS

1. In your food processor, combine the beans with the artichokes and the rest of the ingredients except the oil and pulse well.
2. Add the oil gradually, pulse the mix again, divide into cups and serve as a party dip.

344. Eggplant Dip

PREP TIME
10 mins

COOK TIME
40 mins

SERVINGS
4 people

NUTRITION

Calories 121;
Fat 4.3 g;
Carbs 1.4 g;
Protein 4.3 g

INGREDIENTS

- 1 eggplant, poked with a fork
- 2 tbsp. tahini paste
- 2 tbsp. lemon juice
- 2 garlic cloves, minced
- 1 tbsp. olive oil
- Salt and black pepper to the taste
- 1 tbsp. parsley, chopped

DIRECTIONS

1. Put the eggplant in a roasting pan, bake at 400° F for 40 minutes, cool down, peel and transfer to your food processor.
2. Add the rest of the ingredients except the parsley, pulse well, divide into small bowls and serve as an appetizer with the parsley sprinkled on top.

345. Bulgur Lamb Meatballs

PREP TIME
10 mins

COOK TIME
15 mins

SERVINGS
6 people

NUTRITION

Calories 300;
Fat 9.6 g;
Carbs 22.6 g;
Protein 6.6 g

INGREDIENTS

- 1 and ½ cups Greek yogurt
- ½ tsp. cumin, ground
- 1 cup cucumber, shredded
- ½ tsp. garlic, minced
- A pinch of salt and black pepper
- 1 cup bulgur
- 2 cups water
- 1 lb. lamb, ground
- ¼ cup parsley, chopped
- ¼ cup shallots, chopped
- ½ tsp. allspice, ground
- ½ tsp. cinnamon powder
- 1 tbsp. olive oil

DIRECTIONS

1. In a bowl, combine the bulgur with the water, cover the bowl, leave aside for 10 minutes, drain and transfer to a bowl.
2. Add the meat, the yogurt and the rest of the ingredients except the oil, stir well and shape medium meatballs out of this mix.
3. Heat up a pan with the oil over medium-high heat, add the meatballs, cook them for 7 minutes on each side, arrange them all on a platter and serve as an appetizer.

346. Cucumber Bites

PREP TIME: 10 mins
COOK TIME: 0 mins
SERVINGS: 12 people

INGREDIENTS

- 1 English cucumber, sliced into 32 rounds
- 10 oz. hummus
- 16 cherry tomatoes, halved
- 1 tbsp. parsley, chopped
- 1 oz. feta cheese, crumbled

DIRECTIONS

1. Spread the hummus on each cucumber round, divide the tomato halves on each, sprinkle the cheese and parsley on to and serve as an appetizer.

NUTRITION

Calories 162;
Fat 3.4 g;
Carbs 6.4 g;
Protein 2.4 g

347. Stuffed Avocado

PREP TIME: 10 mins
COOK TIME: 0 mins
SERVINGS: 2 people

INGREDIENTS

- 1 avocado, halved and pitted
- 10 oz. canned tuna, drained
- 2 tbsp. sun-dried tomatoes, chopped
- 1 and ½ tbsp. basil pesto
- 2 tbsp. black olives, pitted and chopped
- Salt and black pepper to the taste
- 2 tsp. pine nuts, toasted and chopped
- 1 tbsp. basil, chopped

DIRECTIONS

1. In a bowl, combine the tuna with the sun-dried tomatoes and the rest of the ingredients except the avocado and stir.
2. Stuff the avocado halves with the tuna mix and serve as an appetizer.

NUTRITION

Calories 233;
Fat 9 g;
Carbs 11.4 g;
Protein 5.6 g

348. Hummus with Ground Lamb

PREP TIME
10 mins

COOK TIME
15 mins

SERVINGS
8 people

NUTRITION

Calories 133;
Fat 9.7 g;
Carbs 6.4 g;
Protein 5

INGREDIENTS

- 10 oz. hummus
- 12 oz. lamb meat, ground
- ½ cup pomegranate seeds
- ¼ cup parsley, chopped
- 1 tbsp. olive oil
- Pita chips for serving

DIRECTIONS

1. Heat up a pan with the oil over medium-high heat, add the meat, and brown for 15 minutes stirring often.
2. Spread the hummus on a platter, spread the ground lamb all over, also spread the pomegranate seeds and the parsley and serve with pita chips as a snack.

349. Wrapped Plums

PREP TIME
5 mins

COOK TIME
0 mins

SERVINGS
8 people

NUTRITION

Calories 30;
Fat 1 g;
Carbs 4 g;
Protein 2 g

INGREDIENTS

- 2 oz. prosciutto, cut into 16 pieces
- 4 plums, quartered
- 1 tbsp. chives, chopped
- A pinch of red pepper flakes, crushed

DIRECTIONS

1. Wrap each plum quarter in a prosciutto slice, arrange them all on a platter, sprinkle the chives and pepper flakes all over and serve.

350. Cucumber Sandwich Bites

PREP TIME 5 mins
COOK TIME 0 mins
SERVINGS 12 people

INGREDIENTS
- 1 cucumber, sliced
- 8 slices whole wheat bread
- 2 tbsp. cream cheese, soft
- 1 tbsp. chives, chopped
- ¼ cup avocado, peeled, pitted and mashed
- 1 tsp. mustard
- Salt and black pepper to the taste

DIRECTIONS
1. Spread the mashed avocado on each bread slice, also spread the rest of the ingredients except the cucumber slices.
2. Divide the cucumber slices on the bread slices, cut each slice in thirds, arrange on a platter and serve as an appetizer.

NUTRITION
Calories 187;
Fat 12.4 g;
Carbs 4.5 g;
Protein 8.2 g

351. Cucumber Rolls

PREP TIME 5 mins
COOK TIME 0 mins
SERVINGS 6 people

INGREDIENTS
- 1 big cucumber, sliced lengthwise
- 1 tbsp. parsley, chopped
- 8 oz. canned tuna, drained and mashed
- Salt and black pepper to the taste
- 1 tsp. lime juice

DIRECTIONS
1. Arrange cucumber slices on a working surface, divide the rest of the ingredients, and roll.
2. Arrange all the rolls on a platter and serve as an appetizer.

NUTRITION
Calories 200;
Fat 6 g;
Carbs 7.6 g;
Protein 3.5 g

352. Olives and Cheese Stuffed Tomatoes

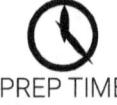
PREP TIME
10 mins

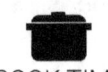
COOK TIME
0 mins

SERVINGS
24 people

INGREDIENTS

- 24 cherry tomatoes, top cut off and insides scooped out
- 2 tbsp. olive oil
- ¼ tsp. red pepper flakes
- ½ cup feta cheese, crumbled
- 2 tbsp. black olive paste
- ¼ cup mint, torn

DIRECTIONS

1. In a bowl, mix the olives paste with the rest of the ingredients except the cherry tomatoes and whisk well. Stuff the cherry tomatoes with this mix, arrange them all on a platter and serve as an appetizer.

NUTRITION

Calories 136;
Fat 8.6 g;
Carbs 5.6 g;
Protein 5.1 g

353. Tomato Salsa

PREP TIME
5 mins

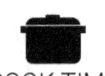
COOK TIME
0 mins

SERVINGS
6 people

INGREDIENTS

- 1 garlic clove, minced
- 4 tbsp. olive oil
- 5 tomatoes, cubed
- 1 tbsp. balsamic vinegar
- ¼ cup basil, chopped
- 1 tbsp. parsley, chopped
- 1 tbsp. chives, chopped
- Salt and black pepper to the taste
- Pita chips for serving

DIRECTIONS

1. In a bowl, mix the tomatoes with the garlic and the rest of the ingredients except the pita chips, stir, divide into small cups and serve with the pita chips on the side.

NUTRITION

Calories 160;
Fat 13.7 g;
Carbs 10.1 g;
Protein 2.2

354. Chili Mango and Watermelon Salsa

PREP TIME
5 mins

COOK TIME
0 mins

SERVINGS
12 people

NUTRITION

Calories 62;
Fat 2g;
Fiber 1.3 g;
Carbs 3.9 g;
Protein 2.3 g

INGREDIENTS

- 1 red tomato, chopped
- Salt and black pepper to the taste
- 1 cup watermelon, seedless, peeled and cubed
- 1 red onion, chopped
- 2 mangos, peeled and chopped
- 2 chili peppers, chopped
- ¼ cup cilantro, chopped
- 3 tbsp. lime juice
- Pita chips for serving

DIRECTIONS

1. In a bowl, mix the tomato with the watermelon, the onion and the rest of the ingredients except the pita chips and toss well. Divide the mix into small cups and serve with pita chips on the side.

355. Creamy Spinach and Shallots Dip

PREP TIME
10 mins

COOK TIME
0 mins

SERVINGS
4 people

NUTRITION

Calories 204;
Fat 11.5 g;
Carbs 4.2 g;
Protein 5.9 g

INGREDIENTS

- 1 lb. spinach, roughly chopped
- 2 shallots, chopped
- 2 tbsp. mint, chopped
- ¾ cup cream cheese, soft
- Salt and black pepper to the taste

DIRECTIONS

1. In a blender, combine the spinach with the shallots and the rest of the ingredients, and pulse well. Divide into small bowls and serve as a party dip.

356. Feta Artichoke Dip

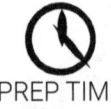
PREP TIME
10 mins

COOK TIME
30 mins

SERVINGS
8 people

NUTRITION

Calories 186;
Fat 12.4 g;
Fiber 0.9 g;
Carbs 2.6 g;
Protein 1.5 g

INGREDIENTS

- 8 oz. artichoke hearts, drained and quartered
- ¾ cup basil, chopped
- ¾ cup green olives, pitted and chopped
- 1 cup parmesan cheese, grated
- 5 oz. feta cheese, crumbled

DIRECTIONS

1. In your food processor, mix the artichokes with the basil and the rest of the ingredients, pulse well, and transfer to a baking dish.
2. Introduce in the oven, bake at 375° F for 30 minutes and serve as a party dip.

357. Avocado Dip

PREP TIME
5 mins

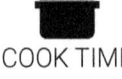
COOK TIME
0 mins

SERVINGS
8 people

NUTRITION

Calories 200;
Fat 14.5 g;
Fiber 3.8 g;
Carbs 8.1 g;
Protein 7.6 g

INGREDIENTS

- ½ cup heavy cream
- 1 green chili pepper, chopped
- Salt and pepper to the taste
- 4 avocados, pitted, peeled and chopped
- 1 cup cilantro, chopped
- ¼ cup lime juice

DIRECTIONS

1. In a blender, combine the cream with the avocados and the rest of the ingredients and pulse well. Divide the mix into bowls and serve cold as a party dip.

358. Goat Cheese and Chives Spread

PREP TIME: 10 mins
COOK TIME: 0 mins
SERVINGS: 4 people

INGREDIENTS
- 2 oz. goat cheese, crumbled
- ¾ cup sour cream
- 2 tbsp. chives, chopped
- 1 tbsp. lemon juice
- Salt and black pepper to the taste
- 2 tbsp. extra virgin olive oil

DIRECTIONS
1. In a bowl, mix the goat cheese with the cream and the rest of the ingredients and whisk really well. Keep in the fridge for 10 minutes and serve as a party spread.

NUTRITION
Calories 220;
Fat 11.5 g;
Carbs 8.9 g;
Protein 5.6 g

---

359. Stuffed Chicken

PREP TIME: 10 mins
COOK TIME: 30 mins
SERVINGS: 4 people

INGREDIENTS
- 4 chicken breasts, skinless, boneless and butterflied
- 1 oz. spring onions, chopped
- ½ lb. white mushrooms, sliced
- 1 tsp. hot paprika
- A pinch of salt and black pepper
- 1 cup tomato sauce

DIRECTIONS
1. Flatten chicken breasts with a meat mallet and place them on a plate.
2. In a bowl, mix the spring onions with the mushrooms, paprika, salt and pepper and stir well.
3. Divide this on each chicken breast half, roll them and secure with a toothpick.
4. Add the tomato sauce in the instant pot, put the chicken rolls inside as well. put the lid on and cook on High for 30 minutes.
5. Release the pressure naturally for 10 minutes, arrange the stuffed chicken breasts on a platter and serve.

NUTRITION
Calories 221,
Fat 12g,
Carbs 6g,
Protein 11g

360. Cinnamon Baby Back Ribs Platter

PREP TIME
10 mins

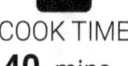
COOK TIME
40 mins

SERVINGS
2 people

NUTRITION

Calories 222,
Fat 12g,
Fiber 4g,
Carbs 6g,
Protein 14g

INGREDIENTS

- 1 rack baby back ribs
- 2 tsp. smoked paprika
- 2 tsp. chili powder
- A pinch of salt and black pepper
- 1 tsp. garlic powder
- 1 tsp. onion powder
- 1 tsp. cinnamon powder
- ½ tsp. cumin seeds
- A pinch of cayenne pepper
- 1 cup tomato sauce
- 3 garlic cloves, minced

DIRECTIONS

1. In your instant pot, combine the baby back ribs with the rest of the ingredients, put the lid on and cook on High for 30 minutes.
2. Release the pressure naturally for 10 minutes, arrange the ribs on a platter and serve as an appetizer.

361. Buttery Carrot Sticks

PREP TIME
10 mins

COOK TIME
15 mins

SERVINGS
4 people

NUTRITION

Calories 142,
Fat 4g,
Carbs 5g,
Protein 7g

INGREDIENTS

- 1 lb. carrot, cut into sticks
- 4 garlic cloves, minced
- ¼ cup chicken stock
- 1 tsp. rosemary, chopped
- A pinch of salt and black pepper
- 2 tbsp. olive oil
- 2 tbsp. ghee, melted

DIRECTIONS

1. Set the instant pot on Sauté mode, add the oil and the ghee, heat them up, add the garlic and brown for 1 minute.
2. Add the rest of the ingredients, put the lid on and cook on High for 14 minutes.
3. Release the pressure naturally for 10 minutes, arrange the carrot sticks on a platter and serve.

362. Cajun Walnuts And Olives Bowls

PREP TIME: 10 mins
COOK TIME: 10 mins
SERVINGS: 2 people

INGREDIENTS

- ½ lb. walnuts, chopped
- A pinch of salt and black pepper
- 1 and ½ cups black olives, pitted
- ½ tbsp. Cajun seasoning
- 2 garlic cloves, minced
- 1 red chili pepper, chopped
- ¼ cup veggie stock
- 2 tbsp. tomato puree

DIRECTIONS

1. In your instant pot, combine the walnuts with the olives and the rest of the ingredients, put the lid on and cook on High 10 minutes.
2. Release the pressure fast for 5 minutes, divide the mix into small bowls and serve as an appetizer.

NUTRITION
Calories 105, Fat 1g, Fiber 1g, Carbs 4g, Protein 7g

363. Mango Salsa

PREP TIME: 10 mins
COOK TIME: 10 mins
SERVINGS: 2 people

INGREDIENTS

- 2 mangoes, peeled and cubed
- ½ tbsp. sweet paprika
- 2 garlic cloves, minced
- 2 tbsp. cilantro, chopped
- 1 tbsp. spring onions, chopped
- 1 cup cherry tomatoes, cubed
- 1 cup avocado, peeled, pitted and cubed
- A pinch of salt and black pepper
- 1 tbsp. olive oil
- ¼ cup tomato puree
- ½ cup kalamata olives, pitted and sliced

DIRECTIONS

1. In your instant pot, combine the mangoes with the paprika and the rest of the ingredients except the cilantro, put the lid on and cook on High for 5 minutes.
2. Release the pressure fast for 5 minutes, divide the mix into small bowls, sprinkle the cilantro on top and serve.

NUTRITION
Calories 123, Fat 4g, Carbs 3g, Protein 5g

364. Hot Asparagus Sticks

PREP TIME
10 mins

COOK TIME
10 mins

SERVINGS
2 people

NUTRITION

Calories 181,
Fat 6g,
Carbs 4g,
Protein 4g

INGREDIENTS

- 1 and ½ lb. asparagus, trimmed
- 2 tbsp. olive oil
- 2 tbsp. cayenne pepper sauce
- A pinch of salt and black pepper
- 1 cup water

DIRECTIONS

1. In a bowl, mix the asparagus with the other ingredients except the water and toss.
2. Put the water in your instant pot, add the steamer basket, put the asparagus sticks inside, put the lid on and cook on High for 6 minutes.
3. Release the pressure fast for 5 minutes, arrange the asparagus on a platter and serve.

365. Pork Bites

PREP TIME
10 mins

COOK TIME
30 mins

SERVINGS
4 people

NUTRITION

Calories 242,
Fat 12g,
Carbs 6g,
Protein 14g

INGREDIENTS

- 1 lb. pork roast, cubed and browned
- 1 tbsp. Italian seasoning
- 1 cup beef stock
- 2 tbsp. water
- 1 tbsp. sweet paprika
- 2 tbsp. tomato sauce
- 1 tbsp. rosemary, chopped

DIRECTIONS

1. In your instant pot, combine the pork cubes with the seasoning and the rest of the ingredients except the rosemary, toss, put the lid on and cook on High for 30 minutes.
2. Release the pressure naturally for 10 minutes, arrange the pork cubes on a platter, sprinkle the rosemary on top and serve.

366. Meatballs Platter

PREP TIME: 10 mins
COOK TIME: 15 mins
SERVINGS: 4 people

NUTRITION
Calories 300;
Fat 15.4 g;
Carbs 22.4 g;
Protein 35 g

INGREDIENTS

- 1 lb. beef meat, ground
- ¼ cup panko breadcrumbs
- A pinch of salt and black pepper
- 3 tbsp. red onion, grated
- ¼ cup parsley, chopped
- 2 garlic cloves, minced
- 2 tbsp. lemon juice
- Zest of 1 lemon, grated
- 1 egg
- ½ tsp. cumin, ground
- ½ tsp. coriander, ground
- ¼ tsp. cinnamon powder
- 2 oz. feta cheese, crumbled

DIRECTIONS

1. In a bowl, mix the beef with the breadcrumbs, salt, pepper and the rest of the ingredients except the cooking spray, stir well and shape medium balls out of this mix.
2. Arrange the meatballs on a baking sheet lined with parchment paper, grease them with cooking spray and bake at 450°F for 15 minutes.
3. Arrange the meatballs on a platter and serve as an appetizer.

---

367. Yogurt Dip

PREP TIME: 10 mins
COOK TIME: 0 mins
SERVINGS: 6 people

NUTRITION
Calories 294;
Fat 18 g;
Carbs 21 g;
Protein 10 g

INGREDIENTS

- 2 cups Greek yogurt
- 2 tbsp. pistachios, toasted and chopped
- A pinch of salt and white pepper
- 2 tbsp. mint, chopped
- 1 tbsp. kalamata olives, pitted and chopped
- ¼ cup za'atar spice
- ¼ cup pomegranate seeds
- 1/3 cup olive oil

DIRECTIONS

1. In a bowl, combine the yogurt with the pistachios and the rest of the ingredients, whisk well, divide into small cups and serve with pita chips on the side.

368. Tomato Bruschetta

PREP TIME 10 mins

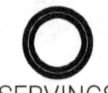
COOK TIME 10 mins

SERVINGS 6 people

NUTRITION

Calories 162;
Fat 4 g;
Fiber 7 g;
Carbs 29 g;
Protein 4 g

INGREDIENTS

- 1 baguette, sliced
- 1/3 cup basil, chopped
- 6 tomatoes, cubed
- 2 garlic cloves, minced
- A pinch of salt and black pepper
- 1 tsp. olive oil
- 1 tbsp. balsamic vinegar
- ½ tsp. garlic powder
- Cooking spray

DIRECTIONS

1. Arrange the baguette slices on a baking sheet lined with parchment paper, grease them with cooking spray and bake at 400° F for 10 minutes.
2. In a bowl, mix the tomatoes with the basil and the remaining ingredients, toss well and leave aside for 10 minutes.
3. Divide the tomato mix on each baguette slice, arrange them all on a platter and serve.

369. Artichoke Flatbread

PREP TIME 10 mins

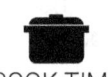
COOK TIME 15 mins

SERVINGS 4 people

NUTRITION

Calories 223;
Fat 11.2 g;
Carbs 15.5 g;
Protein 7.4 g

INGREDIENTS

- 5 tbsp. olive oil
- 2 garlic cloves, minced
- 2 tbsp. parsley, chopped
- 2 round whole wheat flatbreads
- 4 tbsp. parmesan, grated
- ½ cup mozzarella cheese, grated
- 14 oz. canned artichokes, drained and quartered
- 1 cup baby spinach, chopped
- ½ cup cherry tomatoes, halved
- ½ tsp. basil, dried
- Salt and black pepper to the taste

DIRECTIONS

1. In a bowl, mix the parsley with the garlic and 4 tbsp. oil, whisk well and spread this over the flatbreads.
2. Sprinkle the mozzarella and half of the parmesan.
3. In a bowl, mix the artichokes with the spinach, tomatoes, basil, salt, pepper and the rest of the oil, toss and divide over the flatbreads as well.
4. Sprinkle the rest of the parmesan on top, arrange the flatbreads on a baking sheet lined with parchment paper and bake at 425° F for 15 minutes.
5. Serve as an appetizer.

370. Red Pepper Tapenade

PREP TIME: 10 mins
COOK TIME: 0 mins
SERVINGS: 4 people

INGREDIENTS

- 7 oz. roasted red peppers, chopped
- ½ cup parmesan, grated
- 1/3 cup parsley, chopped
- 14 oz. canned artichokes, drained and chopped
- 3 tbsp. olive oil
- ¼ cup capers, drained
- 1 and ½ tbsp. lemon juice
- 2 garlic cloves, minced

DIRECTIONS

1. In your blender, combine the red peppers with the parmesan and the rest of the ingredients and pulse well.
2. Divide into cups and serve as a snack.

NUTRITION
Calories 200; Fat 5.6 g; Carbs 12.4 g; Protein 4.6 g

371. Coriander Falafel

PREP TIME: 10 mins
COOK TIME: 10 mins
SERVINGS: 8 people

INGREDIENTS

- 1 cup canned garbanzo beans, drained and rinsed
- 1 bunch parsley leaves
- 1 yellow onion, chopped
- 5 garlic cloves, minced
- 1 tsp. coriander, ground
- A pinch of salt and black pepper
- ¼ tsp. cayenne pepper
- ¼ tsp. baking soda
- ¼ tsp. cumin powder
- 1 tsp. lemon juice
- 3 tbsp. tapioca flour
- Olive oil for frying

DIRECTIONS

1. In your food processor, combine the beans with the parsley, onion and the rest the ingredients except the oil and the flour and pulse well.
2. Transfer the mix to a bowl, add the flour, stir well, shape 16 balls out of this mix and flatten them a bit.
3. Heat up a pan with some oil over medium-high heat, add the falafels, cook them for 5 minutes on each side, transfer to paper towels, drain excess grease, arrange them on a platter and serve as an appetizer.

NUTRITION
Calories 112; Fat 6.2 g; Carbs 12.3 g; Protein 3.1 g

372. Red Pepper Hummus

PREP TIME
10 mins

COOK TIME
0 mins

SERVINGS
6 people

NUTRITION

Calories 255;
Fat 11.4 g;
Carbs 17.4 g;
Protein 6.5 g

INGREDIENTS

- 6 oz. roasted red peppers, peeled and chopped
- 16 oz. canned chickpeas, drained and rinsed
- ¼ cup Greek yogurt
- 3 tbsp. tahini paste
- Juice of 1 lemon
- 3 garlic cloves, minced 1 tbsp. olive oil
- A pinch of salt and black pepper
- 1 tbsp. parsley, chopped

DIRECTIONS

1. In your food processor, combine the red peppers with the rest of the ingredients except the oil and the parsley and pulse well.
2. Add the oil, pulse again, divide into cups, sprinkle the parsley on top and serve as a party spread.

PIZZA

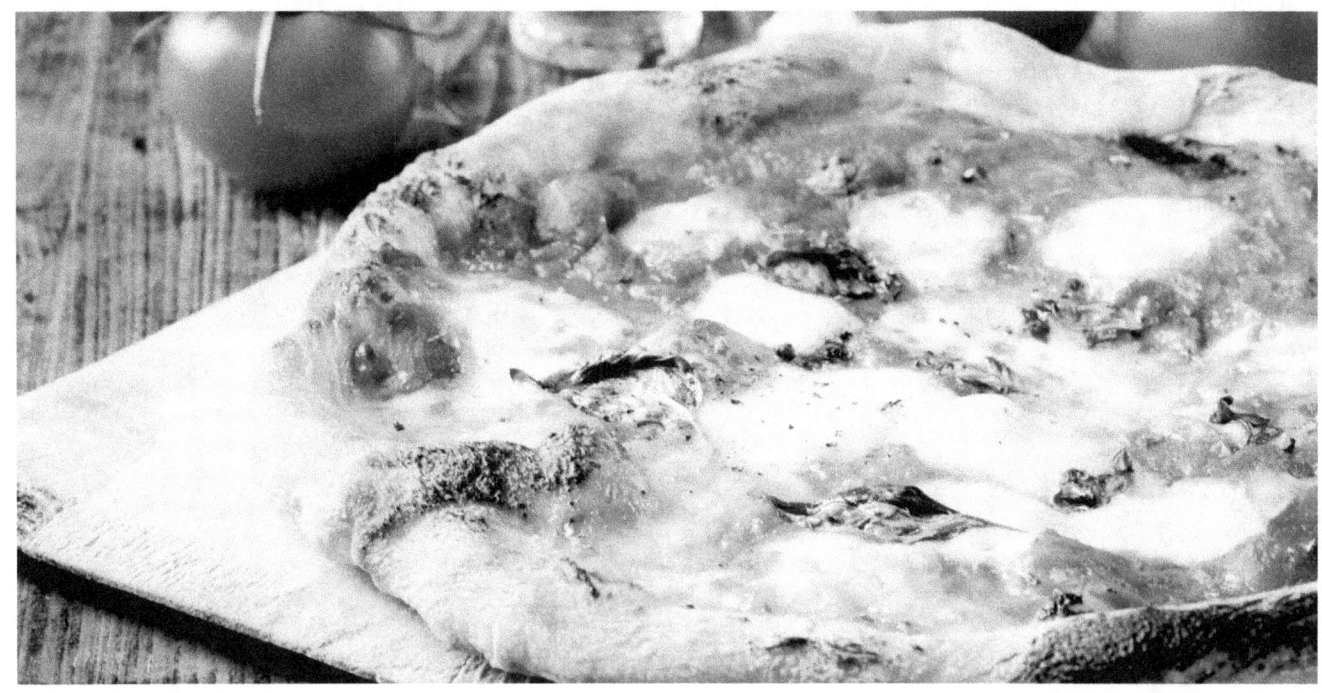

373. White Pizza with Prosciutto and Arugula

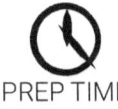
PREP TIME
10 mins

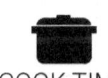
COOK TIME
15 mins

SERVINGS
6 people

NUTRITION

Calories: 273;
Protein: 12.3g;
Carbs: 34g;
Fat: 11g

INGREDIENTS

- 1 lb. prepared pizza dough
- ½ cup ricotta cheese
- 1 tbsp. garlic, minced
- 1 cup grated mozzarella cheese
- 3 oz. prosciutto, thinly sliced
- ½ cup fresh arugula
- ½ tsp. freshly ground black pepper

DIRECTIONS

1. Preheat the oven to 450°F. Roll out the pizza dough on a floured surface.
2. Put the pizza dough on a parchment-lined baking sheet or pizza sheet. Put the dough in the oven and bake for 8 minutes.
3. In a small bowl, mix together the ricotta, garlic, and mozzarella.
4. Remove the pizza dough from the oven and spread the cheese mixture over the top. Bake for another 5 to 6 minutes.
5. Top the pizza with prosciutto, arugula, and pepper; serve warm.

374. Za'atar Pizza

PREP TIME
10 mins

COOK TIME
15 mins

○
SERVINGS
5 people

NUTRITION

Calories: 153;
Protein: 10.3g;
Carbs: 21g;
Fat: 10g

INGREDIENTS

- 1 sheet puff pastry
- ¼ cup extra-virgin olive oil
- 1/3 cup za'atar seasoning

DIRECTIONS

1. Preheat the oven to 350°F.
2. Put the puff pastry on a parchment-lined baking sheet. Cut the pastry into desired slices.
3. Brush the pastry with olive oil. Sprinkle with the za'atar.
4. Put the pastry in the oven and bake for 10 to 12 minutes or until edges are lightly browned and puffed up. Serve warm or at room temperature.

375. Broccoli Cheese Burst Pizza

PREP TIME
20 mins

COOK TIME
5 mins

SERVINGS
6 people

NUTRITION

Calories – 417
Fat – 11g
Carbs – 53g
Fiber – 8
Protein – 19g

INGREDIENTS

- 1 cup mozzarella cheese, shredded
- 2/3 cup ricotta cheese
- 2 tsp. avocado oil
- 1 large whole-wheat pizza crust
- ¼ cup basil, chopped
- 1 ½ cups broccoli florets, chopped
- ½ tsp. garlic powder
- Cornmeal (for dusting)
- 1 ½ cups corn kernels
- Ground black pepper and salt, to taste

DIRECTIONS

1. Preheat your oven at 400°F. Take a baking sheet, line it with parchment paper. Grease it with some avocado oil. (You can also use cooking spray)
2. Spread some cornmeal over the baking sheet
3. In a mixing bowl, combine the corn, broccoli, ricotta, mozzarella, scallions, garlic powder, basil, black pepper and salt.
4. Place the pizza crust on the baking sheet. Add the topping mixture on top and bake until the top is light brown, for 12-15 minutes.
5. Slice and serve warm!

376. Mozzarella Bean Pizza

PREP TIME 10 mins
COOK TIME 15 mins
SERVINGS 6 people

NUTRITION
Calories – 223
Fat – 14g
Carbs – 41g
Fiber – 6g
Protein – 8g

INGREDIENTS
- 2 tbsp. cornmeal
- 1 cup mozzarella
- 1/3 cup barbecue sauce
- 1 roma tomato, diced
- 1 cup black beans
- 1 cup corn kernels
- 1 medium whole-wheat pizza crust

DIRECTIONS
1. Preheat your oven at 400°F. Take a baking sheet, line it with parchment paper. Grease it with some avocado oil. (You can also use cooking spray)
2. Spread some cornmeal over the baking sheet
3. In a bowl, mix together the tomatoes, corn and beans.
4. Place the pizza crust on the baking sheet. Spread the sauce on top; add the topping, and top with the cheese and bake until the cheese melts and the crust edges are golden-brown for 12-15 minutes.
5. Slice and serve warm.

377. Olive Oil Pizza Dough

PREP TIME 10 mins
COOK TIME 15 mins
SERVINGS 5 people

NUTRITION
Calories: 392;
Protein: 8.3g;
Carbs: 44g;
Fat: 6.3g

INGREDIENTS
- Water 2/3 cup
- Wheat flour 2 cups
- Dry yeast 1 tsp.
- Salt 1 tsp.
- 1 tbsp. olive oil

DIRECTIONS
1. Pour the yeast with warm water. Stir the mixture properly so that there are no lumps.
2. Pour 2 cups flour and salt into a large bowl. Add yeast and knead the dough.
3. Put the dough out of the bowl on a dry, floured surface, and continue to knead, adding flour if necessary, until the dough is soft and elastic (about 10 minutes).
4. Lightly grease a large bowl with olive oil. Put the dough in a bowl, turning it so that the entire surface is smeared with oil.
5. Cover with a film and place in a warm, without drafts, place for 1.5 hours (until the dough increases about 2 times).
6. Flatten the dough with your fists. Divide into 2 parts and roll into balls.

378. Crispy Pizza Dough

PREP TIME
10 mins

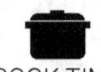
COOK TIME
25 mins

SERVINGS
5 people

NUTRITION

Calories: 253;
Protein: 9.3g;
Carbs: 34g;
Fat: 6.3g

INGREDIENTS

- Wheat flour 2 cups
- 2 tbsp. olive oil
- ½ cup milk
- Chicken egg 2 pieces
- Salt pinch

DIRECTIONS

1. Heat milk, add eggs and butter, stir.
2. Constantly mixing, pour the milk mixture into the flour, add salt
3. Knead the dough for about 10 minutes to make it elastic.

379. Thin Crispy Pizza Dough

PREP TIME
10 mins

COOK TIME
20 mins

SERVINGS
– people

NUTRITION

Calories: 233;
Protein: 10.3g;
Carbs: 34g;
Fat: 5.3g

INGREDIENTS

- Wheat flour 9 oz.
- Cane sugar 0.3 tsp.
- Dry yeast 4 g
- 0.4 tsp. salt
- Water 125 ml

DIRECTIONS

1. Prepare the dough. To do this, mix yeast, sugar and 2 tbsp. of warm water in a bowl. Then add 2 tbsp. of flour, mix well again, cover with a towel and put in a warm place for 30 minutes. Watch the dough, it happens that it is ready in 10 minutes!
2. Pour flour into a bowl, make a depression in the middle. Put the dough in the recess, salt, add about 125 ml of warm water. Knead for about 10-15 minutes until the dough is soft, smooth and elastic. It should not stick to your hands, so you may need to add a little flour or water.
3. Cover the dough with a towel and put in a warm place for 1 hour. It should increase in volume by about half.
4. Making a crunch! Heat the oven to 350°F, grease the pizza dish with olive oil, roll it out with a diameter of about 28 cm, put it in the mold, form the sides (or not), grease with tomato sauce and put in the oven for about 5 minutes.
5. Then remove, distribute the rest of the filling and bake for another 20 minutes. Due to the fact that the dough is slightly baked at the beginning, it will become crispy, but at the same time it will not burn!

380. Yeast Pizza Dough

PREP TIME: 10 mins
COOK TIME: 15 mins
SERVINGS: 5 people

INGREDIENTS
- Wheat flour 2 cups
- Vegetable oil 1 tbsp.
- Fresh yeast 3/4 oz.
- Sugar 1 tsp.
- Salt 1 tsp.

DIRECTIONS
1. In one glass of warm water, dilute 3/4 oz. of yeast (or 1/3 sachet of dry yeast). Leave to stand for 10 minutes.
2. Add 1 tbsp. of vegetable oil, pour all this into 2 cups flour, add salt and sugar.
3. Knead the dough well.

NUTRITION
Calories: 353;
Protein: 10.3g;
Carbs: 34g;
Fat: 5.3g

381. Fresh Sour Cream Pizza Dough

PREP TIME: 10 mins
COOK TIME: 15 mins
SERVINGS: 5 people

INGREDIENTS
- Wheat flour 7 oz.
- Sour cream 7 oz.

DIRECTIONS
1. Knead the dough from flour and sour cream, divide into 3 equal parts, roll each part into a thin circle.
2. Put on a baking sheet, put the filling.

NUTRITION
Calories: 333;
Protein: 10.3g;
Carbs: 21.4g;
Fat: 12.3g

382. Fast, Yeast-Free Pizza Dough

PREP TIME
10 mins

COOK TIME
25 mins

SERVINGS
3 people

NUTRITION

Calories: 468;
Protein: 20.3g;
Carbs: 41g;
Fat: 15.3g

INGREDIENTS

- Wheat flour 12 oz.
- Kefir 250 ml
- Chicken egg 2 pieces
- Olive oil 40 ml
- ¼ tsp. salt
- ¼ tsp. soda

DIRECTIONS

1. Beat eggs with salt in a small bowl.
2. Pour kefir into a large bowl.
3. Add to the kefir soda quenched with vinegar.
4. Pour beaten eggs to kefir, mix well the mixture.
5. Add the flour, I prefer to add it in parts to feel the consistency of the dough. In principle, you can use a blender to prepare the dough, but I prefer to knead this particular dough with my hands.
6. Add olive oil to the dough.
7. Stir the dough. It should be consistency like thick sour cream - liquid, but at the same time it should turn out magnificent - as a result of the reaction of kefir and soda.
8. Lubricate the baking sheet with vegetable oil and pour the quick pizza dough on kefir and put the baking sheet in the oven about 400°F. When the dough is browned, you can spread the filling and bake until cooked.

383. Thin Pizza Dough With Honey

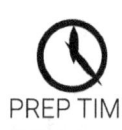
PREP TIME
10 mins

COOK TIME
15 mins

SERVINGS
5 people

NUTRITION

Calories: 386;
Protein: 10.3g;
Carbs: 6.6g;
Fat: 4.3g

INGREDIENTS

- Wheat flour 3 cups
- Water 1 cup
- Dry yeast 12 g
- Honey 1.5 tsp.
- Salt 1 tsp.
- 1 tbsp. olive oil

DIRECTIONS

1. Heat the water to 120°F. Combine half a glass of warm water with yeast (12 g - 1 sachet) and honey.
2. Separately mix flour, salt, oil.
3. Add the honey-yeast mixture and the remaining water. Knead for at least 5 minutes (the dough should not stick to your hands).
4. Allow the dough to rise in a warm place for 30 minutes (cover with a damp towel so that the dough is not weathered).
5. Knead the dough again for 2 minutes, roll into a circle about 30 cm and put on a baking sheet, pre-oiled. The filling is your choice.

384. Pasta (Pizza Dough)

PREP TIME
10 mins

COOK TIME
20 mins

SERVINGS
4 people

NUTRITION

Calories: 562;
Protein: 10.3g;
Carbs: 3.4g;
Fat: 14.3g

INGREDIENTS

- Wheat flour 17 oz.
- Salt ¼ oz.
- Sugar ½ oz.
- Water 300 ml
- Olive oil 50 ml
- Dry yeast 7g

DIRECTIONS

1. Mix the dry ingredients: flour, salt and sugar.
2. In another bowl, mix water (room temperature), yeast and oil.
3. Combine everything and knead the dough.
4. Leave the dough for an hour, cover with a towel.
5. Distribute on a baking sheet, form the base of the pizza.
6. Lubricate with tomato paste, sprinkle with grated mozzarella and fill the pizza as desired (very tasty with mushrooms and prosciutto, or with tuna and olives), garnish with basil leaves.
7. Bake at 390°F for approximately 20–25 minutes.

385. Pizza Dough Without Yeast In Milk

PREP TIME
5 mins

COOK TIME
60 mins

SERVINGS
5 people

NUTRITION

Calories: 453;
Protein: 10.3g;
Carbs: 30.4g;
Fat: 14.3g

INGREDIENTS

- Wheat flour 2 cups
- Milk 125 ml
- Salt 1 tsp.
- Chicken egg 2 pieces
- Sunflower oil 2 tbsp.

DIRECTIONS

1. Making pizza dough without yeast in milk is quite simple. The recipe is designed to prepare a dough, which is enough for two, but only large, baking sheets.
2. Combine flour and salt in one bowl. And in the second butter, milk and eggs, mix well and combine the contents of two bowls in one large container.
3. Wait a few minutes for the whole liquid consistency to soak in the flour, and start mixing the dough. It will take about 15 minutes. Dough, in finished form, should be elastic, soft and smooth.
4. Then you need to take a kitchen towel, of course clean, and soak it in water. As a result, it should be moist, but not wet. Excess fluid must be squeezed out. Wrap the dough in a towel, leave to lie down for 20 minutes.
5. After waiting for the set time, remove the dough and, sprinkling flour on the countertop, roll out, but only very thinly.
6. Place it on a baking sheet and lay out the filling prepared according to your taste preferences. As a result, the finished dough will have an effect that is easy, of course, of puff pastry and has a crispy taste.

386. Puff Pastry Pizza

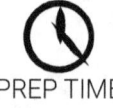
PREP TIME
10 mins

COOK TIME
30 mins

SERVINGS
5 people

NUTRITION

Calories: 253;
Protein: 10.3g;
Carbs: 3.4g;
Fat: 16.3g

INGREDIENTS

- Puff pastry 17 oz.
- Sausages 7 oz.
- Hard cheese 5 oz.
- Tomatoes 4 pieces
- Dill 1 bunch
- Mayonnaise to taste
- Tomato paste to taste
- Champagne Vinegar 150 ml

DIRECTIONS

1. Thaw the dough, roll out, distribute on a baking sheet greased with vegetable oil, make small sides.
2. Sausages cut into rings. Cut the tomatoes into slices. Grate the cheese. Fry the champignons in a pan, add chopped herbs, mix.
3. Grease the dough with tomato paste, put sausages, then tomatoes, grease with mayonnaise, put mushrooms, sprinkle with cheese.
4. Put the pizza in the oven preheated to 360°F

387. Ideal Pizza Dough (On A Large Baking Sheet)

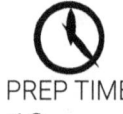
PREP TIME
10 mins

COOK TIME
60 mins

SERVINGS
5 people

NUTRITION

Calories: 193;
Protein: 10.3g;
Carbs: 34g;
Fat: 9.3g

INGREDIENTS

- Wheat flour 13 oz.
- Salt 1.5 tsp.
- Dry yeast 1,799 tsp.
- Sugar 1 tsp.
- Water 200 ml
- 1 tbsp. olive oil
- Dried Basil 1.5 tsp.

DIRECTIONS

1. We cultivate yeast in warm water. There you can add a spoonful of sugar, so the yeast will begin to work faster. Leave them for 10 minutes.
2. Sift the flour through a sieve (leave 2 oz. for the future) in a deep bowl. Add salt, basil, mix.
3. Pour water with yeast into the cavity in the flour and mix thoroughly with a fork.
4. Somewhere in the middle of the process, when the dough becomes less than one whole, add olive oil (you can also sunflower).
5. When the dough is ready (it becomes smooth and elastic), cover with a damp towel and put in heat (you can use the battery) for 30 minutes.
6. Now just lay it on a flour dusted surface and roll out the future pizza to a thickness of 2-3 mm.
7. The main rule of pizza is the maximum possible temperature, minimum time. Therefore, feel free to set the highest temperature that is available in your oven.

388. Vegetable Oil Pizza Dough

PREP TIME 10 mins
COOK TIME 60 mins
SERVINGS 3 people

INGREDIENTS

- Wheat flour 1 cup
- Water 1 cup
- Salt to taste
- Vegetable oil 1 tbsp.
- Dry yeast 10 g

DIRECTIONS

1. We mix water and yeast, leave for 40 minutes so that they disperse. You can add a tbsp. of sugar.
2. Then pour in the oil, add the flour (here already at the request and degree of tightness of the dough - it should be quite tight, but not too much).
3. Knead well and put in a warm place to increase the volume by 2 times.

NUTRITION

Calories: 223;
Protein: 10.3g;
Carbs: 9.4g;
Fat: 5.3g

389. Pizza Dough On Yogurt

PREP TIME 10 mins
COOK TIME 30 mins
SERVINGS 5 people

INGREDIENTS

- Natural yogurt 9 oz.
- Vegetable oil 5 tbsp.
- ½ tsp. salt
- Wheat flour 2.5 cups
- Baking powder 1 tsp.

DIRECTIONS

1. Mix flour, baking powder and salt;
2. Add yogurt and butter, mix everything thoroughly;
3. Preheat the oven to 190 ° C;
4. Lubricate the pan with oil;
5. Roll the dough very thinly and transfer to a baking sheet;
6. Put the filling to taste;
7. Bake for 10-15 minutes.

NUTRITION

Calories: 336;
Protein: 10.3g;
Carbs: 24g;
Fat: 13.3g

390. American Pizza Dough Recipe

PREP TIME
10 mins

COOK TIME
15 mins

SERVINGS
5 people

NUTRITION

Calories: 353;
Protein: 18.3g;
Carbs: 27g;
Fat: 13.3g

INGREDIENTS

- Wheat flour 6 oz.
- Chicken egg 1 piece
- Water 85 ml
- Dry yeast 2 g
- Salt 3 g
- Sugar 10 g
- Sunflower oil 5 ml

DIRECTIONS

1. Combine all dry ingredients.
2. Add water and egg. Mix well.
3. After the dough has become homogeneous, gradually add the butter.
4. Leave the dough for 5 minutes.

391. Eggplant Pizza

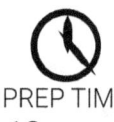
PREP TIME
10 mins

COOK TIME
30 mins

SERVINGS
6 people

NUTRITION

Protein: 8 g
Fat: 20 g
Carbs: 25 g
Calories: 257

INGREDIENTS

- Eggplants (1 large or 2 medium)
- Olive oil (.33 cup)
- Black pepper & salt (as desired)
- Marinara sauce - store-bought/ homemade (1.25 cups)
- Shredded mozzarella cheese (1.5 cups)
- Cherry tomatoes (2 cups - halved)
- Torn basil leaves (.5 cup)

DIRECTIONS

1. Heat the oven to reach 400°F. Prepare a baking sheet with a layer of parchment baking paper.
2. Slice the end/ends off of the eggplant and them it into ¾-inch slices. Arrange the slices on the prepared sheet and brush both sides with olive oil. Dust with pepper and salt to your liking.
3. Roast the eggplant until tender (10 to 12 min.).
4. Transfer the tray from the oven and add two tbsp. of sauce on top of each section. Top it off with the mozzarella and three to five tomato pieces on top.
5. Bake it until the cheese is melted. The tomatoes should begin to blister in about five to seven more minutes.
6. Take the tray from the oven. Serve hot and garnish with a dusting of basil.

392. Mediterranean Whole Wheat Pizza

PREP TIME: 5 mins
COOK TIME: 25 mins
SERVINGS: 4 people

INGREDIENTS
- Whole-wheat pizza crust (1)
- Basil pesto (4 oz. jar)
- Artichoke hearts (.5 cup)
- Kalamata olives (2 tbsp.)
- Pepperoncini (2 tbsp. drained)
- Feta cheese (.25 cup)

DIRECTIONS
1. Program the oven to 450°F.
2. Drain and pull the artichokes to pieces. Slice/chop the pepperoncini and olives.
3. Arrange the pizza crust onto a floured work surface and cover it using pesto. Arrange the artichoke, pepperoncini slices, and olives over the pizza. Lastly, crumble and add the feta.
4. Bake in the hot oven until the cheese has melted, and it has a crispy crust or 10-12 minutes.

NUTRITION
Calories: 277
Protein: 9.7 g
Carbs: 24 g
Fat: 18.6 g

393. Chicken Pizza

PREP TIME: 1 min
COOK TIME: 10 mins
SERVINGS: 4 people

INGREDIENTS
- 2 flatbreads
- 1 tbsp. Greek vinaigrette
- ½ cup feta cheese, crumbled
- ¼ cup Parmesan cheese, grated
- ½ cup water-packed artichoke hearts, rinsed, drained and chopped
- ½ cup olives, pitted and sliced
- ½ cup cooked chicken breast strips, chopped
- 1/8 tsp. dried basil
- 1/8 tsp. dried oregano
- Pinch of ground black pepper
- 1 cup part-skim mozzarella cheese, shredded

DIRECTIONS
1. Preheat the oven to 400°F.
2. Arrange the flatbreads onto a large ungreased baking sheet and coat each with vinaigrette.
3. Top with feta, followed by the Parmesan, veggies and chicken.
4. Sprinkle with dried herbs and black pepper.
5. Top with mozzarella cheese evenly.
6. Bake for about 8-10 minutes or until cheese is melted.
7. Remove from the oven and set aside for about 1-2 minutes before slicing.
8. Cut each flat bread into 2 pieces and serve.

NUTRITION
Calories 393
Fat 22 g
Carbs 20.6 g
Protein 28.9 g

394. Spinach & Feta Pita Bake

PREP TIME
10 mins

COOK TIME
22 mins

SERVINGS
6 people

NUTRITION

Calories: 350
Protein: 11.6 g
Carbs: 24 g
Fat: 17.1g g

INGREDIENTS

- Sun-dried tomato pesto (6 oz. tub)
- Roma - plum tomatoes (2 chopped)
- Whole-wheat pita bread (Six 6-inch)
- Spinach (1 bunch)
- Mushrooms (4 sliced)
- Grated Parmesan cheese (2 tbsp.)
- Crumbled feta cheese (.5 cup)
- Olive oil (3 tbsp.)
- Black pepper (as desired)

DIRECTIONS

1. Set the oven at 350°F.
2. Spread the pesto onto one side of each pita bread and arrange them onto a baking tray (pesto-side up).
3. Rinse and chop the spinach. Top the pitas with spinach, mushrooms, tomatoes, feta cheese, pepper, Parmesan cheese, pepper, and a drizzle of oil.
4. Bake in the hot oven until the pita bread is crispy (12 min.). Slice the pitas into quarters.

395. Beef Pizza

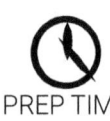
PREP TIME
25 mins

COOK TIME
50 mins

SERVINGS
10 people

NUTRITION

Calories 309
Fat 8.7 g
Carbs 36.4 g
Protein 21.4 g

INGREDIENTS

- For Crust:
- 3 cups all-purpose flour
- 1 tbsp. sugar
- 2¼ tsp. active dry yeast
- 1 tsp. salt
- 2 tbsp. olive oil
- 1 cup warm water
- For Topping:
- 1-lb. ground beef
- 1 medium onion, chopped
- 2 tbsp. tomato paste
- 1 tbsp. ground cumin
- Salt and ground black pepper, as required
- ¼ cup water
- 1 cup fresh spinach, chopped
- 8 oz. artichoke hearts, quartered
- 4 oz. fresh mushrooms, sliced
- 2 tomatoes, chopped
- 4 oz. feta cheese, crumbled

DIRECTIONS

For crust:
1. In the bowl of a stand mixer, fitted with the dough hook, add the flour, sugar, yeast and salt.
2. Add 2 tbsp. of the oil and warm water and knead until a smooth and elastic dough is formed.
3. Make a ball of the dough and set aside for about 15 minutes.
4. Place the dough onto a lightly floured surface and roll into a circle.
5. Place the dough into a lightly, greased round pizza pan and gently, press to fit.
6. Set aside for about 10-15 minutes.
7. Coat the crust with some oil.
8. Preheat the oven to 400°F.

For topping:
1. Heat a nonstick skillet over medium-high heat and cook the beef for about 4-5 minutes.
2. Add the onion and cook for about 5 minutes, stirring frequently.
3. Add the tomato paste, cumin, salt, black pepper and water and stir to combine.
4. Reduce the heat to medium and cook for about 5-10 minutes.
5. Remove from the heat and set aside.
6. Place the beef mixture over the pizza crust and top with the spinach, followed by the artichokes, mushrooms, tomatoes, and Feta cheese.
7. Bake for about 25-30 minutes or until the cheese is melted.
8. Remove from the oven and set aside for about 3-5 minutes before slicing.
9. Cut into desired sized slices and serve.

396. Shrimp Pizza

PREP TIME: 15 mins
COOK TIME: 10 mins
SERVINGS: 1 people

NUTRITION
Calories 482
Fat 18.9 g
Carbs 44.5 g
Protein 33.4 g

INGREDIENTS
- 2 tbsp. spaghetti sauce
- 1 tbsp. pesto sauce
- 1 (6-inch) pita bread
- 2 tbsp. mozzarella cheese, shredded
- 5 cherry tomatoes, halved
- 1/8 cup bay shrimp
- Pinch of garlic powder
- Pinch of dried basil

DIRECTIONS
1. Preheat the oven to 325°F. Lightly, grease a baking sheet.
2. In a bowl, mix together the spaghetti sauce and pesto.
3. Spread the pesto mixture over the pita bread in a thin layer.
4. Top the pita bread with the cheese, followed by the tomatoes and shrimp.
5. Sprinkle with the garlic powder and basil.
6. Arrange the pita bread onto the prepared baking sheet and bake for about 7-10 minutes.
7. Remove from the oven and set aside for about 3-5 minutes before slicing.
8. Cut into desired sized slices and serve.

397. Veggie Pizza

PREP TIME: 20 mins
COOK TIME: 12 mins
SERVINGS: 6 people

NUTRITION
Calories 381
Fat 16.1 g
Carbs 42.4 g
Protein 19.4 g

INGREDIENTS
- 1 (12-inch) prepared pizza crust
- ¼ tsp. Italian seasoning
- ¼ tsp. red pepper flakes, crushed
- 1 cup goat cheese, crumbled
- 1 (14-oz.) can quartered artichoke hearts
- 3 plum tomatoes, sliced into ¼-inch thick size
- 6 kalamata olives, pitted and sliced
- ¼ cup fresh basil, chopped

DIRECTIONS
1. Preheat the oven to 450°F. Grease a baking sheet.
2. Sprinkle the pizza crust with Italian seasoning and red pepper flakes evenly.
3. Place the goat cheese over crust evenly, leaving about ½-inch of the sides.
4. With the back of a spoon, gently press the cheese downwards.
5. Place the artichoke, tomato and olives on top of the cheese.
6. Arrange the pizza crust onto the prepared baking sheet.
7. Bake for about 10-12 minutes or till cheese becomes bubbly.
8. Remove from oven and sprinkle with the basil.
9. Cut into equal sized wedges and serve.

398. Watermelon Feta & Balsamic Pizza

PREP TIME
5 mins

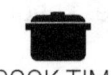
COOK TIME
15 mins

SERVINGS
4 people

NUTRITION

Calories: 90
Protein: 2 g
Fat: 3 g
Carbs 5 g

INGREDIENTS

- Watermelon (1-inch thick from the center)
- Crumbled feta cheese (1 oz.)
- Sliced Kalamata olives (5-6)
- Mint leaves (1 tsp.)
- Balsamic glaze (.5 tbsp.)

DIRECTIONS

1. Slice the widest section of the watermelon in half. Then, slice each half into four wedges.
2. Serve on a round pie dish like a pizza round and cover with the olives, cheese, mint leaves, and glaze.

399. Fruit Pizza

PREP TIME
15 mins

COOK TIME
0 mins

SERVINGS
4 people

NUTRITION

69 Calories,
4.4g Protein,
1.4g Carbs,
5.1g Fat

INGREDIENTS

- 4 watermelon slices
- 1 oz blueberries
- 2 oz goat cheese, crumbled
- 1 tsp. fresh parsley, chopped

DIRECTIONS

1. Put the watermelon slices in the plate in one layer.
2. Then sprinkle them with blueberries, goat cheese, and fresh parsley.

400. Sprouts Pizza

PREP TIME: 25 mins
COOK TIME: 15 mins
SERVINGS: 6 people

INGREDIENTS

- 4 oz wheat flour, whole grain
- 2 tbsp. olive oil
- ¼ tsp. baking powder
- 5 oz chicken fillet, boiled
- 2 oz Mozzarella cheese, shredded
- 1 tomato, chopped
- 2 oz bean sprouts

DIRECTIONS

1. Make the pizza crust: mix wheat flour, olive oil, baking powder, and knead the dough.
2. Roll it up in the shape of pizza crust and transfer in the pizza mold.
3. Then sprinkle it with chopped tomato, shredded chicken, and Mozzarella.
4. Bake the pizza at 365F for 15 minutes.
5. Sprinkle the cooked pizza with bean sprouts and cut into servings.

NUTRITION: 184 Calories, 11.9g Protein, 15.6g Carbs, 8.2g Fat

---

401. Cheese Pinwheels

PREP TIME: 20 mins
COOK TIME: 25 mins
SERVINGS: 4 people

INGREDIENTS

- 1 tsp. chili flakes
- ½ tsp. dried cilantro
- 1 egg, beaten
- 1 tsp. cream cheese
- 1 oz Cheddar cheese, grated
- 6 oz pizza dough

DIRECTIONS

1. Roll up the pizza dough and cut into 6 squares.
2. Sprinkle the dough with dried cilantro, cream cheese, and Cheddar cheese.
3. Roll the dough in the shape of pinwheels, brush with beaten egg and bake in the preheated to 365°F oven for 25 minutes or until the pinwheels are light brown.

NUTRITION: 16 Calories, 3.8g Protein, 12.1g Carbs, 11.2g Fat

402. Ground Meat Pizza

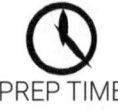
PREP TIME
15 mins

COOK TIME
35 mins

SERVINGS
4 people

NUTRITION

213 Calories,
18g Protein,
17g Carbs,
12.8g Fat

INGREDIENTS

- 7 oz ground beef
- 1 tsp. tomato paste
- ½ tsp. ground black pepper
- 2 egg whites, whisked
- ½ cup Mozzarella cheese, shredded
- 1 tsp. fresh basil, chopped

DIRECTIONS

1. Line the baking tray with baking paper. Preheat the oven to 370F.
2. Mix all ingredients except Mozzarella in the mixing bowl.
3. Then place the mixture in the tray and flatten it to get a thick layer.
4. Top the pizza with Mozzarella cheese and bake in the oven for 35 minutes.
5. Then cut the cooked pizza into the servings.

403. Quinoa Flour Pizza

PREP TIME
15 mins

COOK TIME
15 mins

SERVINGS
6 people

NUTRITION

38 Calories,
2g Protein,
10g Carbs,
8g Fat

INGREDIENTS

- 1 oz pumpkin puree
- 3 tbsp. quinoa flour
- ½ tsp. dried oregano
- 1 cup Mozzarella cheese, shredded
- 1 tomato, chopped
- 1 tsp. olive oil

DIRECTIONS

1. Mix pumpkin puree, quinoa flour, and olive oil. Knead the dough.
2. Roll it up in the shape of pizza crust and transfer in the lined with a baking paper baking tray.
3. Then top the pizza crust with tomato, oregano, and Mozzarella cheese.
4. Bake the pizza at 365°F for 15 minutes.

404. Greek Style Bread with Black Olives

PREP TIME 25 mins
COOK TIME 45 mins
SERVINGS 12 people

NUTRITION
176 Calories,
6.6g Protein,
27g Carbs,
4.6g Fat

INGREDIENTS

- 1 cup black olives, pitted, sliced
- 1 tbsp. avocado oil
- ½ oz fresh yeast
- 4 oz cream cheese
- 2 cup wheat flour, whole grain
- 3 eggs, beaten
- 1 tsp. olive oil, melted
- 1 tsp. sugar

DIRECTIONS

1. In the big bowl combine fresh yeast, sugar, and cream cheese. Stir it until yeast is dissolved.
2. Then add olive oil and eggs. Stir the dough mixture until homogenous and add 1 cup of wheat flour. Mix it up until smooth.
3. Add olives and remaining flour. Add avocado oil and knead the non-sticky dough.
4. Transfer the dough into the non-sticky dough mold.
5. Cook the bread for 65 minutes at 350°F.
6. When the bread is cooked, cool it well and remove it from the mold.
7. Slice the bread.

405. Turkey Flatbread

PREP TIME 15 mins
COOK TIME 30 mins
SERVINGS 8 people

NUTRITION
246 Calories,
20.7g Protein,
25.8g Carbs,
7.3g Fat

INGREDIENTS

- 1 ½ cup ground turkey
- 1 tsp. baking powder
- ¼ cup plain yogurt
- 9 oz wheat flour, whole grain
- 1 tsp. avocado oil
- 1 tsp. tomato paste

DIRECTIONS

1. Make the yeast dough: mix baking powder, plain yogurt, and whole-grain flour.
2. Knead the non-sticky dough and leave it in a warm place for 15 minutes.
3. After this, roll up the dough in the shape of a square and transfer it in the lined baking tray.
4. Bake it at 365°F for 10 minutes.
5. Meanwhile, mix ground turkey, tomato paste, and avocado oil.
6. Spread the ground turkey mixture over the flatbread and bake it at 365f for 20 minutes more.

406. Pepper Flatbread Bites

PREP TIME
20 mins

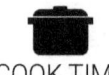
COOK TIME
10 mins

SERVINGS
8 people

INGREDIENTS

- 2 tbsp. olive oil, softened
- 1/3 cup plain yogurt
- 9 oz wheat flour, whole grain
- 1 tsp. olive oil
- 1 cup bell pepper, chopped
- 1 oz Parmesan, grated

DIRECTIONS

1. Mix olive oil and plain yogurt.
2. Then add flour and knead the soft dough.
3. Cut the dough into 8 pieces and roll into the rounds.
4. Then preheat olive oil in the skillet.
5. Put the dough rounds in the skillet and roast for 3 minutes per side.
6. Then top the cooked dough bites with bell pepper and Parmesan.
7. Cook the meal with closed lid for 2 minutes.

NUTRITION

174 Calories,
5.2g Protein,
26.3g Carbs,
5.2g Fat

---

407. Artichoke Pizza

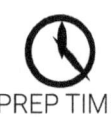
PREP TIME
15 mins

COOK TIME
15 mins

SERVINGS
4 people

INGREDIENTS

- 7 oz pizza crust
- 5 oz artichoke hearts, canned, drained, chopped
- 1 tsp. fresh basil, chopped
- 1 tomato, sliced
- 1 cup Monterey Jack cheese, shredded

DIRECTIONS

1. Line the pizza mold with baking paper.
2. Then put the pizza crust inside.
3. Top it with sliced tomato, canned artichoke hearts, and basil.
4. Then top the pizza with Monterey Jack cheese and transfer in the preheated to 365°F oven.
5. Cook the pizza for 20 minutes.

NUTRITION

247 Calories,
12.1g Protein,
28.2g Carbs,
10.2g Fat

408. 3-Cheese Pizza

PREP TIME: 15 mins
COOK TIME: 10 mins
SERVINGS: 6 people

INGREDIENTS

- 1 pizza crust, cooked
- ½ cup Mozzarella, shredded
- ½ cup Cheddar cheese, shredded
- 2 oz Parmesan, grated
- ¼ cup tomato sauce
- 1 tsp. Italian seasonings

DIRECTIONS

1. Put the pizza crust in the baking pan.
2. Then brush it with tomato sauce and Italian seasonings.
3. After this, sprinkle the pizza with Mozzarella, Cheddar cheese, and Parmesan.
4. Bake the pizza for 10 minutes at 375°F.

NUTRITION

106 Calories, 7g Protein, 6.3g Carbs, 6.1g Fat

---

409. Chickpea Pizza

PREP TIME: 10 mins
COOK TIME: 25 mins
SERVINGS: 4 people

INGREDIENTS

- 4 tbsp. marinara sauce
- 7 oz pizza dough
- 1 tomato, sliced
- 1 red onion, sliced
- 5 oz chickpeas, canned
- ½ cup Mozzarella cheese, shredded

DIRECTIONS

1. Roll up the pizza dough in the shape of pizza crust and transfer in the pizza mold.
2. Then brush the pizza crust with marinara sauce and sprinkle with sliced onion, tomato, and chickpeas.
3. Top the chickpeas with mozzarella cheese and bake the pizza for 25 minutes at 355°F.

NUTRITION

266 Calories, 7.6g Protein, 31.9g Carbs, 12.4g Fat

POULTRY AND MEAT

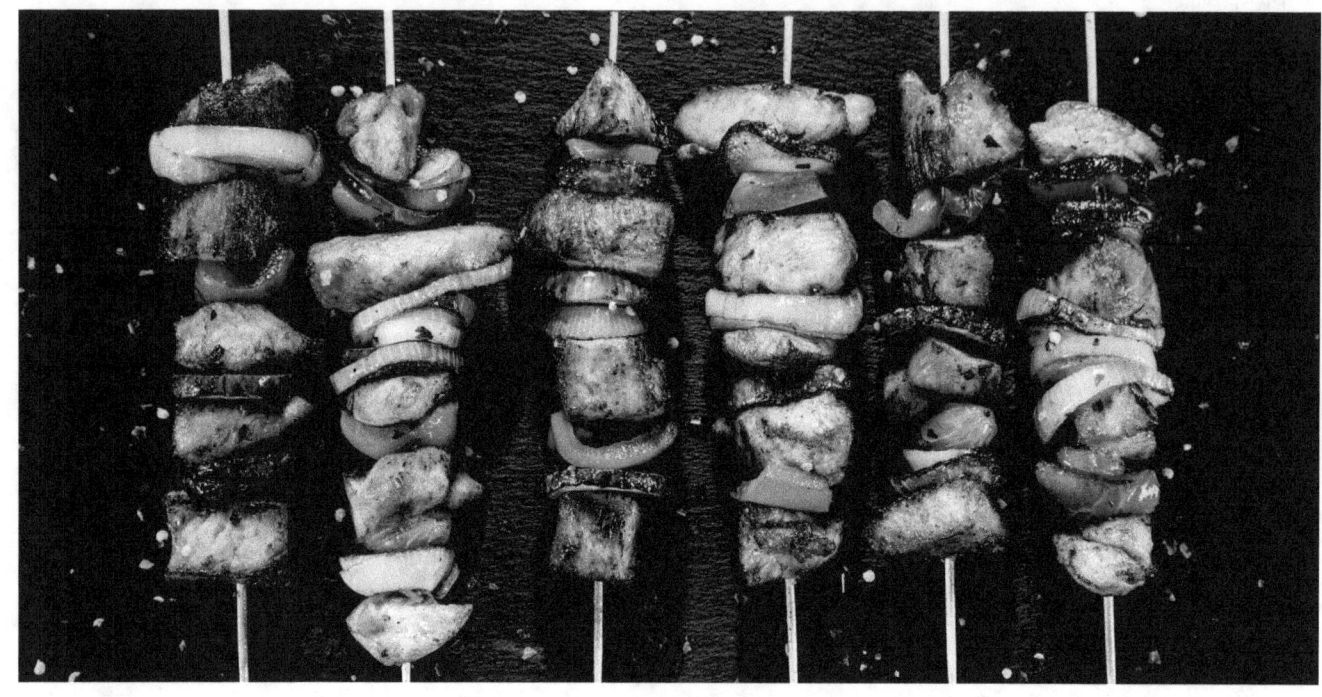

410. Arugula Fig Chicken

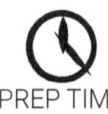
PREP TIME
15 mins

COOK TIME
30 mins

SERVINGS
4 people

NUTRITION

Calories – 364
Fat – 14g
Carbs – 29g
Protein – 31g

INGREDIENTS

- 2 tsp. cornstarch
- 2 clove garlic, crushed
- ¾ cup Mission figs, chopped
- ¼ cup black or green olives, chopped
- 1 bag baby arugula
- ½ cup chicken broth
- 8 skinless chicken thighs
- 2 tsp. olive oil
- 2 tsp. brown sugar
- ½ cup red wine vinegar
- Ground black pepper and salt, to taste

DIRECTIONS

1. Over medium stove flame, heat the oil in a skillet or saucepan (preferably of medium size).
2. Add the chicken, sprinkle with some salt and cook until evenly brown. Set it aside.
3. Add and sauté the garlic.
4. In a mixing bowl, combine the vinegar, broth, cornstarch and sugar. Add the mixture into the pan and simmer until the sauce thickens.
5. Add the figs and olives; simmer for a few minutes. Serve warm with chopped arugula on top.

411. Parmesan Chicken Gratin

PREP TIME 10 mins
COOK TIME 30 mins
SERVINGS 4 people

NUTRITION
Calories 100,
Fat 5.2,
Carbs 6.7,
Protein 8.1

INGREDIENTS
- 2 chicken thighs, skinless, boneless
- 1 tsp. paprika
- 1 tbsp. lemon juice
- ½ tsp. chili flakes
- ¼ tsp. garlic powder
- 3 oz Parmesan, grated
- 1/3 cup milk
- 1 onion, sliced
- 2 oz pineapple, sliced

DIRECTIONS
1. Chop the chicken thighs roughly and sprinkle them with paprika, lemon juice, chili flakes, garlic powder, and mix up well.
2. Arrange the chopped chicken thighs in the baking dish in one layer.
3. Then place sliced onion over the chicken.
4. Add the layer of sliced pineapple.
5. Mix up together milk and Parmesan and pour the liquid over the pineapple,
6. Cover the surface of the baking dish with foil and bake gratin for 30 minutes at 355°F.

412. Chicken Saute

PREP TIME 10 mins
COOK TIME 25 mins
SERVINGS 2 people

NUTRITION
Calories 192,
Fat 7.2 g,
Carbs 14.4 g,
Protein 19.2 g

INGREDIENTS
- 4 oz chicken fillet
- 4 tomatoes, peeled
- 1 bell pepper, chopped
- 1 tsp. olive oil
- 1 cup of water
- 1 tsp. salt
- 1 chili pepper, chopped
- ½ tsp. saffron

DIRECTIONS
1. Pour water in the pan and bring it to boil.
2. Meanwhile, chop the chicken fillet.
3. Add the chicken fillet in the boiling water and cook it for 10 minutes or until the chicken is tender.
4. After this, put the chopped bell pepper and chili pepper in the skillet.
5. Add olive oil and roast the vegetables for 3 minutes.
6. Add chopped tomatoes and mix up well.
7. Cook the vegetables for 2 minutes more.
8. Then add salt and a ¾ cup of water from chicken.
9. Add chopped chicken fillet and mix up.
10. Cook the saute for 10 minutes over the medium heat.

413. Grilled Marinated Chicken

PREP TIME
35 mins

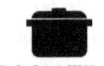
COOK TIME
20 mins

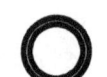
SERVINGS
6 people

NUTRITION

Calories 218,
Fat 8.2 g,
Carbs 0.4 g,
Protein 32.2 g

INGREDIENTS

- 2-lb. chicken breast, skinless, boneless
- 2 tbsp. lemon juice
- 1 tsp. sage
- ½ tsp. ground nutmeg
- ½ tsp. dried oregano
- 1 tsp. paprika
- 1 tsp. onion powder
- 2 tbsp. olive oil
- 1 tsp. chili flakes
- 1 tsp. salt
- 1 tsp. apple cider vinegar

DIRECTIONS

1. Make the marinade: whisk together apple cider vinegar, salt, chili flakes, olive oil, onion powder, paprika, dried oregano, ground nutmeg, sage, and lemon juice.
2. Then rub the chicken with marinade carefully and leave for 25 minutes to marinate.
3. Meanwhile, preheat grill to 385°F.
4. Place the marinated chicken breast in the grill and cook it for 10 minutes from each side.
5. Cut the cooked chicken on the servings.

414. Chicken Fillets with Artichoke Hearts

PREP TIME
10 mins

COOK TIME
30 mins

SERVINGS
3 people

NUTRITION

Calories 267,
Fat 8.2 g,
Carbs 10.4 g,
Protein 35.2 g

INGREDIENTS

- 1 can artichoke hearts, chopped
- 12 oz chicken fillets (3 oz each fillet)
- 1 tsp. avocado oil
- ½ tsp. ground thyme
- ½ tsp. white pepper
- 1/3 cup water
- 1/3 cup shallot, roughly chopped
- 1 lemon, sliced

DIRECTIONS

1. Mix up together chicken fillets, artichoke hearts, avocado oil, ground thyme, white pepper, and shallot.
2. Line the baking tray with baking paper and place the chicken fillet mixture in it.
3. Then add sliced lemon and water.
4. Bake the meal for 30 minutes at 375°F. Stir the ingredients during cooking to avoid burning.

415. Chicken Loaf

PREP TIME
10 mins

COOK TIME
40 mins

SERVINGS
4 people

NUTRITION

Calories 167,
Fat 6.2 g,
Carbs 3.4 g,
Protein 32.2 g

INGREDIENTS

- 2 cups ground chicken
- 1 egg, beaten
- 1 tbsp. fresh dill, chopped
- 1 garlic clove, chopped
- ½ tsp. salt
- 1 tsp. chili flakes
- 1 onion, minced

DIRECTIONS

1. In the mixing bowl combine together all ingredient and mix up until you get smooth mass.
2. Then line the loaf dish with baking paper and put the ground chicken mixture inside.
3. Flatten the surface well.
4. Bake the chicken loaf for 40 minutes at 355°F.
5. Then chill the chicken loaf to the room temperature and remove from the loaf dish. Slice it.

416. Chicken Meatballs with Carrot

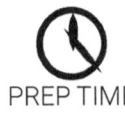
PREP TIME
10 mins

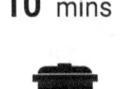
COOK TIME
10 mins

SERVINGS
8 people

NUTRITION

Calories 107,
Fat 4.2 g,
Carbs 4.6 g,
Protein 11.2 g

INGREDIENTS

- 1/3 cup carrot, grated
- 1 onion, diced
- 2 cups ground chicken
- 1 tbsp. semolina
- 1 egg, beaten
- ½ tsp. salt
- 1 tsp. dried oregano
- 1 tsp. dried cilantro
- 1 tsp. chili flakes
- 1 tbsp. coconut oil

DIRECTIONS

1. In the mixing bowl combine together grated carrot, diced onion, ground chicken, semolina, egg, salt, dried oregano, cilantro, and chili flakes.
2. With the help of scooper make the meatballs.
3. Heat up the coconut oil in the skillet.
4. When it starts to shimmer, put meatballs in it.
5. Cook the meatballs for 5 minutes from each side over the medium-low heat.

417. Chicken Burgers

PREP TIME
15 mins

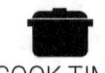
COOK TIME
15 mins

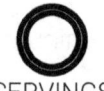
SERVINGS
4 people

NUTRITION

Calories 177,
Fat 5.2 g,
Carbs 10.4 g,
Protein 13.2 g

INGREDIENTS

- 8 oz ground chicken
- 1 cup fresh spinach, blended
- 1 tsp. minced onion
- ½ tsp. salt
- 1 red bell pepper, grinded
- 1 egg, beaten
- 1 tsp. ground black pepper
- 4 tbsp. Panko breadcrumbs

DIRECTIONS

1. In the mixing bowl mix up together ground chicken, blended spinach, minced garlic, salt, grinded bell pepper, egg, and ground black pepper.
2. When the chicken mixture is smooth, make 4 burgers from it and coat them in Panko breadcrumbs.
3. Place the burgers in the non-sticky baking dish or line the baking tray with baking paper.
4. Bake the burgers for 15 minutes at 365F.
5. Flip the chicken burgers on another side after 7 minutes of cooking.

418. Duck Patties

PREP TIME
15 mins

COOK TIME
10 mins

SERVINGS
8 people

NUTRITION

Calories 106,
Fat 5.2 g,
Carbs 6.2 g,
Protein 13.2 g

INGREDIENTS

- 1-lb. duck breast, skinless, boneless
- 1 tsp. semolina
- ½ tsp. cayenne pepper
- 2 eggs, beaten
- 1 tsp. salt
- 1 tbsp. fresh cilantro, chopped
- 1 tbsp. olive oil

DIRECTIONS

1. Chop the duck breast on the tiny pieces (grind it) and combine together with semolina, cayenne pepper, salt, and cilantro. Mix up well.
2. Then add eggs and stir gently.
3. Pour olive oil in the skillet and heat it up.
4. Place the duck mixture in the oil with the help of the spoon to make the shape of small patties.
5. Roast the patties for 3 minutes from each side over the medium heat.
6. Then close the lid and cook patties for 4 minutes more over the low heat.

419. Creamy Chicken Pate

PREP TIME: 2 hours
COOK TIME: 20 mins
SERVINGS: 6 people

INGREDIENTS
- 8 oz chicken liver
- 3 tbsp. butter
- 1 white onion, chopped
- 1 bay leaf
- 1 tsp. salt
- ½ tsp. ground black pepper
- ½ cup of water

DIRECTIONS
1. Place the chicken liver in the saucepan.
2. Add onion, bay leaf, salt, ground black pepper, and water.
3. Mix up the mixture and close the lid.
4. Cook the liver mixture for 20 minutes over the medium heat.
5. Then transfer it in the blender and blend until smooth.
6. Add butter and mix up until it is melted.
7. Pour the pate mixture in the pate ramekin and refrigerate for 2 hours.

NUTRITION
Calories 322, Fat 18.2 g, Carbs 12.7 g, Protein 19.2 g

420. Curry Chicken Drumsticks

PREP TIME: 10 mins
COOK TIME: 30 mins
SERVINGS: 4 people

INGREDIENTS
- 4 chicken drumsticks
- 1 apple, grated
- 1 tbsp. curry paste
- 4 tbsp. milk
- 1 tsp. coconut oil
- 1 tsp. chili flakes
- ½ tsp. minced ginger

DIRECTIONS
1. Mix up together grated apple, curry paste, milk, chili flakes, and minced garlic.
2. Put coconut oil in the skillet and melt it.
3. Add apple mixture and stir well.
4. Then add chicken drumsticks and mix up well.
5. Roast the chicken for 2 minutes from each side.
6. Then preheat oven to 360°F.
7. Place the skillet with chicken drumsticks in the oven and bake for 25 minutes.

NUTRITION
Calories 152, Fat 7.2 g, Carbs 9.4 g, Protein 13.2 g

421. Chicken Enchiladas

PREP TIME
20 mins

COOK TIME
15 mins

SERVINGS
5 people

NUTRITION

Calories 152,
Fat 5.2 g,
Carbs 16.5 g,
Protein 19.6 g

INGREDIENTS

- 5 corn tortillas
- 10 oz chicken breast, boiled, shredded
- 1 tsp. chipotle pepper
- 3 tbsp. green salsa
- ½ tsp. minced garlic
- ½ cup cream
- ¼ cup chicken stock
- 1 cup Mozzarella, shredded
- 1 tsp. butter, softened

DIRECTIONS

1. Mix up together shredded chicken breast, chipotle pepper, green salsa, and minced garlic.
2. Then put the shredded chicken mixture in the center of every corn tortilla and roll them.
3. Spread the baking dish with softened butter from inside and arrange the rolled corn tortillas.
4. Then pour chicken stock and cream over the tortillas.
5. Top them with shredded Mozzarella.
6. Bake the enchiladas for 15 minutes at 365°F.

422. Chicken Fajitas

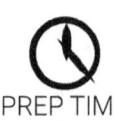
PREP TIME
15 mins

COOK TIME
15 mins

SERVINGS
2 people

NUTRITION

Calories 346,
Fat 14.2 g,
Carbs 23.4 g,
Protein 25.2 g

INGREDIENTS

- 1 bell pepper
- ½ red onion, peeled
- 5 oz chicken fillets
- 1 garlic clove, sliced
- 1 tbsp. olive oil
- 1 tsp. balsamic vinegar
- 1 tsp. chili pepper
- ½ tsp. salt
- 1 tsp. lemon juice
- 2 flour tortillas

DIRECTIONS

1. Cut the bell pepper and chicken fillet on the wedges.
2. Then slice the onion.
3. Pour olive oil in the skillet and heat it up.
4. Add chicken wedges and sprinkle them with chili pepper and salt.
5. Roast the chicken for 4 minutes. Stir it from time to time.
6. After this, add lemon juice and balsamic vinegar. Mix up well.
7. Add bell pepper, onion, and garlic clove.
8. Roast fajitas for 10 minutes over the medium-high heat. Stir it from time to time.
9. Put the cooked fajitas on the tortillas and transfer in the serving plates.

423. Chicken Stroganoff

PREP TIME
10 mins

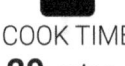
COOK TIME
20 mins

SERVINGS
4 people

NUTRITION

Calories 224,
Fat 9.2 g,
Carbs 7.4 g,
Protein 24.2 g

INGREDIENTS

- 1 cup cremini mushrooms, sliced
- 1 onion, sliced
- 1 tbsp. olive oil
- ½ tsp. thyme
- 1 tsp. salt
- 1 cup Plain yogurt
- 10 oz chicken fillet, chopped

DIRECTIONS

1. Heat up olive oil in the saucepan.
2. Add mushrooms and onion.
3. Sprinkle the vegetables with thyme and salt. Mix up well and cook them for 5 minutes.
4. After this, add chopped chicken fillet and mix up well.
5. Cook the ingredients for 5 minutes more.
6. Then add plain yogurt, mix up well, and close the lid.
7. Cook chicken stroganoff for 10 minutes over the low heat.

424. European Posole

PREP TIME
10 mins

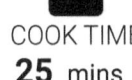
COOK TIME
25 mins

SERVINGS
2 people

NUTRITION

Calories 207,
Fat 8.3 g,
Carbs 6 g,
Protein 25.4 g

INGREDIENTS

- 1 ½ cup water
- 6 oz chicken fillet
- 1 chili pepper, chopped
- 1 onion, diced
- 1 tsp. butter
- ½ tsp. salt
- ½ tsp. paprika
- 1 tbsp. fresh dill, chopped

DIRECTIONS

1. Pour water in the saucepan.
2. Add chicken fillet and salt. Boil it for 15 minutes over the medium heat.
3. Then remove the chicken fillet from water and shred it with the help of the fork.
4. Return it back in the hot water.
5. Melt butter in the skillet and add diced onion. Roast it until light brown and transfer in the shredded chicken.
6. Add paprika, dill, chili pepper, and mix up.
7. Close the lid and simmer Posole for 5 minutes.

425. Mango Chicken Salad

PREP TIME
10 mins

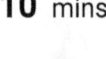
COOK TIME
12 mins

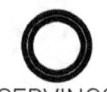
SERVINGS
3 people

NUTRITION

Calories 183,
Fat 5.2 g,
Carbs 17.4 g,
Protein 17.2 g

INGREDIENTS

- 1 cup lettuce, chopped
- 1 cup arugula, chopped
- 1 mango, peeled, chopped
- 8 oz chicken breast, skinless, boneless
- 1 tbsp. lime juice
- 1 tsp. sesame oil
- ½ tsp. salt
- ½ tsp. ground black pepper
- 1 tsp. butter

DIRECTIONS

1. Sprinkle the chicken breast with salt and ground black pepper.
2. Melt butter in the skillet and add chicken breast.
3. Roast it for 10 minutes over the medium heat. Flip it on another side from time to time.
4. Meanwhile, combine together lettuce, arugula, mango, and sesame oil in the salad bowl.
5. Add lime juice.
6. Chop the cooked chicken breast roughly and chill it to the room temperature.
7. Add it in the mango salad and mix up.

426. Chicken Zucchini Boats

PREP TIME
15 mins

COOK TIME
30 mins

SERVINGS
2 people

NUTRITION

Calories 134,
Fat 6.3 g,
Carbs: 7.1g
Protein 13.4 g

INGREDIENTS

- 1 zucchini
- ½ cup ground chicken
- ½ tsp. chipotle pepper
- ½ tsp. tomato sauce
- 1 oz Swiss cheese, shredded
- ½ tsp. salt
- 4 tbsp. water

DIRECTIONS

1. Trim the zucchini and cut it on 2 halves.
2. Remove the zucchini pulp.
3. In the mixing bowl mix up together ground chicken, chipotle pepper, tomato sauce, and salt.
4. Fill the zucchini with chicken mixture and top with Swiss cheese.
5. Place the zucchini boats in the tray. Add water.
6. Bake the boats for 30 minutes at 355°F.

427. Urban Chicken Alfredo

PREP TIME 10 mins
COOK TIME 20 mins
SERVINGS 2 people

NUTRITION
Calories 279,
Fat 14 g,
Carbs: 6.9 g
Protein 26.4 g

INGREDIENTS
- 1 onion, chopped
- 1 sweet red pepper, roasted, chopped
- 1 cup spinach, chopped
- ½ cup cream
- 1 tsp. cream cheese
- 1 tbsp. olive oil
- ½ tsp. ground black pepper
- 8 oz chicken breast, skinless, boneless, sliced

DIRECTIONS
1. Mix up together sliced chicken breast with ground black pepper and put in the saucepan.
2. Add olive oil and mix up.
3. Roast the chicken for 5 minutes over the medium-high heat. Stir it from time to time.
4. After this, add chopped sweet pepper, onion, and cream cheese.
5. Mix up well and bring to boil.
6. Add spinach and cream. Mix up well.
7. Close the lid and cook chicken Alfredo for 10 minutes more over the medium heat.

428. Tender Chicken Quesadilla

PREP TIME 10 mins
COOK TIME 20 mins
SERVINGS 4 people

NUTRITION
Calories 167,
Fat 8.2 g,
Carbs 16.4 g,
Protein 24.2 g

INGREDIENTS
- 2 bread tortillas
- 1 tsp. butter
- 2 tsp. olive oil
- 1 tsp. Taco seasoning
- 6 oz chicken breast, skinless, boneless, sliced
- 1/3 cup Cheddar cheese, shredded
- 1 bell pepper, cut on the wedges

DIRECTIONS
1. Pour 1 tsp. of olive oil in the skillet and add chicken.
2. Sprinkle the meat with Taco seasoning and mix up well.
3. Roast chicken for 10 minutes over the medium heat. Stir it from time to time.
4. Then transfer the cooked chicken in the plate.
5. Add remaining olive oil in the skillet.
6. Then add bell pepper and roast it for 5 minutes. Stir it all the time.
7. Mix up together bell pepper with chicken.
8. Toss butter in the skillet and melt it.
9. Put 1 tortilla in the skillet.
10. Put Cheddar cheese on the tortilla and flatten it.
11. Then add chicken-pepper mixture and cover it with the second tortilla.
12. Roast the quesadilla for 2 minutes from each side.
13. Cut the cooked meal on the halves and transfer in the serving plates.

429. Light Caesar

PREP TIME
10 mins

COOK TIME
10 mins

SERVINGS
4 people

NUTRITION
Calories 134,
Fat 13.3 g,
Carbs 2 g,
Protein 9.4 g

INGREDIENTS
- 4 oz chicken fillet, chopped
- ¼ cup black olives, chopped
- 2 cups lettuce, chopped
- 1 tbsp. mayo sauce
- 1 tsp. lemon juice
- ½ oz Parmesan cheese, shaved
- 1 tsp. olive oil
- ½ tsp. ground black pepper
- ½ tsp. coconut oil

DIRECTIONS
1. Sprinkle the chicken fillet with ground black pepper.
2. Heat up coconut oil and add chopped chicken fillet.
3. Roast it got 10 minutes or until it is cooked. Stir it from time to time.
4. Meanwhile, mix up together black olives, lettuce, Parmesan in the bowl.
5. Make mayo dressing: whisk together mayo sauce, olive oil, and lemon juice.
6. Add the cooked chicken in the salad and shake well.
7. Pour the mayo sauce dressing over the salad.

430. Chicken Parm

PREP TIME
10 mins

COOK TIME
30 mins

SERVINGS
4 people

NUTRITION
Calories 354,
Fat 21.3 g,
Carbs 12 g,
Protein 32.4 g

INGREDIENTS
- 4 chicken steaks (4 oz each steak)
- ½ cup crushed tomatoes
- ¼ cup fresh cilantro
- 1 garlic clove, diced
- ½ cup of water
- 1 onion, diced
- 1 tsp. olive oil
- 3 oz Parmesan, grated
- 3 tbsp. Panko breadcrumbs
- 2 eggs, beaten
- 1 tsp. ground black pepper

DIRECTIONS
1. Pour olive oil in the saucepan.
2. Add garlic and onion. Roast the vegetables for 3 minutes.
3. Then add fresh cilantro, crushed tomatoes, and water.
4. Simmer the mixture for 5 minutes.
5. Meanwhile, mix up together ground black pepper and eggs.
6. Dip the chicken steaks in the egg mixture.
7. Then coat them in Panko breadcrumbs and again in the egg mixture.
8. Coat the chicken steaks in grated Parmesan.
9. Place the prepared chicken steaks in the crushed tomato mixture.
10. Close the lid and cook chicken parm for 20 minutes. Flip the chicken steaks after 10 minutes of cooking.
11. Serve the chicken parm with crushed tomatoes sauce.

431. Chicken Bolognese

PREP TIME
7 mins

COOK TIME
25 mins

SERVINGS
4 people

NUTRITION

Calories 154,
Fat 9.3 g,
Carbs 6 g,
Protein 15.4 g

INGREDIENTS

- 1 cup ground chicken
- 2 oz Parmesan, grated
- 1 tbsp. olive oil
- 2 tbsp. fresh parsley, chopped
- 1 tsp. chili pepper
- 1 tsp. paprika
- ½ tsp. dried oregano
- ¼ tsp. garlic, minced
- ½ tsp. dried thyme
- 1/3 cup crushed tomatoes

DIRECTIONS

1. Heat up olive oil in the skillet.
2. Add ground chicken and sprinkle it with chili pepper, paprika, dried oregano, dried thyme, and parsley. Mix up well.
3. Cook the chicken for 5 minutes and add crushed tomatoes. Mix up well.
4. Close the lid and simmer the chicken mixture for 10 minutes over the low heat.
5. Then add grated Parmesan and mix up.
6. Cook chicken bolognese for 5 minutes more over the medium heat.

432. Jerk Chicken

PREP TIME
10 mins

COOK TIME
30 mins

SERVINGS
2 people

NUTRITION

Calories 139,
Fat 7.3 g,
Carbs 4 g,
Protein 19.4 g

INGREDIENTS

- 2 chicken thighs, skinless, boneless
- 1 tsp. fresh ginger, chopped
- 1 garlic clove, chopped
- ½ spring onion, chopped
- 1 tsp. liquid honey
- 1 tsp. fresh parsley, chopped
- 1 tsp. fresh coriander, chopped
- ¼ tsp. chili flakes
- ¼ tsp. ground black pepper
- 2 tsp. lemon juice

DIRECTIONS

1. Mix up together fresh ginger, garlic, onion, liquid honey, parsley, coriander, chili flakes, and ground black pepper.
2. Rub the chicken thighs with honey mixture generously.
3. Preheat the grill to 385°F.
4. Place the chicken thighs in the grill and cook for 30 minutes. Flip the chicken thighs on another side after 15 minutes of cooking. The cooked jerk chicken should have a brown crust.
5. Sprinkle the cooked chicken with lemon juice.

433. Crack Chicken

PREP TIME
10 mins

COOK TIME
30 mins

SERVINGS
4 people

NUTRITION

Calories 79,
Fat 7.3 g,
Carbs 1 g,
Protein 2.4 g

INGREDIENTS

- 4 chicken thighs, skinless, boneless
- 1 tsp. ground black pepper
- ½ tsp. salt
- 1 tsp. paprika
- ¼ cup Cheddar cheese, shredded
- 1 tbsp. cream cheese
- ½ tsp. garlic powder
- 1 tsp. fresh dill, chopped
- 1 tbsp. butter
- 1 tsp. olive oil
- ½ tsp. ground nutmeg

DIRECTIONS

1. Grease the baking dish with butter.
2. Then heat up olive oil in the skillet.
3. Meanwhile, rub the chicken thighs with ground nutmeg, garlic powder, paprika, and salt. Add ground black pepper.
4. Roast the chicken thighs in the hot oil over the high heat for 2 minutes from each side.
5. Then transfer the chicken thighs in the prepared baking dish.
6. Mix up together Cheddar cheese, cream cheese, and dill.
7. Top every chicken thigh with cheese mixture and bake for 25 minutes at 365°F.

434. Pomegranate Chicken Thighs

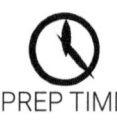
PREP TIME
10 mins

COOK TIME
10 mins

SERVINGS
2 people

NUTRITION

Calories 374,
Fat 21.3 g,
Carbs 9 g,
Protein 30.4 g

INGREDIENTS

- 1 tbsp. pomegranate molasses
- 8 oz chicken thighs (4 oz each chicken thigh)
- ½ tsp. paprika
- 1 tsp. cornstarch
- ½ tsp. chili flakes
- ½ tsp. ground black pepper
- 1 tsp. olive oil
- ½ tsp. lime juice

DIRECTIONS

1. In the shallow bowl mix up together ground black pepper, chili flakes, paprika, and cornstarch.
2. Rub the chicken thighs with spice mixture.
3. Heat up olive oil in the skillet.
4. Add chicken thighs and roast them for 4 minutes from each side over the medium heat.
5. When the chicken thighs are light brown, sprinkle them with pomegranate molasses and roast for 1 minute from each side.

435. Butter Chicken

PREP TIME: 15 mins
COOK TIME: 30 mins
SERVINGS: 5 people

NUTRITION
Calories 254,
Fat 19.3 g,
Carbs 1 g,
Protein 36.4 g

INGREDIENTS
- 1-lb. chicken fillet
- 1/3 cup butter, softened
- 1 tbsp. rosemary
- ½ tsp. thyme
- 1 tsp. salt
- ½ lemon

DIRECTIONS
1. Churn together thyme, salt, and rosemary.
2. Chop the chicken fillet roughly and mix up with churned butter mixture.
3. Place the prepared chicken in the baking dish.
4. Squeeze the lemon over the chicken.
5. Chop the squeezed lemon and add in the baking dish.
6. Cover the chicken with foil and bake it for 20 minutes at 365°F.
7. Then discard the foil and bake the chicken for 10 minutes more.

436. Santa le Skillet Chicken

PREP TIME: 10 mins
COOK TIME: 20 mins
SERVINGS: 4 people

NUTRITION
Calories 184,
Fat 6.3 g,
Carbs 13 g,
Protein 22.4 g

INGREDIENTS
- 12 oz chicken breast, skinless, boneless, chopped
- 1 tbsp. taco seasoning
- 1 tbsp. nut oil
- ½ tsp. cayenne pepper
- ½ tsp. salt
- ½ tsp. garlic, chopped
- ½ red onion, sliced
- 1/3 cup black beans, canned, rinsed
- ½ cup Mozzarella, shredded

DIRECTIONS
1. Rub the chopped chicken breast with taco seasoning, salt, and cayenne pepper.
2. Place the chicken in the skillet, add nut oil and roast it for 10 minutes over the medium heat. Mix up the chicken pieces from time to time to avoid burning.
3. After this, transfer the chicken in the plate.
4. Add sliced onion and garlic in the skillet. Roast the vegetables for 5 minutes. Stir them constantly. Then add black beans and stir well. Cook the ingredients for 2 minute more.
5. Add the chopped chicken and mix up well. Top the meal with Mozzarella cheese.
6. Close the lid and cook the meal for 3 minutes.

437. Tender Lamb Chops

PREP TIME
10 mins

COOK TIME
6 hours

SERVINGS
8 people

INGREDIENTS

- 8 lamb chops
- ½ tsp. dried thyme
- 1 onion, sliced
- 1 tsp. dried oregano
- 2 garlic cloves, minced
- Pepper and salt

DIRECTIONS

1. Add sliced onion into the slow cooker.
2. Combine together thyme, oregano, pepper, and salt. Rub over lamb chops.
3. Place lamb chops in slow cooker and top with garlic.
4. Pour ¼ cup water around the lamb chops.
5. Cover and cook on low for 6 hours.
6. Serve and enjoy.

NUTRITION

Calories 140
Fat 9.9 g
Carbs 5.3 g
Protein 34 g

438. Smoky Pork & Cabbage

PREP TIME
10 mins

COOK TIME
8 hours

SERVINGS
6 people

INGREDIENTS

- 3 lbs pork roast
- 1/2 cabbage head, chopped
- 1 cup water
- 1/3 cup liquid smoke
- 1 tbsp. kosher salt

DIRECTIONS

1. Rub pork with kosher salt and place into the crock pot.
2. Pour liquid smoke over the pork. Add water.
3. Cover and cook on low for 7 hours.
4. Remove pork from crock pot and add cabbage in the bottom of crock pot.
5. Place pork on top of the cabbage.
6. Cover again and cook for 1 hour more.
7. Shred pork with a fork and serve.

NUTRITION

Calories 484
Fat 21.5 g
Carbs 9g
Protein 66 g

439. Seasoned Pork Chops

PREP TIME 10 mins
COOK TIME 4 hours
SERVINGS 4 people

INGREDIENTS

- 4 pork chops
- 2 garlic cloves, minced
- 1 cup chicken broth
- 1 tbsp. poultry seasoning
- 1/4 cup olive oil
- Pepper and salt

DIRECTIONS

1. In a bowl, whisk together olive oil, poultry seasoning, garlic, broth, pepper, and salt.
2. Pour olive oil mixture into the slow cooker then place pork chops to the crock pot.
3. Cover and cook on high for 4 hours. Serve and enjoy.

NUTRITION

Calories 386
Fat 32.9 g
Carbs 3 g
Protein 20 g

440. Beef Stroganoff

PREP TIME 10 mins
COOK TIME 8 hours
SERVINGS 2 people

INGREDIENTS

- 1/2 lb beef stew meat
- 10 oz mushroom soup, homemade
- 1 medium onion, chopped
- 1/2 cup sour cream
- 2.5oz mushrooms, sliced
- Pepper and salt

DIRECTIONS

1. Add all ingredients except sour cream into the crock pot and mix well.
2. Cover and cook on low for 8 hours.
3. Add sour cream and stir well.

NUTRITION

Calories 470
Fat 25 g
Carbs 8.6 g
Protein 49 g

441. Lemon Beef

PREP TIME
10 mins

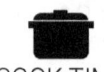
COOK TIME
6 hours

SERVINGS
4 people

INGREDIENTS

- 1 lb beef chuck roast
- 1 fresh lime juice
- 1 garlic clove, crushed
- 1 tsp. chili powder
- 2 cups lemon-lime soda
- 1/2 tsp. salt

DIRECTIONS

1. Place beef chuck roast into the slow cooker.
2. Season roast with garlic, chili powder, and salt.
3. Pour lemon-lime soda over the roast.
4. Cover slow cooker with lid and cook on low for 6 hours. Shred the meat using fork.
5. Add lime juice over shredded roast and serve.

NUTRITION

Calories 355
Fat 16.8 g
Carbs 14 g
Protein 35.5 g

442. Herb Pork Roast

PREP TIME
10 mins

COOK TIME
14 hours

SERVINGS
10 people

INGREDIENTS

- 5 lbs pork roast, boneless or bone-in
- 1 tbsp. dry herb mix
- 4 garlic cloves, cut into slivers
- 1 tbsp. salt

DIRECTIONS

1. Using a sharp knife make small cuts all over meat then insert garlic slivers into the cuts.
2. In a small bowl, mix together Italian herb mix and salt and rub all over pork roast.
3. Place pork roast in the crock pot.
4. Cover and cook on low for 14 hours.
5. Remove meat from crock pot and shred using a fork.
6. Serve and enjoy.

NUTRITION

Calories 327
Fat 8 g
Carbs 0.5 g
Protein 59 g

443. Greek Beef Roast

PREP TIME: 10 mins
COOK TIME: 8 hours
SERVINGS: 6 people

INGREDIENTS
- 2 lbs lean top round beef roast
- 1 tbsp. Italian seasoning
- 6 garlic cloves, minced
- 1 onion, sliced
- 2 cups beef broth
- ½ cup red wine
- 1 tsp. red pepper flakes
- Pepper
- Salt

DIRECTIONS
1. Season meat with pepper and salt and place into the crock pot.
2. Pour remaining ingredients over meat.
3. Cover and cook on low for 8 hours.
4. Shred the meat using fork.
5. Serve and enjoy.

NUTRITION
Calories 231
Fat 6 g
Carbs 4 g
Protein 35 g

444. Tomato Pork Chops

PREP TIME: 10 mins
COOK TIME: 6 hours
SERVINGS: 4 people

INGREDIENTS
- 4 pork chops, bone-in
- 1 tbsp. garlic, minced
- ½ small onion, chopped
- 6 oz can tomato paste
- 1 bell pepper, chopped
- ¼ tsp. red pepper flakes
- 1 tsp. Worcestershire sauce
- 1 tbsp. dried Italian seasoning
- oz can tomatoes, diced
- 2 tsp. olive oil
- ¼ tsp. pepper
- 1 tsp. kosher salt

DIRECTIONS
1. Heat oil in a pan over medium-high heat.
2. Season pork chops with pepper and salt.
3. Sear pork chops in pan until brown from both the sides.
4. Transfer pork chops into the crock pot.
5. Add remaining ingredients over pork chops.
6. Cover and cook on low for 6 hours.
7. Serve and enjoy.

NUTRITION
Calories 325
Fat 23.4 g
Carbs 10 g
Protein 20 g

445. Greek Pork Chops

PREP TIME
10 mins

COOK TIME
6 mins

SERVINGS
8 people

NUTRITION

Calories 324
Fat 26.5 g
Carbs 2.5 g
Protein 18 g

INGREDIENTS

- 8 pork chops, boneless
- 4 tsp. dried oregano
- 2 tbsp. Worcestershire sauce
- 3 tbsp. fresh lemon juice
- ¼ cup olive oil
- 1 tsp. ground mustard
- 2 tsp. garlic powder
- 2 tsp. onion powder
- Pepper
- Salt

DIRECTIONS

1. Whisk together oil, garlic powder, onion powder, oregano, Worcestershire sauce, lemon juice, mustard, pepper, and salt.
2. Place pork chops in a baking dish then pour marinade over pork chops and coat well. Place in refrigerator overnight.
3. Preheat the grill.
4. Place pork chops on hot grill and cook for 3-4 minutes on each side.
5. Serve and enjoy.

446. Pork Cacciatore

PREP TIME
10 mins

COOK TIME
6 hours

SERVINGS
6 people

INGREDIENTS

- 1 ½ lbs pork chops
- 1 tsp. dried oregano
- 1 cup beef broth
- 3 tbsp. tomato paste
- 14 oz can tomatoes, diced
- 2 cups mushrooms, sliced
- 1 small onion, diced
- 1 garlic clove, minced
- 2 tbsp. olive oil
- ¼ tsp. pepper
- ½ tsp. salt

DIRECTIONS

1. Heat oil in a pan over medium-high heat.
2. Add pork chops in pan and cook until brown on both the sides.
3. Transfer pork chops into the crock pot.
4. Pour remaining ingredients over the pork chops.
5. Cover and cook on low for 6 hours.
6. Serve and enjoy.

NUTRITION

Calories 440
Fat 33 g
Carbs 6 g
Protein 28 g

447. Pork with Tomato & Olives

PREP TIME: 10 mins
COOK TIME: 30 mins
SERVINGS: 6 people

INGREDIENTS

- 6 pork chops, boneless and cut into thick slices
- 1/8 tsp. ground cinnamon
- 1/2 cup olives, pitted and sliced
- 8 oz can tomatoes, crushed
- 1/4 cup beef broth
- 2 garlic cloves, chopped
- 1 large onion, sliced
- 1 tbsp. olive oil

DIRECTIONS

1. Heat olive oil in a pan over medium-high heat.
2. Place pork chops in a pan and cook until lightly brown and set aside.
3. Cook garlic and onion in the same pan over medium heat, until onion is softened.
4. Add broth and bring to boil over high heat.
5. Return pork to pan and stir in crushed tomatoes and remaining ingredients.
6. Cover and simmer for 20 minutes.
7. Serve and enjoy.

NUTRITION

Calories 321
Fat 23 g
Carbs 7 g
Protein 19 g

---

448. Pork Roast

PREP TIME: 10 mins
COOK TIME: 95 mins
SERVINGS: 6 people

INGREDIENTS

- 3 lbs pork roast, boneless
- 1 cup water
- 1 onion, chopped
- 3 garlic cloves, chopped
- 1 tbsp. black pepper
- 1 rosemary sprig
- 2 fresh oregano sprigs
- 2 fresh thyme sprigs
- 1 tbsp. olive oil
- 1 tbsp. kosher salt

DIRECTIONS

1. Preheat the oven to 350°F.
2. Season pork roast with pepper and salt.
3. Heat olive oil in a stockpot and sear pork roast on each side, about 4 minutes.
4. Add onion and garlic. Pour in the water, oregano, and thyme and bring to boil for a minute.
5. Cover pot and roast in the preheated oven for 1 1/2 hours.
6. Serve and enjoy.

NUTRITION

Calories 502
Fat 23.8 g
Carbs 3 g
Protein 65 g

449. Easy Beef Kofta

PREP TIME
10 mins

COOK TIME
10 mins

SERVINGS
8 people

NUTRITION

Calories 223
Fat 7.3 g
Carbs 2.5 g
Protein 35 g

INGREDIENTS

- 2 lbs ground beef
- 4 garlic cloves, minced
- 1 onion, minced
- 2 tsp. cumin
- 1 cup fresh parsley, chopped
- ¼ tsp. pepper
- 1 tsp. salt

DIRECTIONS

1. Add all ingredients into the mixing bowl and mix until combined.
2. Roll meat mixture into the kabab shapes and cook in a hot pan for 4-6 minutes on each side or until cooked.
3. Serve and enjoy.

450. Lemon Pepper Pork Tenderloin

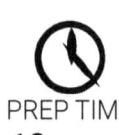

PREP TIME
10 mins

COOK TIME
25 mins

SERVINGS
4 people

NUTRITION

Calories 215
Fat 9.1 g
Carbs 1 g
Protein 30.8 g

INGREDIENTS

- 1 lb pork tenderloin
- 3/4 tsp. lemon pepper
- 2 tsp. dried oregano
- 1 tbsp. olive oil
- 3 tbsp. feta cheese, crumbled
- 3 tbsp. olive tapenade

DIRECTIONS

1. Add pork, oil, lemon pepper, and oregano in a zip-lock bag and rub well and place in a refrigerator for 2 hours.
2. Remove pork from zip-lock bag. Using sharp knife make lengthwise cut through the center of the tenderloin.
3. Spread olive tapenade on half tenderloin and sprinkle with feta cheese.
4. Fold another half of meat over to the original shape of tenderloin.
5. Tie close pork tenderloin with twine at 2-inch intervals.
6. Grill pork tenderloin for 20 minutes.
7. Cut into slices and serve.

451. Jalapeno Lamb Patties

PREP TIME: 10 mins
COOK TIME: 8 mins
SERVINGS: 4 people

INGREDIENTS
- 1 lb ground lamb
- 1 jalapeno pepper, minced
- 5 basil leaves, minced
- 10 mint leaves, minced
- ¼ cup fresh parsley, chopped
- 1 cup feta cheese, crumbled
- 1 tbsp. garlic, minced
- 1 tsp. dried oregano
- ¼ tsp. pepper
- ½ tsp. kosher salt

DIRECTIONS
1. Add all ingredients into the mixing bowl and mix until well combined.
2. Preheat the grill to 450°F.
3. Spray grill with cooking spray.
4. Make four equal shape patties from meat mixture and place on hot grill and cook for 3 minutes. Turn patties to another side and cook for 4 minutes.
5. Serve and enjoy.

NUTRITION
Calories 317
Fat 16 g
Carbs 3 g
Protein 37.5 g

---

452. Basil Parmesan Pork Roast

PREP TIME: 10 mins
COOK TIME: 6 hours
SERVINGS: 8 people

INGREDIENTS
- 2 lbs lean pork roast, boneless
- 1 tbsp. parsley
- ½ cup parmesan cheese, grated
- 28 oz can tomatoes, diced
- 1 tsp. dried oregano
- 1 tsp. dried basil
- 1 tsp. garlic powder
- Pepper
- Salt

DIRECTIONS
1. Add the meat into the crock pot.
2. Mix together tomatoes, oregano, basil, garlic powder, parsley, cheese, pepper, and salt and pour over meat.
3. Cover and cook on low for 6 hours.
4. Serve and enjoy.

NUTRITION
Calories 294
Fat 11.6 g
Carbs 5 g
Protein 38 g

453. Sun-dried Tomato Chuck Roast

PREP TIME
10 mins

COOK TIME
10 hours

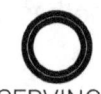
SERVINGS
6 people

INGREDIENTS

- 2 lbs beef chuck roast
- ½ cup beef broth
- ¼ cup sun-dried tomatoes, chopped
- 25 garlic cloves, peeled
- ¼ cup olives, sliced
- 1 tsp. dried Italian seasoning, crushed
- 2 tbsp. balsamic vinegar

DIRECTIONS

1. Place meat into the crock pot.
2. Pour remaining ingredients over meat.
3. Cover and cook on low for 10 hours.
4. Shred the meat using fork.
5. Serve and enjoy.

NUTRITION

Calories 582
Fat 43 g
Carbs 5 g
Protein 40g

454. Lemon Lamb Leg

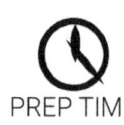
PREP TIME
10 mins

COOK TIME
8 hours

SERVINGS
12 people

INGREDIENTS

- 4 lbs lamb leg, boneless and slice of Fat
- 1 tbsp. rosemary, crushed
- 1/4 cup water
- 1/4 cup lemon juice
- 1 tsp. black pepper
- 1/4 tsp. salt

DIRECTIONS

1. Place lamb into the crock pot.
2. Add remaining ingredients into the crock pot over the lamb.
3. Cover and cook on low for 8 hours.
4. Remove lamb from crock pot and sliced.
5. Serve and enjoy.

NUTRITION

Calories 275
Fat 10.2 g
Carbs 0.4 g
Protein 42 g

455. Lamb Stew

PREP TIME
10 mins

COOK TIME
8 hours

SERVINGS
2 people

NUTRITION

Calories 297
Fat 20.3 g
Carbs 5.4 g
Protein 21 g

INGREDIENTS

- 1/2 lb lamb, boneless and cubed
- 1/4 cup green olives, sliced
- 2 tbsp. lemon juice
- 1/2 onion, chopped
- 2 garlic cloves, minced
- 2 fresh thyme sprigs
- 1/4 tsp. turmeric
- 1/2 tsp. pepper
- 1/4 tsp. salt

DIRECTIONS

1. Add all ingredients into the crock pot and stir well.
2. Cover and cook on low for 8 hours. Stir well and serve.

456. Flavorful Beef Stew

PREP TIME
10 mins

COOK TIME
125 mins

SERVINGS
4 people

NUTRITION

Calories 630
Fat 20.3 g
Carbs 7 g
Protein 69.2 g

INGREDIENTS

- 2 lbs beef chuck, diced into chunks
- 3 thyme sprigs
- 2 bay leaves
- oz olives, pitted
- 3 cups red wine
- 2 garlic cloves, chopped
- 2 tbsp. olive oil
- Pepper
- Salt

DIRECTIONS

1. Season meat with pepper and salt.
2. Heat oil in a pan over high heat.
3. Add meat in hot oil and sear for 3-4 minutes on each side.
4. Add bay leaves, half red wine, garlic, and thyme. Bring to boil, turn heat to low and simmer for 90 minutes. Remove pan from heat.
5. Add olives and remaining red wine. Stir well.
6. Return pan on heat and simmer for 30 minutes more.
7. Serve hot and enjoy.

457. Herb Ground Beef

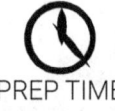
PREP TIME
10 mins

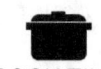
COOK TIME
15 mins

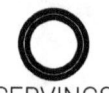
SERVINGS
4 people

NUTRITION

Calories 215
Fat 7.2 g
Carbs 1 g
Protein 34 g

INGREDIENTS

- 1 lb ground beef
- ½ tsp. dried parsley
- ½ tsp. dried basil
- ½ tsp. dried oregano
- 1 tsp. garlic, minced
- 1 tbsp. olive oil
- 1 tsp. pepper
- ¼ tsp. nutmeg
- ½ tsp. dried thyme
- ½ tsp. dried rosemary
- 1 tsp. salt

DIRECTIONS

1. Heat oil in a pan over medium heat.
2. Add ground meat to the pan and fry until cooked.
3. Add remaining ingredients and stir well.
4. Serve and enjoy.

458. Olive Feta Beef

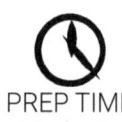
PREP TIME
10 mins

COOK TIME
6 hours

SERVINGS
8 people

NUTRITION

Calories 370
Fat 14 g
Carbs 9 g
Protein 49.1 g

INGREDIENTS

- 2 lbs beef stew meat, cut into half-inch pieces
- 1 cup olives, pitted and cut in half
- 30 oz can tomatoes, diced
- 1/2 cup feta cheese, crumbled
- 1/4 tsp. pepper
- 1/2 tsp. salt

DIRECTIONS

1. Add all ingredients into the crock pot and stir well.
2. Cover and cook on high for 6 hours.
3. Season with pepper and salt.
4. Stir well and serve.

459. Italian Beef Casserole

PREP TIME: 10 mins
COOK TIME: 90 mins
SERVINGS: 6 people

INGREDIENTS

- 1 lb lean stew beef, cut into chunks
- 3 tsp. paprika
- 4 oz black olives, sliced
- 7 oz can tomatoes, chopped
- 1 tbsp. tomato puree
- 1/4 tsp. garlic powder
- 2 tsp. herb de Provence
- 2 cups beef stock
- 2 tbsp. olive oil

DIRECTIONS

1. Preheat the oven to 350°F.
2. Heat oil in a pan over medium heat.
3. Add meat to the pan and cook until brown.
4. Add stock, olives, tomatoes, tomato puree, garlic powder, herb de Provence, and paprika. Stir well and bring to boil.
5. Transfer meat mixture to the casserole dish.
6. Cover and cook in preheated oven for 1 1/2 hours.
7. Serve and enjoy.

NUTRITION
Calories 228
Fat 11.6 g
Carbs 6 g
Protein 26 g

---

460. Roasted Sirloin Steak

PREP TIME: 10 mins
COOK TIME: 30 mins
SERVINGS: 6 people

INGREDIENTS

- 2 lbs sirloin steak, cut into 1" cubes
- 2 garlic cloves, minced
- 3 tbsp. fresh lemon juice
- 1 tsp. dried oregano
- 1/4 cup water
- 1/4 cup olive oil
- 2 cups fresh parsley, chopped
- 1/2 tsp. pepper
- 1 tsp. salt

DIRECTIONS

1. Add all ingredients except beef into the large bowl and mix well.
2. Pour bowl mixture into the large zip-lock bag.
3. Add beef to the bag and shake well and refrigerate for 1 hour.
4. Preheat the oven 400°F.
5. Place marinated beef on a baking tray and bake in preheated oven for 30 minutes.
6. Serve and enjoy.

NUTRITION
Calories 365
Fat 18.1 g
Carbs 2 g
Protein 46.6 g

461. Easy Pork Kabobs

PREP TIME
10 mins

COOK TIME
4 hours **20** mins

SERVINGS
6 people

INGREDIENTS

- 2 lbs pork tenderloin, cut into 1-inch cubes
- 1 onion, chopped
- ½ cup olive oil
- ½ cup red wine vinegar
- 2 tbsp. fresh parsley, chopped
- 2 garlic cloves, chopped
- Pepper
- Salt

DIRECTIONS

1. In a large zip-lock bag, mix together red wine vinegar, parsley, garlic, onion, and oil.
2. Add meat to bag and marinate in the refrigerator for overnight.
3. Remove marinated pork from refrigerator and thread onto soaked wooden skewers. Season with pepper and salt.
4. Preheat the grill over high heat.
5. Grill pork for 3-4 minutes on each side.
6. Serve and enjoy.

NUTRITION

Calories 375
Fat 22 g
Carbs 7.5 g
Protein 58.5 g

462. Meatballs

PREP TIME
10 mins

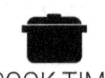
COOK TIME
4 hours

SERVINGS
6 people

INGREDIENTS

- 1 egg
- 2 tbsp. fresh parsley, chopped
- 1 garlic clove, minced
- ½ lb ground beef
- ½ lb ground pork
- 14 oz can tomatoes, crushed
- 2 tbsp. fresh basil, chopped
- ¼ tsp. pepper
- ½ tsp. salt

DIRECTIONS

1. In a mixing bowl, mix together beef, pork, egg, parsley, garlic, pepper, and salt until well combined.
2. Make small balls from meat mixture.
3. Arrange meatballs into the slow cooker.
4. Pour crushed tomatoes, basil, pepper, and salt over meatballs.
5. Cover and cook on low for 4 hours.
6. Serve and enjoy.

NUTRITION

Calories 150
Fat 4 g
Carbs 4 g
Protein 24 g

463. Baked Patties

PREP TIME
10 mins

COOK TIME
15 mins

SERVINGS
4 people

NUTRITION

Calories 112
Fat 4.3 g
Carbs 1.3 g
Protein 16 g

INGREDIENTS

- 1 lb ground lamb
- 1 tsp. ground coriander
- 1 tsp. ground cumin
- ¼ cup fresh parsley, chopped
- ¼ cup onion, minced
- ¼ tsp. cayenne pepper
- ½ tsp. ground allspice
- 1 tsp. ground cinnamon
- 1 tbsp. garlic, minced
- ¼ tsp. pepper
- 1 tsp. kosher salt

DIRECTIONS

1. Preheat the oven to 450°F.
2. Add all ingredients into the large bowl and mix until well combined.
3. Make small balls from meat mixture and place on a baking tray and lightly flatten the meatballs with back on spoon.
4. Bake in preheated oven for 12-15 minutes.
5. Serve and enjoy.

464. Keto Beef Patties

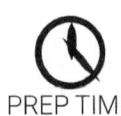
PREP TIME
10 mins

COOK TIME
8 mins

SERVINGS
5 people

NUTRITION

Calories 188
Fat 6.6 g
Carbs 1.7 g
Protein 28.9 g

INGREDIENTS

- 1 lb ground beef
- 1 egg, lightly beaten
- 3 tbsp. almond flour
- 1 small onion, grated
- 2 tbsp. fresh parsley, chopped
- 1 tsp. dry oregano
- 1 tsp. dry mint
- Pepper
- Salt

DIRECTIONS

1. Add all ingredients into the mixing bowl and mix until combined.
2. Make small patties from the meat mixture.
3. Heat grill pan over medium-high heat.
4. Place patties in a hot pan and cook for 4-5 minutes on each side.
5. Serve and enjoy.

465. Tender & Juicy Lamb Roast

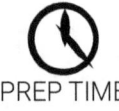
PREP TIME
10 mins

COOK TIME
8 hours

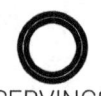
SERVINGS
8 people

INGREDIENTS

- 4 lbs lamb roast, boneless
- ½ tsp. thyme
- 1 tsp. oregano
- 4 garlic cloves, cut into slivers
- ½ tsp. marjoram
- ¼ tsp. pepper
- 2 tsp. salt

DIRECTIONS

1. Using a sharp knife make small cuts all over meat then insert garlic slivers into the cuts.
2. In a small bowl, mix together marjoram, thyme, oregano, pepper, and salt and rub all over lamb roast.
3. Place lamb roast into the slow cooker.
4. Cover and cook on low for 8 hours.
5. Serve and enjoy.

NUTRITION

Calories 605
Fat 48 g
Carbs 0.7 g
Protein 36 g

466. Basil Cheese Pork Roast

PREP TIME
10 mins

COOK TIME
6 hours

SERVINGS
8 people

INGREDIENTS

- 2 lbs lean pork roast, boneless
- 1 tsp. garlic powder
- 1 tbsp. parsley
- ½ cup cheddar cheese, grated
- 30 oz can tomatoes, diced
- 1 tsp. dried oregano
- 1 tsp. dried basil
- Pepper
- Salt

DIRECTIONS

1. Add the meat into the crock pot.
2. Mix together tomatoes, oregano, basil, garlic powder, parsley, cheese, pepper, and salt and pour over meat.
3. Cover and cook on low for 6 hours.
4. Serve and enjoy.

NUTRITION

Calories 260
Fat 9 g
Carbs 5.5 g
Protein 35 g

467. Feta Lamb Patties

PREP TIME: 10 mins
COOK TIME: 12 mins
SERVINGS: 4 people

INGREDIENTS

- 1 lb ground lamb
- 1/2 tsp. garlic powder
- 1/2 cup feta cheese, crumbled
- 1/4 cup mint leaves, chopped
- 1/4 cup roasted red pepper, chopped
- 1/4 cup onion, chopped
- Pepper
- Salt

DIRECTIONS

1. Add all ingredients into the bowl and mix until well combined.
2. Spray pan with cooking spray and heat over medium-high heat.
3. Make small patties from meat mixture and place on hot pan and cook for 6-7 minutes on each side.
4. Serve and enjoy.

NUTRITION
Calories 270
Fat 12 g
Carbs 2.9 g
Protein 34.9 g

---

468. BBQ Pulled Chicken

PREP TIME: 10 mins
COOK TIME: 45 mins
SERVINGS: 6 people

INGREDIENTS

- 1.5-lb. chicken breast, skinless, boneless
- 2 tbsp. BBQ sauce
- 1 tbsp. butter
- 1 tsp. Dijon mustard
- 1 tbsp. olive oil
- 1 tsp. cream cheese
- 1 tsp. salt
- 1 tsp. cayenne pepper

DIRECTIONS

1. Sprinkle the chicken breast with cayenne pepper, salt, and olive oil.
2. Place it in the baking tray and bake for 35 minutes at 365°F. Flip it from time to time to avoid burning.
3. When the chicken breast is cooked, transfer it on the chopping board and shred with the help of the fork.
4. Put the shredded chicken in the saucepan.
5. Add butter, cream cheese, mustard, and BBQ sauce. Mix up gently and heat it up until boiling.
6. Remove the cooked meal from the heat and stir well.

NUTRITION
Calories 154,
Fat 7.3 g,
Carbs 2 g,
Protein 24.4 g

469. Flavorful Lemon Chicken Tacos

PREP TIME
10 mins

COOK TIME
4 hours

SERVINGS
8 people

INGREDIENTS

- 2 lbs chicken breasts, boneless
- oz salsa
- 1 tbsp. taco seasoning, homemade
- 2 fresh lime juice
- 1/4 cup fresh parsley, chopped
- 1/4 tsp. red chili powder
- Pepper
- Salt

DIRECTIONS

1. Place chicken into the crockpot.
2. Pour ingredients over the chicken.
3. Cover and cook on high for 4 hours.
4. Shred the chicken using a fork and serve.

NUTRITION

Calories 235
Fat 8 g
Carbs 5 g
Protein 30 g

470. Crisp Chicken Carnitas

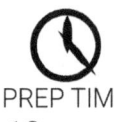
PREP TIME
10 mins

COOK TIME
4 hours

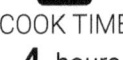
SERVINGS
8 people

INGREDIENTS

- 2 lbs chicken breasts, skinless and boneless
- 1/4 cup fresh parsley, chopped
- 1 tbsp. garlic, minced
- 2 tsp. cumin powder
- 2 tbsp. fresh lime juice
- 1 tbsp. chili powder
- 1/2 tsp. salt

DIRECTIONS

1. Add chicken into the crockpot.
2. Pour remaining ingredients over the chicken.
3. Cover and cook on high for 4 hours.
4. Shred the chicken using a fork.
5. Transfer shredded chicken on a baking tray and broil for 5 minutes.
6. Serve and enjoy.

NUTRITION

Calories 225
Fat 8.7 g
Carbs 2.1 g
Protein 33.2 g

471. Cilantro Lime Chicken Salad

PREP TIME: 10 mins
COOK TIME: 5 mins
SERVINGS: 2 people

INGREDIENTS

- 1 1/2 cups cooked chicken, shredded
- 2 tbsp. fresh lime juice
- 2 tbsp. fresh cilantro, chopped
- 2 tbsp. green onion, sliced
- 1 tsp. chili powder
- Pepper
- Salt

DIRECTIONS

1. Add all ingredients into the medium bowl and mix well. Season with pepper and salt.

NUTRITION

Calories 113
Fat 2 g
Carbs 1 g
Protein 20 g

---

472. Shredded Turkey Breast

PREP TIME: 10 mins
COOK TIME: 8 hours
SERVINGS: 10 people

INGREDIENTS

- 4 lbs turkey breast, skinless, boneless, and halves
- 1 1/2 tbsp. taco seasoning, homemade
- 12 oz chicken stock
- 1/2 cup butter, cubed
- Pepper
- Salt

DIRECTIONS

1. Place turkey breast into the crockpot.
2. Pour remaining ingredients over turkey breast.
3. Cover and cook on low for 8 hours.
4. Shred turkey breast with a fork.
5. Serve and enjoy.

NUTRITION

Calories 327
Fat 15.4 g
Carbs 11.8 g
Protein 34.3 g

473. Delicious Chicken Tenders

PREP TIME
10 mins

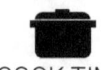
COOK TIME
15 mins

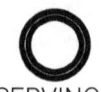
SERVINGS
4 people

INGREDIENTS

- 1 1/2 lbs chicken tenders
- 2 tbsp. BBQ sauce, homemade & sugar-free
- 1 tbsp. olive oil
- 1 tsp. poultry seasoning
- Pepper
- Salt

DIRECTIONS

1. Add all ingredients except oil in a zip-lock bag. Seal bag and place in the fridge for 2 hours.
2. Heat oil in a pan over medium heat.
3. Place marinated chicken tenders on the hot pan and cook until lightly browned and cooked.
4. Serve and enjoy.

NUTRITION

Calories 366
Fat 15 g
Carbs 3 g
Protein 2 oz.

474. Grilled Pesto Chicken

PREP TIME
10 mins

COOK TIME
10 mins

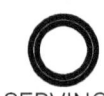
SERVINGS
6 people

INGREDIENTS

- 1 1/2 lbs chicken breasts, skinless, boneless, and slice
- 1/4 cup pesto
- 1/2 cup mozzarella cheese, shredded
- Pepper
- Salt

DIRECTIONS

1. Place chicken into the large bowl.
2. Add pesto, pepper, and salt over chicken and coat well. Cover and place in the fridge for 2 hours.
3. Heat grill over medium-high heat.
4. Place marinated chicken on hot grill and cook until completely done.
5. Sprinkle cheese over chicken.
6. Serve and enjoy.

NUTRITION

Calories 300
Fat 14 g
Carbs 1 g
Protein 40 g

475. Easy & Tasty Salsa Chicken

PREP TIME 10 mins
COOK TIME 2 hours
SERVINGS 6 people

INGREDIENTS
- 1 1/2 lbs chicken tenders, skinless
- 1/4 tsp. garlic powder
- 1/8 tsp. ground cumin
- 1/8 tsp. oregano
- 15 oz salsa
- 1/4 tsp. onion powder
- 1/4 tsp. chili powder
- Pepper
- Salt

DIRECTIONS
1. Place chicken tenders into the crockpot.
2. Pour remaining ingredients over chicken.
3. Cover and cook on high for 2 hours.
4. Shred the chicken using a fork and serve.

NUTRITION
Calories 235
Fat 8 g
Carbs 5 g
Protein 35 g

476. Tender Turkey Breast

PREP TIME 10 mins
COOK TIME 4 hours
SERVINGS 8 people

INGREDIENTS
- 4 lbs turkey breast, bone-in
- 1/2 cup chicken stock
- 6 garlic cloves, peeled
- 3 fresh rosemary sprigs
- Pepper
- Salt

DIRECTIONS
1. Place turkey breast into the crockpot. Season with pepper and salt.
2. Add stock, garlic, and rosemary on top.
3. Cover and cook on low for 4 hours.
4. Serve and enjoy.

NUTRITION
Calories 235
Fat 3.5 g
Carbs 10 g
Protein 39 g

477. Chicken Bacon Salad

PREP TIME
10 mins

COOK TIME
5 mins

SERVINGS
3 people

INGREDIENTS

- 2 cups cooked chicken, shredded
- 1 cup cheddar cheese, shredded
- 1 cup celery, chopped
- 1/2 cup sour cream
- 1/4 cup mayonnaise
- 1/2 cup bacon, crumbles
- 3 green onions, sliced
- 1/4 cup onion, chopped
- Pepper
- Salt

DIRECTIONS

1. Add all ingredients into the large bowl and mix until well combined.
2. Serve and enjoy.

NUTRITION

Calories 482
Fat 31.3 g
Carbs 9.9 g
Protein 39.6 g

478. Green Salsa Chicken

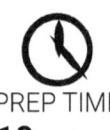
PREP TIME
10 mins

COOK TIME
3 hours

SERVINGS
6 people

INGREDIENTS

- 1 lb chicken breasts, skinless and boneless
- 15 oz green salsa
- Pepper
- Salt

DIRECTIONS

1. Add all ingredients into the crock pot.
2. Cover and cook on high for 3 hours.
3. Shred the chicken using fork.
4. Serve and enjoy.

NUTRITION

Calories 166
Fat 6 g
Carbs 3 g
Protein 22 g

479. Chicken Chili

PREP TIME: 10 mins
COOK TIME: 6 hours
SERVINGS: 4 people

NUTRITION
Calories 265
Fat 8.9 g
Carbs 11.1 g
Protein 34.9 g

INGREDIENTS

- 1 lb chicken breasts, skinless and boneless
- 14 oz can tomato, diced
- 2 cups of water
- 1 jalapeno pepper, chopped
- 1 poblano pepper, chopped
- 12 oz can green chilies
- 1/2 tsp. paprika
- 1/2 tsp. dried sage
- 1/2 tsp. cumin
- 1 tsp. dried oregano
- 1/2 cup dried chives
- 1 tsp. sea salt

DIRECTIONS

1. Add all ingredients into the crockpot and stir well.
2. Cover and cook on low for 6 hours.
3. Shred the chicken using a fork.
4. Stir well and serve.

480. Tasty Chicken Kabobs

PREP TIME: 10 mins
COOK TIME: 10 mins
SERVINGS: 4 people

NUTRITION
Calories 228
Fat 7.8 g
Carbs 1.3 g
Protein 36.2 g

INGREDIENTS

- 1 1/2 lbs chicken breast, boneless & cut into 1-inch pieces
- 1 tsp. dried oregano
- 1 tbsp. fresh lime juice
- 1 tbsp. olive oil
- 1/2 tsp. pepper
- 1/2 tsp. sea salt

DIRECTIONS

1. Add chicken into the mixing bowl. Pour remaining ingredients over chicken and coat well and place it in the refrigerator overnight.
2. Heat grill over medium heat.
3. Thread marinated chicken onto the skewers.
4. Place chicken skewers onto the hot grill and cook for 8-10 minutes.
5. Serve and enjoy.

481. Cheesy Salsa Chicken

PREP TIME
10 mins

COOK TIME
6 hours

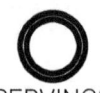
SERVINGS
6 people

INGREDIENTS

- 2 lbs chicken breasts, cut into cubes
- 2 cups cheddar cheese, shredded
- 2 tbsp. taco seasoning
- 2 cups salsa
- Pepper
- Salt

DIRECTIONS

1. Add all ingredients except cheese into the crock pot.
2. Cover and cook on low for 5 hours 30 minutes.
3. Add cheese and stir well and cook for 30 minutes more.
4. Stir and serve.

NUTRITION

Calories 463
Fat 23.8 g
Carbs 5.9 g
Protein 54.5 g

482. Ranch Chicken Salad

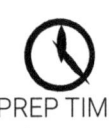
PREP TIME
10 mins

COOK TIME
5 mins

SERVINGS
4 people

INGREDIENTS

- 3 cups cooked chicken, shredded
- 1/2 cup green onion, chopped
- 3/4 cup carrots, chopped
- 1 1/2 cups celery, chopped
- 1/2 cup mayonnaise
- 1/4 sweet onion, diced
- 1 tbsp. ranch seasoning
- 4 tbsp. hot sauce
- Pepper
- Salt

DIRECTIONS

1. In a small bowl, mix together hot sauce, ranch seasoning, and mayonnaise.
2. Add remaining ingredients into the large bowl and mix well.
3. Pour hot sauce mixture over salad and mix well.
4. Serve and enjoy.

NUTRITION

Calories 275
Fat 13 g
Carbs 12 g
Protein 20 g

483. Harissa Chicken

INGREDIENTS

- 1 lb chicken breasts, skinless and boneless
- 1 cup harissa sauce
- 1/4 tsp. garlic powder
- 1/2 tsp. ground cumin
- 1/4 tsp. onion powder
- 1/2 tsp. kosher salt

DIRECTIONS

1. Season chicken with garlic powder, onion powder, cumin, and salt.
2. Place chicken into the crockpot. Pour harissa sauce over chicken.
3. Cover and cook on low for 4 hours.
4. Shred the chicken using a fork.
5. Serve and enjoy.

PREP TIME: 10 mins
COOK TIME: 4 hours
SERVINGS: 4 people

NUTRITION
Calories 230
Fat 10 g
Carbs 2 g
Protein 33 g

---

484. Almond Cranberry Chicken Salad

INGREDIENTS

- 1 lb cooked chicken, shredded
- 1/4 tsp. garlic powder
- 1 celery stalk, chopped
- 1/4 cup almonds, sliced
- 1/4 cup cranberries, dried
- 1/4 cup mayonnaise
- 1/4 cup sour cream
- 1/4 tsp. onion powder
- 1/4 tsp. pepper
- 1/2 tsp. salt

DIRECTIONS

1. Add all ingredients into the mixing bowl and mix well.
2. Place in refrigerator for 1-2 hours.
3. Serve and enjoy.

PREP TIME: 10 mins
COOK TIME: 5 mins
SERVINGS: 4 people

NUTRITION
Calories 175
Fat 12 g
Carbs 6 g
Protein 8 g

485. Simple Baked Chicken Breasts

PREP TIME
10 mins

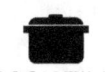
COOK TIME
45 mins

SERVINGS
6 people

NUTRITION

Calories 435
Fat 27 g
Carbs 2 g
Protein 43 g

INGREDIENTS

- 6 chicken breasts, skinless and boneless
- 1/2 cup olive oil
- 1/4 cup soy sauce
- 1 tbsp. oregano
- 2 tbsp. fresh lemon juice
- 1 tsp. garlic salt

DIRECTIONS

1. Add all ingredients into the large zip-lock bag. Seal bag and shake well and place in the fridge for 3-4 hours.
2. Preheat the oven to 350 F.
3. Place marinated chicken into a baking dish and bake for 45 minutes.
4. Serve and enjoy.

FISH AND SEAFOOD

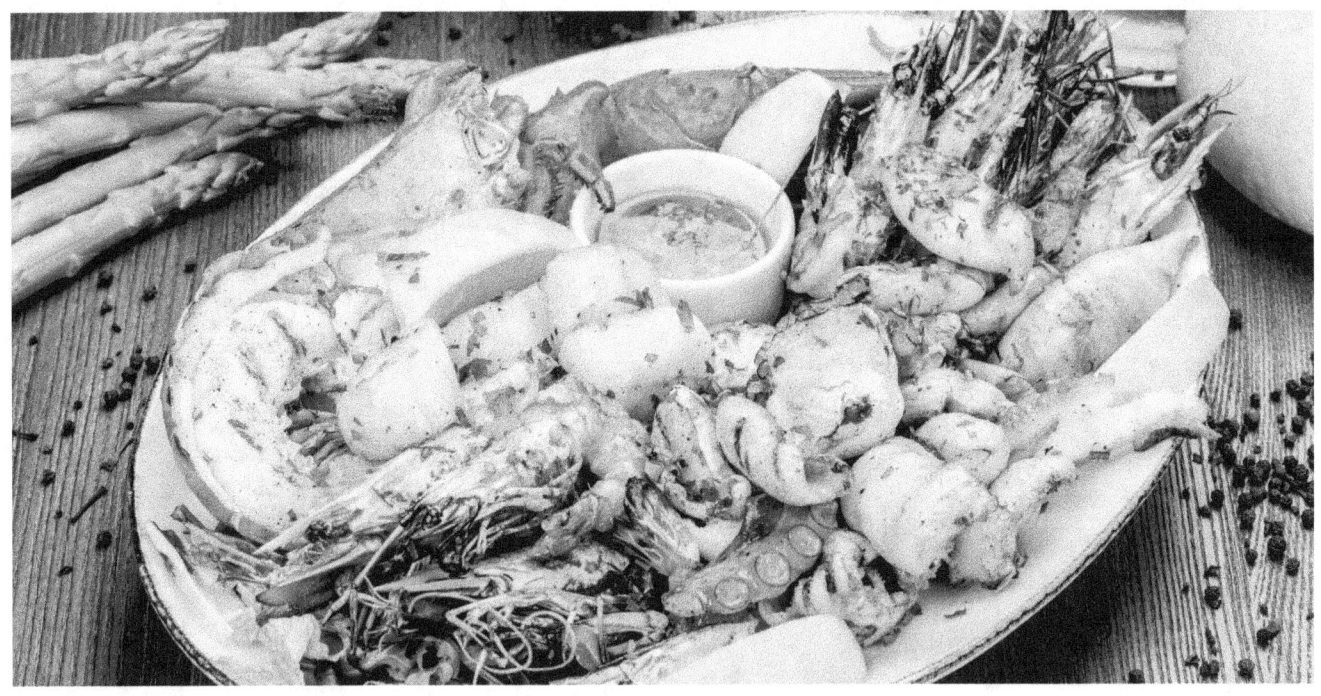

486. Baked Cod Fillets with Ghee Sauce

PREP TIME: 10 mins
COOK TIME: 15 mins
SERVINGS: 2 people

NUTRITION
Calories: 200;
Fat: 12g;
Protein: 21g;
Carbs: 2g

INGREDIENTS

- Pepper and salt to taste
- 2 tbsp. minced parsley
- 1 lemon, sliced into ¼-inch thick circles
- 1 lemon, juiced and zested
- 4 garlic cloves, crushed, peeled, and minced
- ¼ cup melted ghee
- 4 Cod fillets

DIRECTIONS

1. Bring oven to 425o°F.
2. Mix parsley, lemon juice, lemon zest, garlic, and melted ghee in a small bowl. Mix well and then season with pepper and salt to taste.
3. Prepare a large baking dish by greasing it with cooking spray.
4. Evenly lay the cod fillets on the greased dish. Season generously with pepper and salt.
5. Pour the bowl of garlic-ghee sauce from step 2 on top of cod fillets. Top the cod fillets with the thinly sliced lemon.
6. Pop in the preheated oven and bake until flaky, around 13 to 15 minutes. Remove from oven, transfer to dishes, serve, and enjoy.

487. Avocado Peach Salsa on Grilled Swordfish

PREP TIME
15 mins

COOK TIME
12 mins

SERVINGS
2 people

NUTRITION

Calories: 416;
Carbs: 21g;
Protein: 30g;
Fat: 23.5g

INGREDIENTS

- 1 garlic clove, minced
- 1 lemon juice
- 1 tbsp. apple cider vinegar
- 1 tbsp. coconut oil
- 1 tsp. honey
- 2 swordfish fillets (around 4oz each)
- Pinch cayenne pepper
- Pinch of pepper and salt
- Salsa Ingredients:
- ¼ red onion, finely chopped
- ½ cup cilantro, finely chopped
- 1 avocado, halved and diced
- 1 garlic clove, minced
- 2 peaches, seeded and diced
- Juice of 1 lime
- Salt to taste

DIRECTIONS

1. In a shallow dish, mix all swordfish marinade ingredients except fillet. Mix well then add fillets to marinate. Place in refrigerator for at least an hour.
2. Meanwhile create salsa by mixing all salsa ingredients in a medium bowl. Put in the refrigerator to cool.
3. Preheat grill and grill fish on medium fire after marinating until cooked around 4 minutes per side.
4. Place each cooked fillet on one serving plate, top with half of salsa, serve and enjoy.

488. Breaded and Spiced Halibut

PREP TIME
10 mins

COOK TIME
15 mins

SERVINGS
4 people

NUTRITION

Calories: 336.4;
Protein: 25.3g;
Fat: 25.3g;
Carbs: 4.1g

INGREDIENTS

- ¼ cup chopped fresh chives
- ¼ cup chopped fresh dill
- ¼ tsp. ground black pepper
- ¾ cup panko breadcrumbs
- 1 tbsp. extra-virgin olive oil
- 1 tsp. finely grated lemon zest
- 1 tsp. sea salt
- 1/3 cup chopped fresh parsley
- 4 pieces of 6-oz halibut fillets

DIRECTIONS

1. Line a baking sheet with foil, grease with cooking spray and preheat oven to 400°F.
2. In a small bowl, mix black pepper, sea salt, lemon zest, olive oil, chives, dill, parsley and breadcrumbs. If needed add more salt to taste. Set aside.
3. Meanwhile, wash halibut fillets on cold tap water. Dry with paper towels and place on prepared baking sheet.
4. Generously spoon crumb mixture onto halibut fillets. Ensure that fillets are covered with crumb mixture. Press down on crumb mixture onto each fillet.
5. Pop into the oven and bake for 10-15 minutes or until fish is flaky and crumb topping are already lightly browned.

489. Berries and Grilled Calamari

PREP TIME: 10 mins
COOK TIME: 5 mins
SERVINGS: 4 people

NUTRITION
Calories: 567;
Fat: 24.5g;
Protein: 54.8g;
Carbs: 30.6g

INGREDIENTS

- ¼ cup dried cranberries
- ¼ cup extra virgin olive oil
- ¼ cup olive oil
- ¼ cup sliced almonds
- ½ lemon, juiced
- ¾ cup blueberries
- 1 ½ lb. calamari tube, cleaned
- 1 granny smith apple, sliced thinly
- 1 tbsp. fresh lemon juice
- 2 tbsp. apple cider vinegar
- 6 cups fresh spinach
- Freshly grated pepper to taste
- Sea salt to taste

DIRECTIONS

1. In a small bowl, make the vinaigrette by mixing well the tbsp. of lemon juice, apple cider vinegar, and extra virgin olive oil. Season with pepper and salt to taste. Set aside.
2. Turn on the grill to medium fire and let the grates heat up for a minute or two.
3. In a large bowl, add olive oil and the calamari tube. Season calamari generously with pepper and salt.
4. Place seasoned and oiled calamari onto heated grate and grill until cooked or opaque. This is around two minutes per side.
5. As you wait for the calamari to cook, you can combine almonds, cranberries, blueberries, spinach, and the thinly sliced apple in a large salad bowl. Toss to mix.
6. Remove cooked calamari from grill and transfer on a chopping board. Cut into ¼-inch thick rings and throw into the salad bowl.
7. Drizzle with vinaigrette and toss well to coat salad. Serve and enjoy!

490. Coconut Salsa on Chipotle Fish Tacos

PREP TIME: 10 mins
COOK TIME: 10 mins
SERVINGS: 4 people

NUTRITION
Calories: 477;
Protein: 35.0g;
Fat: 12.4g;
Carbs: 57.4g

INGREDIENTS

- ¼ cup chopped fresh cilantro
- ½ cup seeded and finely chopped plum tomato
- 1 cup peeled and finely chopped mango
- 1 lime cut into wedges
- 1 tbsp. chipotle Chile powder
- 1 tbsp. safflower oil
- 1/3 cup finely chopped red onion
- 10 tbsp. fresh lime juice, divided
- 4 6-oz boneless, skinless cod fillets
- 5 tbsp. dried unsweetened shredded coconut
- 8 pcs of 6-inch tortillas, heated

DIRECTIONS

1. Whisk well Chile powder, oil, and 4 tbsp. lime juice in a glass baking dish. Add cod and marinate for 12 – 15 minutes. Turning once halfway through the marinating time.
2. Make the salsa by mixing coconut, 6 tbsp. lime juice, cilantro, onions, tomatoes and mangoes in a medium bowl. Set aside.
3. On high, heat a grill pan. Place cod and grill for four minutes per side turning only once.
4. Once cooked, slice cod into large flakes and evenly divide onto tortilla.
5. Evenly divide salsa on top of cod and serve with a side of lime wedges.

491. Baked Cod Crusted with Herbs

PREP TIME
5 mins

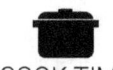
COOK TIME
10 mins

SERVINGS
4 people

NUTRITION

Calories: 137;
Protein: 5g;
Fat: 2g;
Carbs: 21g

INGREDIENTS

- ¼ cup honey
- ¼ tsp. salt
- ½ cup panko
- ½ tsp. pepper
- 1 tbsp. extra virgin olive oil
- 1 tbsp. lemon juice
- 1 tsp. dried basil
- 1 tsp. dried parsley
- 1 tsp. rosemary
- 4 pieces of 4-oz cod fillets

DIRECTIONS

1. With olive oil, grease a 9 x 13-inch baking pan and preheat oven to 375oF.
2. In a zip top bag mix panko, rosemary, salt, pepper, parsley and basil.
3. Evenly spread cod fillets in prepped dish and drizzle with lemon juice.
4. Then brush the fillets with honey on all sides. Discard remaining honey if any.
5. Then evenly divide the panko mixture on top of cod fillets.
6. Pop in the oven and bake for ten minutes or until fish is cooked.
7. Serve and enjoy.

492. Cajun Garlic Shrimp Noodle Bowl

PREP TIME
10 mins

COOK TIME
15 mins

SERVINGS
2 people

NUTRITION

Calories: 712;
Fat: 30.0g;
Protein: 97.8g;
Carbs: 20.2g

INGREDIENTS

- ½ tsp. salt
- 1 onion, sliced
- 1 red pepper, sliced
- 1 tbsp. butter
- 1 tsp. garlic granules
- 1 tsp. onion powder
- 1 tsp. paprika
- 2 large zucchinis, cut into noodle strips
- 20 jumbo shrimps, shells removed and deveined
- 3 cloves garlic, minced
- 3 tbsp. ghee
- A dash of cayenne pepper
- A dash of red pepper flakes

DIRECTIONS

1. Prepare the Cajun seasoning by mixing the onion powder, garlic granules, pepper flakes, cayenne pepper, paprika and salt. Toss in the shrimp to coat in the seasoning.
2. In a skillet, heat the ghee and sauté the garlic. Add in the red pepper and onions and continue sautéing for 4 minutes.
3. Add the Cajun shrimp and cook until opaque. Set aside.
4. In another pan, heat the butter and sauté the zucchini noodles for three minutes.
5. Assemble by the placing the Cajun shrimps on top of the zucchini noodles.

493. Crazy Saganaki Shrimp

PREP TIME: 10 mins
COOK TIME: 10 mins
SERVINGS: 4 people

NUTRITION
Calories: 310;
Protein: 49.7g;
Fat: 6.8g;
Carbs: 8.4g

INGREDIENTS
- ¼ tsp. salt
- ½ cup Chardonnay
- ½ cup crumbled Greek feta cheese
- 1 medium bulb. fennel, cored and finely chopped
- 1 small Chile pepper, seeded and minced
- 1 tbsp. extra virgin olive oil
- 12 jumbo shrimps, peeled and deveined with tails left on
- 2 tbsp. lemon juice, divided
- 5 scallions sliced thinly
- Pepper to taste

DIRECTIONS
1. In medium bowl, mix salt, lemon juice and shrimp.
2. On medium fire, place a saganaki pan (or large nonstick saucepan) and heat oil.
3. Sauté Chile pepper, scallions, and fennel for 4 minutes or until starting to brown and is already soft.
4. Add wine and sauté for another minute.
5. Place shrimps on top of fennel, cover and cook for 4 minutes or until shrimps are pink.
6. Remove just the shrimp and transfer to a plate.
7. Add pepper, feta and 1 tbsp. lemon juice to pan and cook for a minute or until cheese begins to melt.
8. To serve, place cheese and fennel mixture on a serving plate and top with shrimps.

494. Creamy Bacon-Fish Chowder

PREP TIME: 10 mins
COOK TIME: 30 mins
SERVINGS: 8 people

NUTRITION
Calories: 400;
Carbs: 34.5g;
Protein: 20.8g;
Fat: 19.7g

INGREDIENTS
- 1 1/2 lbs. cod
- 1 1/2 tsp. dried thyme
- 1 large onion, chopped
- 1 medium carrot, coarsely chopped
- 1 tbsp. butter, cut into small pieces
- 1 tsp. salt, divided
- 3 1/2 cups baking potato, peeled and cubed
- 3 slices uncooked bacon
- 3/4 tsp. freshly ground black pepper, divided
- 4 1/2 cups water
- 4 bay leaves
- 4 cups 2% reduced-fat milk

DIRECTIONS
1. In a large skillet, add the water and bay leaves and let it simmer. Add the fish. Cover and let it simmer some more until the flesh flakes easily with fork. Remove the fish from the skillet and cut into large pieces. Set aside the cooking liquid.
2. Place Dutch oven in medium heat and cook the bacon until crisp. Remove the bacon and reserve the bacon drippings. Crush the bacon and set aside.
3. Stir potato, onion and carrot in the pan with the bacon drippings, cook over medium heat for 10 minutes. Add the cooking liquid, bay leaves, 1/2 tsp. salt, 1/4 tsp. pepper and thyme, let it boil. Lower the heat and let simmer for 10 minutes. Add the milk and butter, simmer until the potatoes becomes tender, but do not boil. Add the fish, 1/2 tsp. salt, 1/2 tsp. pepper. Remove the bay leaves.
4. Serve sprinkled with the crushed bacon.

495. Crisped Coco-Shrimp with Mango Dip

PREP TIME
10 mins

COOK TIME
20 mins

SERVINGS
4 people

NUTRITION

Calories: 294.2;
Protein: 26.6g;
Fat: 7g;
Carbs: 31.2g

INGREDIENTS

- 1 cup shredded coconut
- 1 lb. raw shrimp, peeled and deveined
- 2 egg whites
- 4 tbsp. tapioca starch
- Pepper and salt to taste
- Mango Dip Ingredients:
- 1 cup mango, chopped
- 1 jalapeño, thinly minced
- 1 tsp. lime juice
- 1/3 cup coconut milk
- 3 tsp. raw honey

DIRECTIONS

1. Preheat oven to 400°F.
2. Ready a pan with wire rack on top.
3. In a medium bowl, add tapioca starch and season with pepper and salt.
4. In a second medium bowl, add egg whites and whisk.
5. In a third medium bowl, add coconut.
6. To ready shrimps, dip first in tapioca starch, then egg whites, and then coconut. Place dredged shrimp on wire rack. Repeat until all shrimps are covered.
7. Pop shrimps in the oven and roast for 10 minutes per side.
8. Meanwhile make the dip by adding all ingredients in a blender. Puree until smooth and creamy. Transfer to a dipping bowl.
9. Once shrimps are golden brown, serve with mango dip.

496. Cucumber-Basil Salsa on Halibut Pouches

PREP TIME
10 mins

COOK TIME
17 mins

SERVINGS
4 people

NUTRITION

Calories: 335.4;
Protein: 20.2g;
Fat: 16.3g;
Carbs: 22.1g

INGREDIENTS

- 1 lime, thinly sliced into 8 pieces
- 2 cups mustard greens, stems removed
- 2 tsp. olive oil
- 4 – 5 radishes trimmed and quartered
- 4 4-oz skinless halibut filets
- 4 large fresh basil leaves
- Cayenne pepper to taste – optional
- Pepper and salt to taste
- Salsa Ingredients:
- 1 ½ cups diced cucumber
- 1 ½ finely chopped fresh basil leaves
- 2 tsp. fresh lime juice
- Pepper and salt to taste

DIRECTIONS

1. Preheat oven to 400°F.
2. Prepare parchment papers by making 4 pieces of 15 x 12-inch rectangles. Lengthwise, fold in half and unfold pieces on the table.
3. Season halibut fillets with pepper, salt and cayenne—if using cayenne.
4. Just to the right of the fold going lengthwise, place ½ cup of mustard greens. Add a basil leaf on center of mustard greens and topped with 1 lime slice. Around the greens, layer ¼ of the radishes. Drizzle with ½ tsp. of oil, season with pepper and salt. Top it with a slice of halibut fillet.
5. Just as you would make a calzone, fold parchment paper over your filling and crimp the edges of the parchment paper beginning from one end to the other end. To seal the end of the crimped parchment paper, pinch it.
6. Repeat process to remaining ingredients until you have 4 pieces of parchment papers filled with halibut and greens.
7. Place pouches in a baking pan and bake in the oven until halibut is flaky, around 15 to 17 minutes.
8. While waiting for halibut pouches to cook, make your salsa by mixing all salsa ingredients in a medium bowl.
9. Once halibut is cooked, remove from oven and make a tear on top. Be careful of the steam as it is very hot. Equally divide salsa and spoon ¼ of salsa on top of halibut through the slit you have created.

497. Curry Salmon with Mustard

PREP TIME 10 mins
COOK TIME 8 mins
SERVINGS 4 people

INGREDIENTS

- ¼ tsp. ground red pepper or chili powder
- ¼ tsp. ground turmeric
- ¼ tsp. salt
- 1 tsp. honey
- 1/8 tsp. garlic powder or 1 clove garlic minced
- 2 teaspoon. whole grain mustard
- 4 pcs 6-oz salmon fillets

DIRECTIONS

1. In a small bowl mix well salt, garlic powder, red pepper, turmeric, honey and mustard.
2. Preheat oven to broil and grease a baking dish with cooking spray.
3. Place salmon on baking dish with skin side down and spread evenly mustard mixture on top of salmon.
4. Pop in the oven and broil until flaky around 8 minutes.

NUTRITION

Calories: 324;
Fat: 18.9 g;
Protein: 34 g;
Carbs: 2.9 g

498. Dijon Mustard and Lime Marinated Shrimp

PREP TIME 10 mins
COOK TIME 10 mins
SERVINGS 8 people

INGREDIENTS

- ½ cup fresh lime juice, plus lime zest as garnish
- ½ cup rice vinegar
- ½ tsp. hot sauce
- 1 bay leaf
- 1 cup water
- 1 lb. uncooked shrimp, peeled and deveined
- 1 medium red onion, chopped
- 2 tbsp. capers
- 2 tbsp. Dijon mustard
- 3 whole cloves

DIRECTIONS

1. Mix hot sauce, mustard, capers, lime juice and onion in a shallow baking dish and set aside.
2. Bring to a boil in a large saucepan bay leaf, cloves, vinegar and water.
3. Once boiling, add shrimps and cook for a minute while stirring continuously.
4. Drain shrimps and pour shrimps into onion mixture.
5. For an hour, refrigerate while covered the shrimps.
6. Then serve shrimps cold and garnished with lime zest.

NUTRITION

Calories: 232.2;
Protein: 17.8g;
Fat: 3g;
Carbs: 15g

499. Dill Relish on White Sea Bass

PREP TIME 10 mins

COOK TIME 12 mins

SERVINGS 4 people

NUTRITION
Calories: 115;
Protein: 7g;
Fat: 1g;
Carbs: 12g

INGREDIENTS
- 1 ½ tbsp. chopped white onion
- 1 ½ tsp. chopped fresh dill
- 1 lemon, quartered
- 1 tsp. Dijon mustard
- 1 tsp. lemon juice
- 1 tsp. pickled baby capers, drained
- 4 pieces of 4-oz white sea bass fillets

DIRECTIONS
1. Preheat oven to 375°F.
2. Mix lemon juice, mustard, dill, capers and onions in a small bowl.
3. Prepare four aluminum foil squares and place 1 fillet per foil.
4. Squeeze a lemon wedge per fish.
5. Evenly divide into 4 the dill spread and drizzle over fillet.
6. Close the foil over the fish securely and pop in the oven.
7. Bake for 10 to 12 minutes or until fish is cooked through.
8. Remove from foil and transfer to a serving platter, serve and enjoy.

500. Garlic Roasted Shrimp with Zucchini Pasta

PREP TIME 10 mins

COOK TIME 10 mins

SERVINGS 2 people

NUTRITION
Calories: 299;
Fat: 23.2g;
Protein: 14.3g;
Carbs: 10.9g

INGREDIENTS
- 2 medium-sized zucchinis, cut into thin strips or spaghetti noodles
- Salt and pepper to taste
- 1 lemon, zested and juiced
- 2 garlic cloves, minced
- 2 tbsp. ghee, melted
- 2 tbsp. olive oil
- 8 oz. shrimps, cleaned and deveined

DIRECTIONS
1. Preheat the oven to 400°F.
2. In a mixing bowl, mix all ingredients except the zucchini noodles. Toss to coat the shrimp.
3. Bake for 10 minutes until the shrimps turn pink.
4. Add the zucchini pasta then toss.

501. Easy Seafood French Stew

PREP TIME 10 mins
COOK TIME 45 mins
SERVINGS 12 people

NUTRITION
Calories: 348;
Carbs: 20.0g;
Protein: 31.8g;
Fat: 15.2g

INGREDIENTS

- Pepper and Salt
- 1/2 lb. littleneck clams
- 1/2 lb. mussels
- 1 lb. shrimp, peeled and deveined
- 1 large lobster
- 2 lbs. assorted small whole fresh fish, scaled and cleaned
- 2 tbsp. parsley, finely chopped
- 2 tbsp. garlic, chopped
- 1 cup fennel, julienned
- Juice and zest of one orange
- 3 cups tomatoes, peeled, seeded, and chopped
- 1 cup leeks, julienned
- Pinch of Saffron
- Stew Ingredients:
- 1 cup white wine
- Water
- 1 lb. fish bones
- 2 sprigs thyme
- 8 peppercorns
- 1 bay leaf
- 3 cloves garlic
- Salt and pepper
- 1/2 cup chopped celery
- 1/2 cup chopped onion
- 2 tbsp. olive oil

DIRECTIONS

1. Do the stew: Heat oil in a large saucepan. Sauté the celery and onions for 3 minutes. Season with pepper and salt. Stir in the garlic and cook for about a minute. Add the thyme, peppercorns, and bay leaves. Stir in the wine, water and fish bones. Let it boil then before reducing to a simmer. Take the pan off the fire and strain broth into another container.
2. For the Bouillabaisse: Bring the strained broth to a simmer and stir in the parsley, leeks, orange juice, orange zest, garlic, fennel, tomatoes and saffron. Sprinkle with pepper and salt. Stir in the lobsters and fish. Let it simmer for eight minutes before stirring in the clams, mussels and shrimps. For six minutes, allow to cook while covered before seasoning again with pepper and salt.
3. Assemble in a shallow dish all the seafood and pour the broth over it.

502. Fresh and No-Cook Oysters

PREP TIME 10 mins
COOK TIME 5 mins
SERVINGS 4 people

NUTRITION
Calories: 247;
Protein: 29g;
Fat: 7g;
Carbs: 17g

INGREDIENTS

- 2 lemons
- 24 medium oysters
- tabasco sauce

DIRECTIONS

1. If you are a newbie when it comes to eating oysters, then I suggest that you blanch the oysters before eating.
2. For some, eating oysters raw is a great way to enjoy this dish because of the consistency and juiciness of raw oysters. Plus, adding lemon juice prior to eating the raw oysters cooks it a bit.
3. So, to blanch oysters, bring a big pot of water to a rolling boil. Add oysters in batches of 6-10 pieces. Leave on boiling pot of water between 3-5 minutes and remove oysters right away. To eat oysters, squeeze lemon juice on oyster on shell, add tabasco as desired and eat.

503. Easy Broiled Lobster Tails

PREP TIME
10 mins

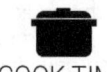
COOK TIME
10 mins

SERVINGS
2 people

NUTRITION

Calories: 175.6;
Protein: 23g;
Fat: 10g;
Carbs: 18.4g

INGREDIENTS

- 1 6-oz frozen lobster tails
- 1 tbsp. olive oil
- 1 tsp. lemon pepper seasoning

DIRECTIONS

1. Preheat oven broiler.
2. With kitchen scissors, cut thawed lobster tails in half lengthwise.
3. Brush with oil the exposed lobster meat. Season with lemon pepper.
4. Place lobster tails in baking sheet with exposed meat facing up.
5. Place on top broiler rack and broil for 10 minutes until lobster meat is lightly browned on the sides and center meat is opaque. Serve and enjoy.

504. Ginger Scallion Sauce over Seared Ahi

PREP TIME
10 mins

COOK TIME
6 mins

SERVINGS
4 people

NUTRITION

Calories: 247;
Protein: 29g;
Fat: 1g;
Carbs: 8g

INGREDIENTS

- 1 bunch scallions, bottoms removed, finely chopped
- 1 tbsp. rice wine vinegar
- 1 tbsp.. Bragg's liquid amino
- 16-oz ahi tuna steaks
- 2 tbsp.. fresh ginger, peeled and grated
- 3 tbsp.. coconut oil, melted
- Pepper and salt to taste

DIRECTIONS

1. In a small bowl mix together vinegar, 2 tbsp.. oil, soy sauce, ginger and scallions. Put aside.
2. On medium fire, place a large saucepan and heat remaining oil. Once oil is hot and starts to smoke, sear tuna until deeply browned or for two minutes per side.
3. Place seared tuna on a serving platter and let it stand for 5 minutes before slicing into 1-inch thick strips.
4. Drizzle ginger-scallion mixture over seared tuna, serve and enjoy.

505. Healthy Poached Trout

PREP TIME 10 mins
COOK TIME 10 mins
SERVINGS 2 people

INGREDIENTS

- 1 8-oz boneless, skin on trout fillet
- 2 cups chicken broth or water
- 2 leeks, halved
- 6-8 slices lemon
- salt and pepper to taste

DIRECTIONS

1. On medium fire, place a large nonstick skillet and arrange leeks and lemons on pan in a layer. Cover with soup stock or water and bring to a simmer.
2. Meanwhile, season trout on both sides with pepper and salt. Place trout on simmering pan of water. Cover and cook until trout is flaky, around 8 minutes.
3. In a serving platter, spoon leek and lemons on bottom of plate, top with trout and spoon sauce into plate. Serve and enjoy.

NUTRITION

Calories: 360.2;
Protein: 13.8g;
Fat: 7.5g;
Carbs: 51.5g

506. Leftover Salmon Salad Power Bowls

PREP TIME 10 mins
COOK TIME 10 mins
SERVINGS 1 people

INGREDIENTS

- ½ cup raspberries
- ½ cup zucchini, sliced
- 1 lemon, juice squeezed
- 1 tbsp. balsamic glaze
- 2 sprigs of thyme, chopped
- 2 tbsp. olive oil
- 4 cups seasonal greens
- 4 oz. leftover grilled salmon
- Salt and pepper to taste

DIRECTIONS

1. Heat oil in a skillet over medium flame and sauté the zucchini. Season with salt and pepper to taste.
2. In a mixing bowl, mix all ingredients together.
3. Toss to combine everything.
4. Sprinkle with nut cheese.

NUTRITION

Calories: 450.3;
Fat: 35.5 g;
Protein: 23.4g;
Carbs: 9.3 g

507. Lemon-Garlic Baked Halibut

PREP TIME 10 mins

COOK TIME 15 mins

SERVINGS 2 people

INGREDIENTS
- 1 large garlic clove, minced
- 1 tbsp. chopped flat leaf parsley
- 1 tsp. olive oil
- 2 5-oz boneless, skin-on halibut fillets
- 2 tsp. lemon zest
- Juice of ½ lemon, divided
- Salt and pepper to taste

DIRECTIONS
1. Grease a baking dish with cooking spray and preheat oven to 400oF.
2. Place halibut with skin touching the dish and drizzle with olive oil.
3. Season with pepper and salt.
4. Pop into the oven and bake until flaky around 12-15 minutes.
5. Remove from oven and drizzle with remaining lemon juice, serve and enjoy with a side of salad greens.

NUTRITION
Calories: 315.3;
Protein: 14.1g;
Fat: 10.5g;
Carbs: 36.6g

508. Minty-Cucumber Yogurt Topped Grilled Fish

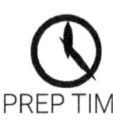
PREP TIME 10 mins

COOK TIME 2 mins

SERVINGS 4 people

INGREDIENTS
- ¼ cup 2% plain Greek yogurt
- ¼ tsp. + 1/8 tsp. salt
- ¼ tsp. black pepper
- ½ green onion, finely chopped
- ½ tsp. dried oregano
- 1 tbsp. finely chopped fresh mint leaves
- 3 tbsp. finely chopped English cucumber
- 4 5-oz cod fillets
- Cooking oil as needed

DIRECTIONS
1. Brush grill grate with oil and preheat grill to high.
2. Season cod fillets on both sides with pepper, ¼ tsp. salt and oregano.
3. Grill cod for 3 minutes per side or until cooked to desired doneness.
4. Mix thoroughly 1/8 tsp. salt, onion, mint, cucumber and yogurt in a small bowl. Serve cod with a dollop of the dressing. This dish can be paired with salad greens or brown rice.

NUTRITION
Calories: 253.5;
Protein: 25.5g;
Fat: 1g;
Carbs: 5g

509. One-Pot Seafood Chowder

PREP TIME
10 mins

COOK TIME
10 mins

SERVINGS
3 people

NUTRITION

Calories: 532;
Carbs: 92.5g;
Protein: 25.3g;
Fat: 6.7g

INGREDIENTS

- 3 cans coconut milk
- 1 tbsp. garlic, minced
- Salt and pepper to taste
- 3 cans clams, chopped
- 2 cans shrimps, canned
- 1 package fresh shrimps, shelled and deveined
- 1 can corn, drained
- 4 large potatoes, diced
- 2 carrots, peeled and chopped
- 2 celery stalks, chopped

DIRECTIONS

1. Place all ingredients in a pot and give a good stir to mix everything.
2. Close the lid and turn on the heat to medium.
3. Bring to a boil and allow to simmer for 10 minutes.
4. Place in individual containers.
5. Put a label and store in the fridge.
6. Allow to warm at room temperature before heating in the microwave oven.

510. Orange Rosemary Seared Salmon

PREP TIME
10 mins

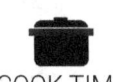
COOK TIME
10 mins

SERVINGS
4 people

NUTRITION

Calories: 493;
Fat: 17.9g;
Protein: 66.7g;
Carbs: 12.8g

INGREDIENTS

- ½ cup chicken stock
- 1 cup fresh orange juice
- 1 tbsp. coconut oil
- 1 tbsp. tapioca starch
- 2 garlic cloves, minced
- 2 tbsp. fresh lemon juice
- 2 tsp. fresh rosemary, minced
- 2 tsp. orange zest
- 4 salmon fillets, skins removed
- Salt and pepper to taste

DIRECTIONS

1. Season the salmon fillet on both sides.
2. In a skillet, heat coconut oil over medium high heat. Cook the salmon fillets for 5 minutes on each side. Set aside.
3. In a mixing bowl, combine the orange juice, chicken stock, lemon juice and orange zest.
4. In the skillet, sauté the garlic and rosemary for 2 minutes and pour the orange juice mixture. Bring to a boil. Lower the heat to medium low and simmer. Season with salt and pepper to taste.
5. Pour the sauce all over the salmon fillet then serve.

511. Orange Herbed Sauced White Bass

PREP TIME
10 mins

COOK TIME
33 mins

SERVINGS
6 people

NUTRITION

Calories: 312.42;
Protein: 84.22;
Fat: 23.14;
Carbs: 33.91g

INGREDIENTS

- ¼ cup thinly sliced green onions
- ½ cup orange juice
- 1 ½ tbsp. fresh lemon juice
- 1 ½ tbsp. olive oil
- 1 large onion, halved, thinly sliced
- 1 large orange, unpeeled, sliced
- 3 tbsp. chopped fresh dill
- 6 3-oz skinless white bass fillets
- Additional unpeeled orange slices

DIRECTIONS

1. Grease a 13 x 9-inch glass baking dish and preheat oven to 400oF.
2. Arrange orange slices in single layer on baking dish, top with onion slices, seasoned with pepper and salt plus drizzled with oil.
3. Pop in the oven and roast for 25 minutes or until onions are tender and browned.
4. Remove from oven and increased oven temperature to 450oF.
5. Push onion and orange slices on sides of dish and place bass fillets in middle of dish. Season with 1 ½ tbsp. dill, pepper and salt. Arrange onions and orange slices on top of fish and pop into the oven.
6. Roast for 8 minutes or until salmon is opaque and flaky.
7. In a small bowl, mix 1 ½ tbsp. dill, lemon juice, green onions and orange juice.
8. Transfer salmon to a serving plate, discard roasted onions, drizzle with the newly made orange sauce and garnish with fresh orange slices. Serve and enjoy.

512. Pan Fried Tuna with Herbs and Nut

PREP TIME
10 mins

COOK TIME
5 mins

SERVINGS
4 people

NUTRITION

Calories: 272;
Fat: 9.7 g;
Protein: 42 g;
Carbs: 4.2 g

INGREDIENTS

- ¼ cup almonds, chopped finely
- ¼ cup fresh tangerine juice
- ½ tsp. fennel seeds, chopped finely
- ½ tsp. ground pepper, divided
- ½ tsp. sea salt, divided
- 1 tbsp. olive oil
- 2 tbsp.. fresh mint, chopped finely
- 2 tbsp.. red onion, chopped finely
- 4 pieces of 6-oz Tuna steak cut in half

DIRECTIONS

1. Mix fennel seeds, olive oil, mint, onion, tangerine juice and almonds in small bowl. Season with ¼ each of pepper and salt.
2. Season fish with the remaining pepper and salt.
3. On medium high fire, place a large nonstick fry pan and grease with cooking spray.
4. Pan fry tuna until desired doneness is reached or for one minute per side.
5. Transfer cooked tuna in serving plate, drizzle with dressing and serve.

513. Paprika Salmon and Green Beans

PREP TIME: 10 mins
COOK TIME: 20 mins
SERVINGS: 3 people

INGREDIENTS

- ¼ cup olive oil
- ½ tbsp. onion powder
- ½ tsp. bouillon powder
- ½ tsp. cayenne pepper
- 1 tbsp. smoked paprika
- 1-lb. green beans
- 2 tsp. minced garlic
- 3 tbsp. fresh herbs
- 6 oz. of salmon steak
- Salt and pepper to taste

DIRECTIONS

1. Preheat the oven to 400°F.
2. Grease a baking sheet and set aside.
3. Heat a skillet over medium low heat and add the olive oil. Sauté the garlic, smoked paprika, fresh herbs, cayenne pepper and onion powder. Stir for a minute then let the mixture sit for 5 minutes. Set aside.
4. Put the salmon steaks in a bowl and add salt and the paprika spice mixture. Rub to coat the salmon well.
5. Place the salmon on the baking sheet and cook for 18 minutes.
6. Meanwhile, blanch the green beans in boiling water with salt.
7. Serve the beans with the salmon.

NUTRITION

Calories: 945.8;
Fat: 66.6 g;
Protein: 43.5 g;
Carbs: 43.1 g

514. Pecan Crusted Trout

PREP TIME: 10 mins
COOK TIME: 12 mins
SERVINGS: 4 people

INGREDIENTS

- ½ cup crushed pecans
- ½ tsp. grated fresh ginger
- 1 egg, beaten
- 1 tsp. crush dried rosemary
- 1 tsp. salt
- 4 4-oz trout fillets
- Black pepper to taste
- Cooking spray
- Whole wheat flour, as needed

DIRECTIONS

1. Grease baking sheet lightly with cooking spray and preheat oven to 400oF.
2. In a shallow bowl, combine black pepper, salt, rosemary and pecans. In another shallow bowl, add whole wheat flour. In a third bowl, add beaten egg.
3. To prepare fish, dip in flour until covered well. Shake off excess flour. Then dip into beaten egg until coated well. Let excess egg drip off before dipping trout fillet into pecan crumbs. Press the trout lightly onto pecan crumbs to make it stick to the fish.
4. Place breaded fish onto prepared pan. Repeat process for remaining fillets.
5. Pop into the oven and bake for 10 to 12 minutes or until fish is flaky.

NUTRITION

Calories: 329;
Fat: 19g;
Protein: 26.95g;
Carbs: 3g

515. Pesto and Lemon Halibut

PREP TIME
10 mins

COOK TIME
10 mins

SERVINGS
4 people

NUTRITION

Calories: 277.4;
Fat: 13g;
Protein: 38.7g;
Carbs: 1.4g

INGREDIENTS

- 1 tbsp. fresh lemon juice
- 1 tbsp. lemon rind, grated
- 2 garlic cloves, peeled
- 2 tbsp. olive oil
- ¼ cup Parmesan Cheese, freshly grated
- 2/3 cups firmly packed basil leaves
- 1/8 tsp. freshly ground black pepper
- ¼ tsp. salt, divided
- 4 pcs 6-oz halibut fillets

DIRECTIONS

1. Preheat grill to medium fire and grease grate with cooking spray.
2. Season fillets with pepper and 1/8 tsp. salt. Place on grill and cook until halibut is flaky around 4 minutes per side.
3. Meanwhile, make your lemon pesto by combining lemon juice, lemon rind, garlic, olive oil, Parmesan cheese, basil leaves and remaining salt in a blender. Pulse mixture until finely minced but not pureed.
4. Once fish is done cooking, transfer to a serving platter, pour over the lemon pesto sauce, serve and enjoy.

516. Red Peppers & Pineapple Topped Mahi-Mahi

PREP TIME
10 mins

COOK TIME
30 mins

SERVINGS
4 people

NUTRITION

Calories: 302;
Protein: 43.1g;
Fat: 4.8g;
Carbs: 22.0g

INGREDIENTS

- ¼ tsp. black pepper
- ¼ tsp. salt
- 1 cup whole wheat couscous
- 1 red bell pepper, diced
- 2 1/3 cups low sodium chicken broth
- 2 cups chopped fresh pineapple
- 2 tbsp.. chopped fresh chives
- 2 teaspoon. olive oil
- 4 pieces of skinless, boneless mahi mahi (dolphin fish) fillets (around 4-oz each)

DIRECTIONS

1. On high fire, add 1 1/3 cups broth to a small saucepan and heat until boiling. Once boiling, add couscous. Turn off fire, cover and set aside to allow liquid to be fully absorbed around 5 minutes.
2. On medium high fire, place a large nonstick saucepan and heat oil.
3. Season fish on both sides with pepper and salt. Add mahi mahi to hot pan and pan fry until golden around one minute each side. Once cooked, transfer to plate.
4. On same pan, sauté bell pepper and pineapples until soft, around 2 minutes on medium high fire.
5. Add couscous to pan along with chives, and remaining broth.
6. On top of the mixture in pan, place fish. With foil, cover pan and continue cooking until fish is steaming and tender underneath the foil, around 3-5 minutes.

517. Roasted Halibut with Banana Relish

PREP TIME 10 mins
COOK TIME 12 mins
SERVINGS 4 people

NUTRITION
Calories: 245.7;
Protein: 15.3g;
Fat: 6g;
Carbs: 21g

INGREDIENTS
- ¼ cup cilantro
- ½ tsp. freshly grated orange zest
- ½ tsp. kosher salt, divided
- 1 lb. halibut or any deep-water fish
- 1 tsp. ground coriander, divided into half
- 2 oranges (peeled, segmented and chopped)
- 2 ripe bananas, diced
- 2 tbsp. lime juice

DIRECTIONS
1. In a pan, prepare the fish by rubbing ½ tsp. coriander and ¼ tsp. kosher salt.
2. Place in a baking sheet with cooking spray and bake for 8 to 12 minutes inside a 450°F preheated oven.
3. Prepare the relish by stirring the orange zest, bananas, chopped oranges, lime juice, cilantro and the rest of the salt and coriander in a medium bowl.
4. Spoon the relish over the roasted fish.
5. Serve and enjoy.

518. Roasted Pollock Fillet with Bacon and Leeks

PREP TIME 10 mins
COOK TIME 30 mins
SERVINGS 2 people

NUTRITION
Calories: 442;
Carbs: 13.6 g;
Protein: 42.9 g;
Fat: 24 g

INGREDIENTS
- ¼ cup olive oil
- ½ cup white wine
- 1 ½ lbs. Pollock fillets
- 1 sprig fresh thyme
- 1 tbsp. chopped fresh thyme
- 2 tbsp.. olive oil
- 4 leeks, sliced

DIRECTIONS
1. Grease a 9x13 baking dish and preheat oven to 400°F F.
2. In baking pan add olive oil and leeks. Toss to combine.
3. Pop into the oven and roast for 10 minutes.
4. Remove from oven; add white wine and 1 tbsp. chopped thyme. Return to oven and roast for another 10 minutes.
5. Remove pan from oven and add fish on top. With a spoon, spoon olive oil mixture onto fish until coated fully. Return to oven and roast for another ten minutes.
6. Remove from oven, garnish with a sprig of thyme and serve.

519. Scallops in Wine 'n Olive Oil

PREP TIME
10 mins

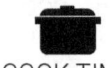
COOK TIME
8 mins

SERVINGS
4 people

NUTRITION

Calories: 205.2;
Fat: 8 g;
Protein: 28.6 g;
Carbs: 4.7 g

INGREDIENTS

- ¼ tsp. salt
- ½ cup dry white wine
- 1 ½ lbs. large sea scallops
- 1 ½ tsp. chopped fresh tarragon
- 2 tbsp. olive oil
- Black pepper – optional

DIRECTIONS

1. On medium high fire, place a large nonstick fry pan and heat oil.
2. Add scallops and fry for 3 minutes per side or until edges are lightly browned. Transfer to a serving plate.
3. On same pan, add salt, tarragon and wine while scraping pan to loosen browned bits.
4. Turn off fire.
5. Pour sauce over scallops and serve.

520. Seafood Stew Cioppino

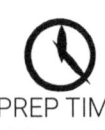
PREP TIME
10 mins

COOK TIME
40 mins

SERVINGS
6 people

NUTRITION

Calories: 371;
Carbs: 15.5 g;
Protein: 62 g;
Fat: 6.8 g

INGREDIENTS

- ¼ cup Italian parsley, chopped
- ¼ tsp. dried basil
- ¼ tsp. dried thyme
- ½ cup dry white wine like pinot grigio
- ½ lb. King crab legs, cut at each joint
- ½ onion, chopped
- ½ tsp. red pepper flakes (adjust to desired spiciness)
- 1 28-oz can crushed tomatoes
- 1 lb. mahi mahi, cut into ½-inch cubes
- 1 lb. raw shrimp
- 1 tbsp. olive oil
- 2 bay leaves
- 2 cups clam juice
- 50 live clams, washed
- 6 cloves garlic, minced
- Pepper and salt to taste

DIRECTIONS

1. On medium fire, place a stockpot and heat oil.
2. Add onion and for 4 minutes sauté until soft.
3. Add bay leaves, thyme, basil, red pepper flakes and garlic. Cook for a minute while stirring a bit.
4. Add clam juice and tomatoes. Once simmering, place fire to medium low and cook for 20 minutes uncovered.
5. Add white wine and clams. Cover and cook for 5 minutes or until clams have slightly opened.
6. Stir pot then add fish pieces, crab legs and shrimps. Do not stir soup to maintain the fish's shape. Cook while covered for 4 minutes or until clams are fully opened; fish and shrimps are opaque and cooked.
7. Season with pepper and salt to taste.
8. Transfer Cioppino to serving bowls and garnish with parsley before serving.

521. Simple Cod Piccata

PREP TIME: 10 mins
COOK TIME: 15 mins
SERVINGS: 3 people

INGREDIENTS

- ¼ cup capers, drained
- ½ tsp. salt
- ¾ cup chicken stock
- 1/3 cup almond flour
- 1-lb. cod fillets, patted dry
- 2 tbsp. fresh parsley, chopped
- 2 tbsp. grapeseed oil
- 3 tbsp. extra-virgin oil
- 3 tbsp. lemon juice

DIRECTIONS

1. In a bowl, combine the almond flour and salt.
2. Dredge the fish in the almond flour to coat. Set aside.
3. Heat a little bit of olive oil to coat a large skillet. Heat the skillet over medium high heat. Add grapeseed oil. Cook the cod for 3 minutes on each side to brown. Remove from the plate and place on a paper towel-lined plate.
4. In a saucepan, mix together the chicken stock, capers and lemon juice. Simmer to reduce the sauce to half. Add the remaining grapeseed oil.
5. Drizzle the fried cod with the sauce and sprinkle with parsley.

NUTRITION
Calories: 277.1;
Fat: 28.3 g;
Protein: 21.9 g;
Carbs: 3.7 g

522. Smoked Trout Tartine

PREP TIME: 10 mins
COOK TIME: 0 mins
SERVINGS: 4 people

INGREDIENTS

- ½ 15-oz can cannellini beans
- ½ cup diced roasted red peppers
- ¾ lb. smoked trout, flaked into bite-sized pieces
- 1 stalk celery, finely chopped
- 1 tbsp. extra virgin olive oil
- 1 tsp. chopped fresh dill
- 1 tsp. Dijon mustard
- 2 tbsp. capers, rinsed and drained
- 2 tbsp. freshly squeezed lemon juice
- 2 tsp. minced onion
- 4 large whole grain bread, toasted
- Dill sprigs – for garnish
- Pinch of sugar

DIRECTIONS

1. Mix sugar, mustard, olive oil and lemon juice in a big bowl.
2. Add the rest of the ingredients except for toasted bread.
3. Toss to mix well.
4. Evenly divide fish mixture on top of bread slices and garnish with dill sprigs.
5. Serve and enjoy.

NUTRITION
Calories: 348.1;
Protein: 28.2 g;
Fat: 10.1g;
Carbs: 36.1g

523. Steamed Mussels Thai Style

PREP TIME
10 mins

COOK TIME
15 mins

SERVINGS
4 people

NUTRITION

Calories: 407.2;
Protein: 43.4g;
Fat: 21.2g;
Carbs: 10.8g

INGREDIENTS

- ¼ cup minced shallots
- ½ tsp. Madras curry
- 1 cup dry white wine
- 1 small bay leaf
- 1 tbsp. chopped fresh basil
- 1 tbsp. chopped fresh cilantro
- 1 tbsp. chopped fresh mint
- 2 lbs. mussel, cleaned and debearded
- 2 tbsp. butter
- 4 medium garlic cloves, minced

DIRECTIONS

1. In a large heavy bottomed pot, on medium high fire add to pot the curry powder, bay leaf, wine plus the minced garlic and shallots. Bring to a boil and simmer for 3 minutes.
2. Add the cleaned mussels, stir, cover, and cook for 3 minutes.
3. Stir mussels again, cover, and cook for another 2 or 3 minutes. Cooking is done when majority of shells have opened.
4. With a slotted spoon, transfer cooked mussels in a large bowl. Discard any unopened mussels.
5. Continue heating pot with sauce. Add butter and the chopped herbs.
6. Season with pepper and salt to taste.
7. Once good, pour over mussels, serve and enjoy.

524. Tasty Tuna Scaloppine

PREP TIME
10 mins

COOK TIME
10 mins

SERVINGS
4 people

NUTRITION

Calories: 405;
Protein: 27.5g;
Fat: 11.9g;
Carbs: 27.5

INGREDIENTS

- ¼ cup chopped almonds
- ¼ cup fresh tangerine juice
- ½ tsp. fennel seeds
- ½ tsp. ground black pepper, divided
- ½ tsp. salt
- 1 tbsp. extra virgin olive oil
- 2 tbsp. chopped fresh mint
- 2 tbsp. chopped red onion
- 4 6-oz sushi-grade Yellowfin tuna steaks, each split in half horizontally
- Cooking spray

DIRECTIONS

1. In a small bowl mix fennel seeds, olive oil, mint, onion, tangerine juice, almonds, ¼ tsp. pepper and ¼ tsp. salt. Combine thoroughly.
2. Season fish with remaining salt and pepper.
3. On medium high fire, place a large nonstick pan and grease with cooking spray. Pan fry fish in two batches cooking each side for a minute.
4. Fish is best served with a side of salad greens or a half cup of cooked brown rice.

525. Thyme and Lemon on Baked Salmon

PREP TIME
10 mins

COOK TIME
25 mins

SERVINGS
2 people

NUTRITION
Calories: 684.4;
Protein: 94.3g;
Fat: 32.7g;
Carbs: 4.3g

INGREDIENTS
- 1 32-oz salmon fillet
- 1 lemon, sliced thinly
- 1 tbsp. capers
- 1 tbsp. fresh thyme
- Olive oil for drizzling
- Pepper and salt to taste

DIRECTIONS
1. In a foil line baking sheet, place a parchment paper on top.
2. Place salmon with skin side down on parchment paper.
3. Season generously with pepper and salt.
4. Place capers on top of fillet. Cover with thinly sliced lemon.
5. Garnish with thyme.
6. Pop in cold oven and bake for 25 minutes at 400°F settings.
7. Serve right away and enjoy.

526. Warm Caper Tapenade on Cod

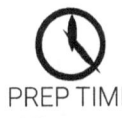
PREP TIME
10 mins

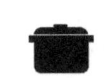
COOK TIME
30 mins

SERVINGS
4 people

NUTRITION
Calories: 107;
Fat: 2.9g;
Protein: 17.6g;
Carbs: 2.0g

INGREDIENTS
- ¼ cup chopped cured olives
- ¼ tsp. freshly ground pepper
- 1 ½ tsp. chopped fresh oregano
- 1 cup halved cherry tomatoes
- 1 lb. cod fillet
- 1 tbsp. capers, rinsed and chopped
- 1 tbsp. minced shallot
- 1 tsp. balsamic vinegar
- 3 tsp. extra virgin olive oil, divided

DIRECTIONS
1. Grease baking sheet with cooking spray and preheat oven to 450oF.
2. Place cod on prepared baking sheet. Rub with 2 tsp. oil and season with pepper.
3. Roast in oven for 15 to 20 minutes or until cod is flaky.
4. While waiting for cod to cook, on medium fire, place a small fry pan and heat 1 tsp. oil.
5. Sauté shallots for a minute.
6. Add tomatoes and cook for two minutes or until soft.
7. Add capers and olives. Sauté for another minute.
8. Add vinegar and oregano. Turn off fire and stir to mix well.
9. Evenly divide cod into 4 serving and place on a plate.
10. 1 To serve, top cod with Caper-Olive-Tomato Tapenade and enjoy.

527. Yummy Salmon Panzanella

PREP TIME
10 mins

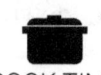
COOK TIME
10 mins

SERVINGS
4 people

NUTRITION

Calories: 383;
Fat: 20.6g;
Protein: 34.8g;
Carbs: 13.6g

INGREDIENTS

- ¼ cup thinly sliced fresh basil
- ¼ cup thinly sliced red onion
- ¼ tsp. freshly ground pepper, divided
- ½ tsp. salt
- 1 lb. center cut salmon, skinned and cut into 4 equal portions
- 1 medium cucumber, peeled, seeded, and cut into 1-inch slices
- 1 tbsp. capers, rinsed and chopped
- 2 large tomatoes, cut into 1-inch pieces
- 2 thick slices day old whole grain bread, sliced into 1-inch cubes
- 3 tbsp. extra virgin olive oil
- 3 tbsp. red wine vinegar
- 8 Kalamata olives, pitted and chopped

DIRECTIONS

1. Grease grill grate and preheat grill to high.
2. In a large bowl, whisk 1/8 tsp. pepper, capers, vinegar, and olives. Add oil and whisk well.
3. Stir in basil, onion, cucumber, tomatoes, and bread.
4. Season both sides of salmon with remaining pepper and salt.
5. Grill on high for 4 minutes per side.
6. Into 4 plates, evenly divide salad, top with grilled salmon, and serve.

528. Fish and Orzo

PREP TIME
10 mins

COOK TIME
35 mins

SERVINGS
4 people

NUTRITION

Calories 402,
Fat 21g,
Fiber 8g,
Carbs 21g,
Protein 31g

INGREDIENTS

- 1 tsp. garlic, minced
- 1 tsp. red pepper, crushed
- 2 shallots, chopped
- 1 tbsp. olive oil
- 1 tsp. anchovy paste
- 1 tbsp. oregano, chopped
- 2 tbsp. black olives, pitted and chopped
- 2 tbsp. capers, drained
- 15 oz. canned tomatoes, crushed
- A pinch of salt and black pepper
- 4 cod fillets, boneless
- 1 oz. feta cheese, crumbled
- 1 tbsp. parsley, chopped
- 3 cups chicken stock
- 1 cup orzo pasta
- Zest of 1 lemon, grated

DIRECTIONS

1. Heat up a pan with the oil over medium heat, add the garlic, red pepper and the shallots and sauté for 5 minutes.
2. Add the anchovy paste, oregano, black olives, capers, tomatoes, salt and pepper, stir and cook for 5 minutes more.
3. Add the cod fillets, sprinkle the cheese and the parsley on top, introduce in the oven and bake at 375°F for 15 minutes more.
4. Meanwhile, put the stock in a pot, bring to a boil over medium heat, add the orzo and the lemon zest, bring to a simmer, cook for 10 minutes, fluff with a fork, and divide between plates.
5. Top each serving with the fish mix and serve.

529. Baked Sea Bass

PREP TIME: 10 mins
COOK TIME: 12 mins
SERVINGS: 4 people

INGREDIENTS

- 4 sea bass fillets, boneless
- Sal and black pepper to the taste
- 2 cups potato chips, crushed
- 1 tbsp. mayonnaise

DIRECTIONS

1. Season the fish fillets with salt and pepper, brush with the mayonnaise and dredge each in the potato chips.
2. Arrange the fillets on a baking sheet lined with parchment paper and bake at 400°F for 12 minutes.
3. Divide the fish between plates and serve with a side salad.

NUTRITION

Calories 228, Fat 8.6g, Fiber 0.6g, Carbs 9.3g, Protein 25g

---

530. Fish and Tomato Sauce

PREP TIME: 10 mins
COOK TIME: 30 mins
SERVINGS: 4 people

INGREDIENTS

- 4 cod fillets, boneless
- 2 garlic cloves, minced
- 2 cups cherry tomatoes, halved
- 1 cup chicken stock
- A pinch of salt and black pepper
- ¼ cup basil, chopped

DIRECTIONS

1. Put the tomatoes, garlic, salt and pepper in a pan, heat up over medium heat and cook for 5 minutes.
2. Add the fish and the rest of the ingredients, bring to a simmer, cover the pan and cook for 25 minutes.
3. Divide the mix between plates and serve.

NUTRITION

Calories 180, Fat 1.9g, Fiber 1.4g, Carbs 5.3g, Protein 33.8g

531. Halibut and Quinoa Mix

PREP TIME
10 mins

COOK TIME
12 mins

SERVINGS
4 people

NUTRITION

Calories 364,
Fat 15.4g,
Fiber 11.2g,
Carbs 56.4g,
Protein 24.5g

INGREDIENTS

- 4 halibut fillets, boneless
- 2 tbsp. olive oil
- 1 tsp. rosemary, dried
- 2 tsp. cumin, ground
- 1 tbsp. coriander, ground
- 2 tsp. cinnamon powder
- 2 tsp. oregano, dried
- A pinch of salt and black pepper
- 2 cups quinoa, cooked
- 1 cup cherry tomatoes, halved
- 1 avocado, peeled, pitted and sliced
- 1 cucumber, cubed
- ½ cup black olives, pitted and sliced
- Juice of 1 lemon

DIRECTIONS

1. In a bowl, combine the fish with the rosemary, cumin, coriander, cinnamon, oregano, salt and pepper and toss.
2. Heat up a pan with the oil over medium heat, add the fish, and sear for 2 minutes on each side.
3. Introduce the pan in the oven and bake the fish at 425°F for 7 minutes.
4. Meanwhile, in a bowl, mix the quinoa with the remaining ingredients, toss and divide between plates.
5. Add the fish next to the quinoa mix and serve right away.

532. Lemon and Dates Barramundi

PREP TIME
10 mins

COOK TIME
12 mins

SERVINGS
2 people

NUTRITION

Calories 232,
Fat 16.5g,
Fiber 11.1g,
Carbs 24.8g,
Protein 6.5g

INGREDIENTS

- 2 barramundi fillets, boneless
- 1 shallot, sliced
- 4 lemon slices
- Juice of ½ lemon
- Zest of 1 lemon, grated
- 2 tbsp. olive oil
- 6 oz. baby spinach
- ¼ cup almonds, chopped
- 4 dates, pitted and chopped
- ¼ cup parsley, chopped
- Salt and black pepper to the taste

DIRECTIONS

1. Season the fish with salt and pepper and arrange on 2 parchment paper pieces.
2. Top the fish with the lemon slices, drizzle the lemon juice, and then top with the other ingredients except the oil.
3. Drizzle 1 tbsp. oil over each fish mix, wrap the parchment paper around the fish shaping to packets and arrange them on a baking sheet.
4. Bake at 400°F for 12 minutes, cool the mix a bit, unfold, divide everything between plates and serve.

533. Fish Cakes

PREP TIME: 10 mins
COOK TIME: 10 mins
SERVINGS: 6 people

NUTRITION
Calories 288, Fat 12.8g, Fiber 10.2g, Carbs 22.2g, Protein 6.8g

INGREDIENTS

- 20 oz. canned sardines, drained and mashed well
- 2 garlic cloves, minced
- 2 tbsp. dill, chopped
- 1 yellow onion, chopped
- 1 cup panko breadcrumbs
- 1 egg, whisked
- A pinch of salt and black pepper
- 2 tbsp. lemon juice
- 5 tbsp. olive oil

DIRECTIONS

1. In a bowl, combine the sardines with the garlic, dill and the rest of the ingredients except the oil, stir well and shape medium cakes out of this mix.
2. Heat up a pan with the oil over medium-high heat, add the fish cakes, cook for 5 minutes on each side.
3. Serve the cakes with a side salad.

534. Catfish Fillets and Rice

PREP TIME: 10 mins
COOK TIME: 55 mins
SERVINGS: 2 people

NUTRITION
Calories 261, Fat 17.6g, Fiber 12.2g, Carbs 24.8g, Protein 12.5g

INGREDIENTS

- 2 catfish fillets, boneless
- 2 tbsp. Italian seasoning
- 2 tbsp. olive oil
- For the rice:
- 1 cup brown rice
- 2 tbsp. olive oil
- 1 and ½ cups water
- ½ cup green bell pepper, chopped
- 2 garlic cloves, minced
- ½ cup white onion, chopped
- 2 tsp. Cajun seasoning
- ½ tsp. garlic powder
- Salt and black pepper to the taste

DIRECTIONS

1. Heat up a pot with 2 tbsp. oil over medium heat, add the onion, garlic, garlic powder, salt and pepper and sauté for 5 minutes.
2. Add the rice, water, bell pepper and the seasoning, bring to a simmer and cook over medium heat for 40 minutes.
3. Heat up a pan with 2 tbsp. oil over medium heat, add the fish and the Italian seasoning, and cook for 5 minutes on each side.
4. Divide the rice between plates, add the fish on top and serve.

535. Halibut Pan

PREP TIME
10 mins

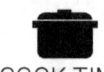
COOK TIME
20 mins

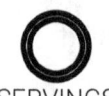
SERVINGS
4 people

NUTRITION

Calories 253,
Fat 8g,
Fiber 1g,
Carbs 5g,
Protein 28g

INGREDIENTS

- 4 halibut fillets, boneless
- 1 red bell pepper, chopped
- 2 tbsp. olive oil
- 1 yellow onion, chopped
- 4 garlic cloves, minced
- ½ cup chicken stock
- 1 tsp. basil, dried
- ½ cup cherry tomatoes, halved
- 1/3 cup kalamata olives, pitted and halved
- Salt and black pepper to the taste

DIRECTIONS

1. Heat up a pan with the oil over medium heat, add the fish, cook for 5 minutes on each side and divide between plates.
2. Add the onion, bell pepper, garlic and tomatoes to the pan, stir and sauté for 3 minutes.
3. Add salt, pepper and the rest of the ingredients, toss, cook for 3 minutes more, divide next to the fish and serve.

536. Baked Shrimp Mix

PREP TIME
10 mins

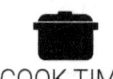
COOK TIME
32 mins

SERVINGS
4 people

NUTRITION

Calories 341,
Fat 19g,
Fiber 9g,
Carbs 34g,
Protein 10g

INGREDIENTS

- 4 gold potatoes, peeled and sliced
- 2 fennel bulbs, trimmed and cut into wedges
- 2 shallots, chopped
- 2 garlic cloves, minced
- 3 tbsp. olive oil
- ½ cup kalamata olives, pitted and halved
- 2 lb. shrimp, peeled and deveined
- 1 tsp. lemon zest, grated
- 2 tsp. oregano, dried
- 4 oz. feta cheese, crumbled
- 2 tbsp. parsley, chopped

DIRECTIONS

1. In a roasting pan, combine the potatoes with 2 tbsp. oil, garlic and the rest of the ingredients except the shrimp, toss, introduce in the oven and bake at 450°F for 25 minutes.
2. Add the shrimp, toss, bake for 7 minutes more, divide between plates and serve.

537. Shrimp and Lemon Sauce

PREP TIME: 10 mins
COOK TIME: 15 mins
SERVINGS: 4 people

NUTRITION
Calories 237, Fat 15.3g, Fiber 4.6g, Carbs 15.4g, Protein 7.6g

INGREDIENTS

- 1 lb. shrimp, peeled and deveined
- 1/3 cup lemon juice
- 4 egg yolks
- 2 tbsp. olive oil
- 1 cup chicken stock
- Salt and black pepper to the taste
- 1 cup black olives, pitted and halved
- 1 tbsp. thyme, chopped

DIRECTIONS

1. In a bowl, mix the lemon juice with the egg yolks and whisk well.
2. Heat up a pan with the oil over medium heat, add the shrimp and cook for 2 minutes on each side and transfer to a plate.
3. Heat up a pan with the stock over medium heat, add some of this over the egg yolks and lemon juice mix and whisk well.
4. Add this over the rest of the stock, also add salt and pepper, whisk well and simmer for 2 minutes.
5. Add the shrimp and the rest of the ingredients, toss and serve right away.

538. Shrimp and Beans Salad

PREP TIME: 10 mins
COOK TIME: 4 mins
SERVINGS: 4 people

NUTRITION
Calories 207, Fat 12.3g, Fiber 6.6g, Carbs 15.4g, Protein 8.7g

INGREDIENTS

- 1 lb. shrimp, peeled and deveined
- 30 oz. canned cannellini beans, drained and rinsed
- 2 tbsp. olive oil
- 1 cup cherry tomatoes, halved
- 1 tsp. lemon zest, grated
- ½ cup red onion, chopped
- 4 handfuls baby arugula
- A pinch of salt and black pepper
- For the dressing:
- 3 tbsp. red wine vinegar
- 2 garlic cloves, minced
- ½ cup olive oil

DIRECTIONS

1. Heat up a pan with 2 tbsp. oil over medium-high heat, add the shrimp and cook for 2 minutes on each side.
2. In a salad bowl, combine the shrimp with the beans and the rest of the ingredients except the ones for the dressing and toss.
3. In a separate bowl, combine the vinegar with ½ cup oil and the garlic and whisk well.
4. Pour over the salad, toss and serve right away.

539. Pecan Salmon Fillets

PREP TIME
10 mins

COOK TIME
15 mins

SERVINGS
6 people

INGREDIENTS

- 3 tbsp. olive oil
- 3 tbsp. mustard
- 5 tsp. honey
- 1 cup pecans, chopped
- 6 salmon fillets, boneless
- 1 tbsp. lemon juice
- 3 tsp. parsley, chopped
- Salt and pepper to the taste

DIRECTIONS

1. In a bowl, mix the oil with the mustard and honey and whisk well.
2. Put the pecans and the parsley in another bowl.
3. Season the salmon fillets with salt and pepper, arrange them on a baking sheet lined with parchment paper, brush with the honey and mustard mix and top with the pecans mix.
4. Introduce in the oven at 400°F, bake for 15 minutes, divide between plates, drizzle the lemon juice on top and serve.

NUTRITION

Calories 282,
Fat 15.5g,
Fiber 8.5g,
Carbs 20.9g,
Protein 16.8g

540. Salmon and Broccoli

PREP TIME
10 mins

COOK TIME
20 mins

SERVINGS
4 people

INGREDIENTS

- 2 tbsp. balsamic vinegar
- 1 broccoli head, florets separated
- 4 pieces salmon fillets, skinless
- 1 big red onion, roughly chopped
- 1 tbsp. olive oil
- Sea salt and black pepper to the taste

DIRECTIONS

1. In a baking dish, combine the salmon with the broccoli and the rest of the ingredients, introduce in the oven and bake at 390°F for 20 minutes.
2. Divide the mix between plates and serve.

NUTRITION

Calories 302,
Fat 15.5g,
Fiber 8.5g,
Carbs 18.9g,
Protein 19.8g

541. Salmon and Peach Pan

PREP TIME: 10 mins
COOK TIME: 11 mins
SERVINGS: 4 people

INGREDIENTS

- 1 tbsp. balsamic vinegar
- 1 tsp. thyme, chopped
- 1 tbsp. ginger, grated
- 2 tbsp. olive oil
- Sea salt and black pepper to the taste
- 3 peaches, cut into medium wedges
- 4 salmon fillets, boneless

DIRECTIONS

1. Heat up a pan with the oil over medium-high heat, add the salmon and cook for 3 minutes on each side.
2. Add the vinegar, the peaches and the rest of the ingredients, cook for 5 minutes more, divide everything between plates and serve.

NUTRITION

Calories 293, Fat 17.1g, Fiber 4.1g, Carbs 26.4g, Protein 24.5g

---

542. Tarragon Cod Fillets

PREP TIME: 10 mins
COOK TIME: 12 mins
SERVINGS: 4 people

INGREDIENTS

- 4 cod fillets, boneless
- ¼ cup capers, drained
- 1 tbsp. tarragon, chopped
- Sea salt and black pepper to the taste
- 2 tbsp. olive oil
- 2 tbsp. parsley, chopped
- 1 tbsp. olive oil
- 1 tbsp. lemon juice

DIRECTIONS

1. Heat up a pan with the oil over medium-high heat, add the fish and cook for 3 minutes on each side.
2. Add the rest of the ingredients, cook everything for 7 minutes more, divide between plates and serve.

NUTRITION

Calories 162, Fat 9.6g, Fiber 4.3g, Carbs 12.4g, Protein 16.5g

543. Salmon and Radish Mix

PREP TIME
10 mins

COOK TIME
15 mins

SERVINGS
4 people

NUTRITION

Calories 274, Fat 14.5g, Fiber 3.5g, Carbs 8.5g, Protein 22.3g

INGREDIENTS

- 2 tbsp. olive oil
- 1 tbsp. balsamic vinegar
- 1 and ½ cup chicken stock
- 4 salmon fillets, boneless
- 2 garlic cloves, minced
- 1 tbsp. ginger, grated
- 1 cup radishes, grated
- ¼ cup scallions, chopped

DIRECTIONS

1. Heat up a pan with the oil over medium-high heat, add the salmon, cook for 4 minutes on each side and divide between plates
2. Add the vinegar and the rest of the ingredients to the pan, toss gently, cook for 10 minutes, add over the salmon and serve.

544. Smoked Salmon and Watercress Salad

PREP TIME
5 mins

COOK TIME
0 mins

SERVINGS
4 people

NUTRITION

Calories 244, Fat 16.7g, Fiber 4.5g, Carbs 22.5g, Protein 15.6g

INGREDIENTS

- 2 bunches watercress
- 1 lb. smoked salmon, skinless, boneless and flaked
- 2 tsp. mustard
- ¼ cup lemon juice
- ½ cup Greek yogurt
- Salt and black pepper to the taste
- 1 big cucumber, sliced
- 2 tbsp. chives, chopped

DIRECTIONS

1. In a salad bowl, combine the salmon with the watercress and the rest of the ingredients toss and serve right away.

545. Salmon and Corn Salad

PREP TIME 5 mins
COOK TIME 0 mins
SERVINGS 4 people

INGREDIENTS

- ½ cup pecans, chopped
- 2 cups baby arugula
- 1 cup corn
- ¼ lb. smoked salmon, skinless, boneless and cut into small chunks
- 2 tbsp. olive oil
- 2 tbsp. lemon juice
- Sea salt and black pepper to the taste

DIRECTIONS

1. In a salad bowl, combine the salmon with the corn and the rest of the ingredients, toss and serve right away.

NUTRITION
Calories 284, Fat 18.4g, Fiber 5.4g, Carbs 22.6g, Protein 17.4g

546. Cod and Mushrooms Mix

PREP TIME 10 mins
COOK TIME 25 mins
SERVINGS 4 people

INGREDIENTS

- 2 cod fillets, boneless
- 4 tbsp. olive oil
- 4 oz. mushrooms, sliced
- Sea salt and black pepper to the taste
- 12 cherry tomatoes, halved
- 8 oz. lettuce leaves, torn
- 1 avocado, pitted, peeled and cubed
- 1 red chili pepper, chopped
- 1 tbsp. cilantro, chopped
- 2 tbsp. balsamic vinegar
- 1 oz. feta cheese, crumbled

DIRECTIONS

1. Put the fish in a roasting pan, brush it with 2 tbsp. oil, sprinkle salt and pepper all over and broil under medium-high heat for 15 minutes. Meanwhile, heat up a pan with the rest of the oil over medium heat, add the mushrooms, stir and sauté for 5 minutes.
2. Add the rest of the ingredients, toss, cook for 5 minutes more and divide between plates.
3. Top with the fish and serve right away.

NUTRITION
Calories 257, Fat 10g, Fiber 3.1g, Carbs 24.3g, Protein 19.4g

547. Sesame Shrimp Mix

PREP TIME 10 mins

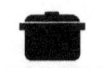
COOK TIME 0 mins

SERVINGS 4 people

NUTRITION

Calories 177, Fat 9g, Fiber 7.1g, Carbs 14.3g, Protein 9.4g

INGREDIENTS

- 2 tbsp. lime juice
- 3 tbsp. teriyaki sauce
- 2 tbsp. olive oil
- 8 cups baby spinach
- 14 oz. shrimp, cooked, peeled and deveined
- 1 cup cucumber, sliced
- 1 cup radish, sliced
- ¼ cup cilantro, chopped
- 2 tsp. sesame seeds, toasted

DIRECTIONS

1. In a bowl, mix the shrimp with the lime juice, spinach and the rest of the ingredients, toss and serve cold.

548. Creamy Curry Salmon

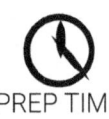
PREP TIME 10 mins

COOK TIME 20 mins

SERVINGS 2 people

NUTRITION

Calories 284, Fat 14.1g, Fiber 8.5g, Carbs 26.7g, Protein 31.4g

INGREDIENTS

- 2 salmon fillets, boneless and cubed
- 1 tbsp. olive oil
- 1 tbsp. basil, chopped
- Sea salt and black pepper to the taste
- 1 cup Greek yogurt
- 2 tsp. curry powder
- 1 garlic clove, minced
- ½ tsp. mint, chopped

DIRECTIONS

1. Heat up a pan with the oil over medium-high heat, add the salmon and cook for 3 minutes.
2. Add the rest of the ingredients, toss, cook for 15 minutes more, divide between plates and serve.

549. Mahi Mahi and Pomegranate Sauce

PREP TIME
10 mins

COOK TIME
10 mins

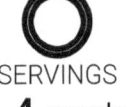
SERVINGS
4 people

NUTRITION

Calories 224,
Fat 11.1g,
Fiber 5.5g,
Carbs 16.7g,
Protein 11.4g

INGREDIENTS

- 1 and ½ cups chicken stock
- 1 tbsp. olive oil
- 4 mahi mahi fillets, boneless
- 4 tbsp. tahini paste
- Juice of 1 lime
- Seeds from 1 pomegranate
- 1 tbsp. parsley, chopped

DIRECTIONS

1. Heat up a pan with the oil over medium-high heat, add the fish and cook for 3 minutes on each side.
2. Add the rest of the ingredients, flip the fish again, cook for 4 minutes more, divide everything between plates and serve.

550. Smoked Salmon and Veggies Mix

PREP TIME
10 mins

COOK TIME
20 mins

SERVINGS
4 people

NUTRITION

Calories 301,
Fat 5.9g,
Fiber 11.9g,
Carbs 26.4g,
Protein 22.4g

INGREDIENTS

- 3 red onions, cut into wedges
- ¾ cup green olives, pitted and halved
- 3 red bell peppers, roughly chopped
- ½ tsp. smoked paprika
- Salt and black pepper to the taste
- 3 tbsp. olive oil
- 4 salmon fillets, skinless and boneless
- 2 tbsp. chives, chopped

DIRECTIONS

1. In a roasting pan, combine the salmon with the onions and the rest of the ingredients, introduce in the oven and bake at 390°F for 20 minutes.
2. Divide the mix between plates and serve.

551. Salmon and Mango Mix

PREP TIME
10 mins

COOK TIME
25 mins

SERVINGS
2 people

INGREDIENTS

- 2 salmon fillets, skinless and boneless
- Salt and pepper to the taste
- 2 tbsp. olive oil
- 2 garlic cloves, minced
- 2 mangos, peeled and cubed
- 1 red chili, chopped
- 1 small piece ginger, grated
- Juice of 1 lime
- 1 tbsp. cilantro, chopped

DIRECTIONS

1. In a roasting pan, combine the salmon with the oil, garlic and the rest of the ingredients except the cilantro, toss, introduce in the oven at 350°F and bake for 25 minutes.
2. Divide everything between plates and serve with the cilantro sprinkled on top.

NUTRITION

Calories 251, Fat 15.9g, Fiber 5.9g, Carbs 26.4g, Protein 12.4g

552. Salmon and Creamy Endives

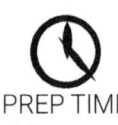
PREP TIME
10 mins

COOK TIME
15 mins

SERVINGS
4 people

INGREDIENTS

- 4 salmon fillets, boneless
- 2 endives, shredded
- Juice of 1 lime
- Salt and black pepper to the taste
- ¼ cup chicken stock
- 1 cup Greek yogurt
- ¼ cup green olives pitted and chopped
- ¼ cup fresh chives, chopped
- 3 tbsp. olive oil

DIRECTIONS

1. Heat up a pan with half of the oil over medium heat, add the endives and the rest of the ingredients except the chives and the salmon, toss, cook for 6 minutes and divide between plates.
2. Heat up another pan with the rest of the oil, add the salmon, season with salt and pepper, cook for 4 minutes on each side, add next to the creamy endives mix, sprinkle the chives on top and serve.

NUTRITION

Calories 266, Fat 13.9g, Fiber 11.1g, Carbs 23.8g, Protein 17.5g

553. Trout and Tzatziki Sauce

PREP TIME: 10 mins
COOK TIME: 10 mins
SERVINGS: 4 people

NUTRITION
Calories 393, Fat 18.5g, Fiber 6.5g, Carbs 18.3g, Protein 39.6g

INGREDIENTS

- Juice of ½ lime
- Salt and black pepper to the taste
- 1 and ½ tsp. coriander, ground
- 1 tsp. garlic, minced
- 4 trout fillets, boneless
- 1 tsp. sweet paprika
- 2 tbsp. avocado oil
- For the sauce:
- 1 cucumber, chopped
- 4 garlic cloves, minced
- 1 tbsp. olive oil
- 1 tsp. white vinegar
- 1 and ½ cups Greek yogurt
- A pinch of salt and white pepper

DIRECTIONS

1. Heat up a pan with the avocado oil over medium-high heat, add the fish, salt, pepper, lime juice, 1 tsp. garlic and the paprika, rub the fish gently and cook for 4 minutes on each side.
2. In a bowl, combine the cucumber with 4 garlic cloves and the rest of the ingredients for the sauce and whisk well.
3. Divide the fish between plates, drizzle the sauce all over and serve with a side salad.

554. Parsley Trout and Capers

PREP TIME: 10 mins
COOK TIME: 10 mins
SERVINGS: 4 people

NUTRITION
Calories 308, Fat 17g, Fiber 1g, Carbs 3g, Protein 16g

INGREDIENTS

- 4 trout fillets, boneless
- 3 oz. tomato sauce
- A handful parsley, chopped
- 2 tbsp. olive oil
- Salt and black pepper to the taste

DIRECTIONS

1. Heat up a pan with the oil over medium-high heat, add the fish, salt and pepper and cook for 3 minutes on each side.
2. Add the rest of the ingredients, cook everything for 4 minutes more.
3. Divide everything between plates and serve.

555. Baked Trout and Fennel

PREP TIME
10 mins

COOK TIME
22 mins

SERVINGS
4 people

INGREDIENTS

- 1 fennel bulb, sliced
- 2 tbsp. olive oil
- 1 yellow onion, sliced
- 3 tsp. Italian seasoning
- 4 rainbow trout fillets, boneless
- ¼ cup panko breadcrumbs
- ½ cup kalamata olives, pitted and halved
- Juice of 1 lemon

DIRECTIONS

1. Spread the fennel the onion and the rest of the ingredients except the trout and the breadcrumbs on a baking sheet lined with parchment paper, toss them and cook at 400°F for 10 minutes.
2. Add the fish dredged in breadcrumbs and seasoned with salt and pepper and cook it at 400°F for 6 minutes on each side.
3. Divide the mix between plates and serve.

NUTRITION

Calories 306,
Fat 8.9g,
Fiber 11.1g,
Carbs 23.8g,
Protein 14.5g

556. Lemon Rainbow Trout

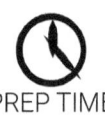
PREP TIME
10 mins

COOK TIME
15 mins

SERVINGS
2 people

INGREDIENTS

- 2 rainbow trout
- Juice of 1 lemon
- 3 tbsp. olive oil
- 4 garlic cloves, minced
- A pinch of salt and black pepper

DIRECTIONS

1. Line a baking sheet with parchment paper, add the fish and the rest of the ingredients and rub.
2. Bake at 400°F for 15 minutes, divide between plates and serve with a side salad.

NUTRITION

Calories 321,
Fat 19g,
Fiber 5g,
Carbs 6g,
Protein 35g

557. Trout and Peppers Mix

PREP TIME: 10 mins
COOK TIME: 20 mins
SERVINGS: 4 people

INGREDIENTS

- 4 trout fillets, boneless
- 2 tbsp. kalamata olives, pitted and chopped
- 1 tbsp. capers, drained
- 2 tbsp. olive oil
- A pinch of salt and black pepper
- 1 and ½ tsp. chili powder
- 1 yellow bell pepper, chopped
- 1 red bell pepper, chopped
- 1 green bell pepper, chopped

DIRECTIONS

1. Heat up a pan with the oil over medium-high heat, add the trout, salt and pepper and cook for 10 minutes.
2. Flip the fish, add the peppers and the rest of the ingredients, cook for 10 minutes more, divide the whole mix between plates and serve.

NUTRITION

Calories 572, Fat 17.4g, Fiber 6g, Carbs 71g, Protein 33.7g

FRUITS, SWEETS AND DESSERTS

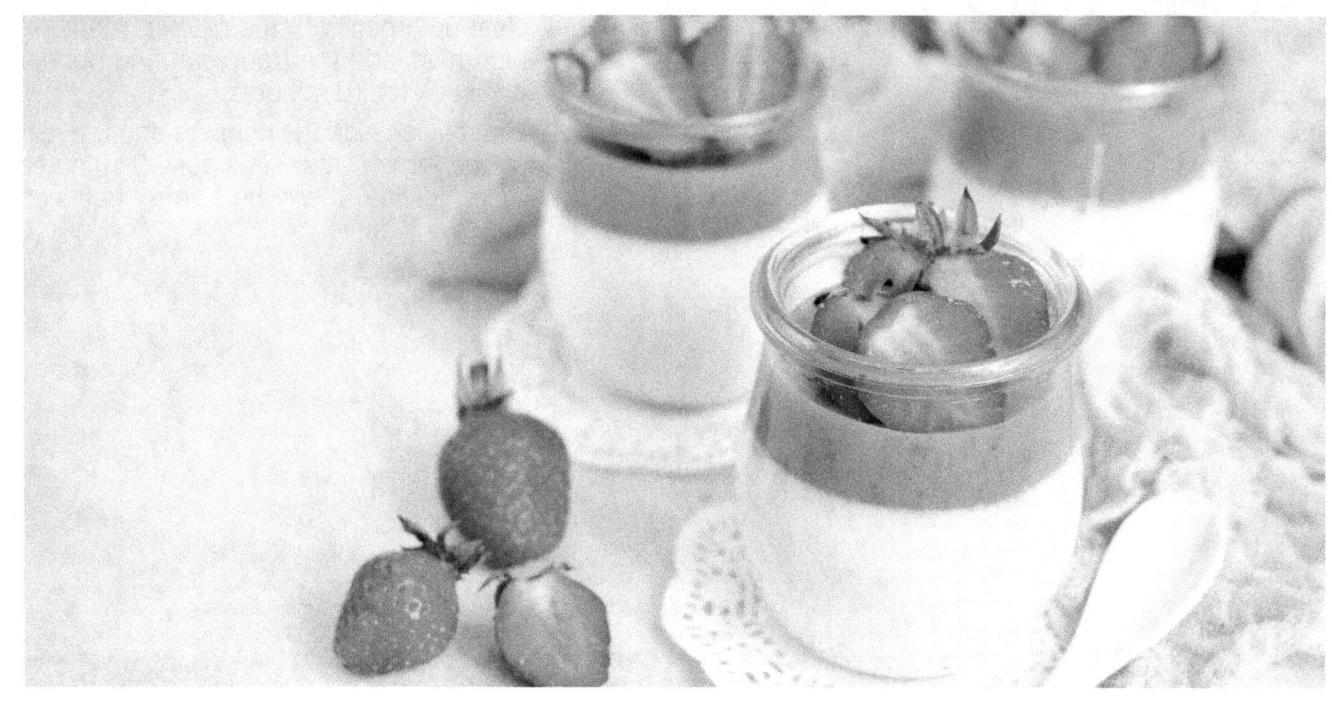

558. Banana Shake Bowls

PREP TIME
5 mins

COOK TIME
0 mins

SERVINGS
4 people

INGREDIENTS

- 4 medium bananas, peeled
- 1 avocado, peeled, pitted and mashed
- ¾ cup almond milk
- ½ tsp. vanilla extract

DIRECTIONS

1. In a blender, combine the bananas with the avocado and the other ingredients, pulse, divide into bowls and keep in the fridge until serving.

NUTRITION

Calories 185
Fat 4.3g
Carbs 6g
Protein 6.45g

559. Cold Lemon Squares

INGREDIENTS

- 1 cup avocado oil + a drizzle
- 2 bananas, peeled and chopped
- 1 tbsp. honey
- ¼ cup lemon juice
- A pinch of lemon zest, grated

DIRECTIONS

1. In your food processor, mix the bananas with the rest of the ingredients, pulse well and spread on the bottom of a pan greased with a drizzle of oil.
2. Introduce in the fridge for 30 minutes, slice into squares and serve.

PREP TIME 30 mins
COOK TIME 0 mins
SERVINGS 4 people

NUTRITION

Calories 136g
Fat 11.2g
Carbs 7g
Protein 1.1g

---

560. Blackberry and Apples Cobbler

INGREDIENTS

- ¾ cup stevia
- 6 cups blackberries
- ¼ cup apples, cored and cubed
- ¼ tsp. baking powder
- 1 tbsp. lime juice
- ½ cup almond flour
- ½ cup water
- 3 and ½ tbsp. avocado oil
- Cooking spray

DIRECTIONS

1. In a bowl, mix the berries with half of the stevia and lemon juice, sprinkle some flour all over, whisk and pour into a baking dish greased with cooking spray.
2. In another bowl, mix flour with the rest of the sugar, baking powder, the water and the oil, and stir the whole thing with your hands.
3. Spread over the berries, introduce in the oven at 375°F and bake for 30 minutes.
4. Serve warm.

PREP TIME 10 mins
COOK TIME 30 mins
SERVINGS 6 people

NUTRITION

Calories 221
Fat 6.3g
Carbs 6g
Protein 9g

561. Black Tea Cake

PREP TIME
10 mins

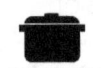
COOK TIME
35 mins

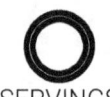
SERVINGS
8 people

INGREDIENTS

- 6 tbsp. black tea powder
- 2 cups almond milk, warmed up
- 1 cup avocado oil
- 2 cups stevia
- 4 eggs
- 2 tsp. vanilla extract
- 3 and ½ cups almond flour
- 1 tsp. baking soda
- 3 tsp. baking powder

DIRECTIONS

1. In a bowl, combine the almond milk with the oil, stevia and the rest of the ingredients and whisk well.
2. Pour this into a cake pan lined with parchment paper, introduce in the oven at 350°F and bake for 35 minutes.
3. Leave the cake to cool down, slice and serve.

NUTRITION

Calories 200
Fat 6.4g
Carbs 6.5g
Protein 5.4g

562. Green Tea and Vanilla Cream

PREP TIME
2 hours

COOK TIME
0 mins

SERVINGS
4 people

INGREDIENTS

- 14 oz. almond milk, hot
- 2 tbsp. green tea powder
- 14 oz. heavy cream
- 3 tbsp. stevia
- 1 tsp. vanilla extract
- 1 tsp. gelatin powder

DIRECTIONS

1. In a bowl, combine the almond milk with the green tea powder and the rest of the ingredients, whisk well, cool down, divide into cups and keep in the fridge for 2 hours before serving.

NUTRITION

Calories 120
Fat 3g
Carbs 7g
Protein 4g

563. Figs Pie

PREP TIME: 10 mins
COOK TIME: 60 mins
SERVINGS: 8 people

INGREDIENTS
- ½ cup stevia
- 6 figs, cut into quarters
- ½ tsp. vanilla extract
- 1 cup almond flour
- 4 eggs, whisked

DIRECTIONS
1. Spread the figs on the bottom of a springform pan lined with parchment paper.
2. In a bowl, combine the other ingredients, whisk and pour over the figs,
3. Bake at 375 digress F for 1 hour, flip the pie upside down when it's done and serve.

NUTRITION
Calories 200
Fat 4.4g
Carbs 7.6g
Protein 8g

---

564. Cherry Cream

PREP TIME: 2 hours
COOK TIME: 0 mins
SERVINGS: 4 people

INGREDIENTS
- 2 cups cherries, pitted and chopped
- 1 cup almond milk
- ½ cup whipping cream
- 3 eggs, whisked
- 1/3 cup stevia
- 1 tsp. lemon juice
- ½ tsp. vanilla extract

DIRECTIONS
1. In your food processor, combine the cherries with the milk and the rest of the ingredients, pulse well, divide into cups and keep in the fridge for 2 hours before serving.

NUTRITION
Calories 200
Fat 4.5g
Carbs 5.6g
Protein 3.4g

565. Strawberries Cream

PREP TIME
10 mins

COOK TIME
20 mins

SERVINGS
4 people

NUTRITION

Calories 152
Fat 4.4g
Carbs 5.1g
Protein 0.8g

INGREDIENTS

- ½ cup stevia
- 2 lb. strawberries, chopped
- 1 cup almond milk
- Zest of 1 lemon, grated
- ½ cup heavy cream
- 3 egg yolks, whisked

DIRECTIONS

1. Heat up a pan with the milk over medium-high heat, add the stevia and the rest of the ingredients, whisk well, simmer for 20 minutes, divide into cups and serve cold.

566. Apples and Plum Cake

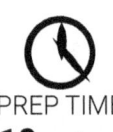
PREP TIME
10 mins

COOK TIME
40 mins

SERVINGS
4 people

NUTRITION

Calories 209
Fat 6.4g
Carbs 8g
Protein 6.6g

INGREDIENTS

- 7 oz. almond flour
- 1 egg, whisked
- 5 tbsp. stevia
- 3 oz. warm almond milk
- 2 lb. plums, pitted and cut into quarters
- 2 apples, cored and chopped
- Zest of 1 lemon, grated
- 1 tsp. baking powder

DIRECTIONS

1. In a bowl, mix the almond milk with the egg, stevia, and the rest of the ingredients except the cooking spray and whisk well.
2. Grease a cake pan with the oil, pour the cake mix inside, introduce in the oven and bake at 350°F for 40 minutes.
3. Cool down, slice and serve.

567. Cinnamon Chickpeas Cookies

PREP TIME: 10 mins
COOK TIME: 20 mins
SERVINGS: 12 people

INGREDIENTS

- 1 cup canned chickpeas, drained, rinsed and mashed
- 2 cups almond flour
- 1 tsp. cinnamon powder
- 1 tsp. baking powder
- 1 cup avocado oil
- ½ cup stevia
- 1 egg, whisked
- 2 tsp. almond extract
- 1 cup raisins
- 1 cup coconut, unsweetened and shredded

DIRECTIONS

1. In a bowl, combine the chickpeas with the flour, cinnamon and the other ingredients, and whisk well until you obtain a dough.
2. Scoop tbsp. of dough on a baking sheet lined with parchment paper, introduce them in the oven at 350°F and bake for 20 minutes.
3. Leave them to cool down for a few minutes and serve.

NUTRITION

Calories 200
Fat 4.5g
Carbs 9.5g
Protein 2.4g

568. Cocoa Brownies

PREP TIME: 10 mins
COOK TIME: 20 mins
SERVINGS: 8 people

INGREDIENTS

- 30 oz. canned lentils, rinsed and drained
- 1 tbsp. honey
- 1 banana, peeled and chopped
- ½ tsp. baking soda
- 4 tbsp. almond butter
- 2 tbsp. cocoa powder
- Cooking spray

DIRECTIONS

1. In a food processor, combine the lentils with the honey and the other ingredients except the cooking spray and pulse well.
2. Pour this into a pan greased with cooking spray, spread evenly, introduce in the oven at 375°F and bake for 20 minutes.
3. Cut the brownies and serve cold.

NUTRITION

Calories 200
Fat 4.5g
Carbs 8.7g
Protein 4.3g

569. Cardamom Almond Cream

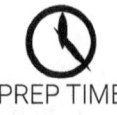
PREP TIME 30 mins

COOK TIME 0 mins

SERVINGS 4 people

INGREDIENTS
- Juice of 1 lime
- ½ cup stevia
- 1 and ½ cups water
- 3 cups almond milk
- ½ cup honey
- 2 tsp. cardamom, ground
- 1 tsp. rose water
- 1 tsp. vanilla extract

DIRECTIONS
1. In a blender, combine the almond milk with the cardamom and the rest of the ingredients, pulse well, divide into cups and keep in the fridge for 30 minutes before serving.

NUTRITION
Calories 283
Fat 11.8g
Carbs 4.7g
Protein 7.1g

570. Banana Cinnamon Cupcakes

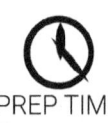
PREP TIME 10 mins

COOK TIME 20 mins

SERVINGS 4 people

INGREDIENTS
- 4 tbsp. avocado oil
- 4 eggs
- ½ cup orange juice
- 2 tsp. cinnamon powder
- 1 tsp. vanilla extract
- 2 bananas, peeled and chopped
- ¾ cup almond flour
- ½ tsp. baking powder
- Cooking spray

DIRECTIONS
1. In a bowl, combine the oil with the eggs, orange juice and the other ingredients except the cooking spray, whisk well, pour in a cupcake pan greased with the cooking spray, introduce in the oven at 350°F and bake for 20 minutes.
2. Cool the cupcakes down and serve.

NUTRITION
Calories 142
Fat 5.8g
Carbs 5.7g
Protein 1.6g

571. Rhubarb and Apples Cream

PREP TIME: 10 mins
COOK TIME: 0 mins
SERVINGS: 6 people

INGREDIENTS
- 3 cups rhubarb, chopped
- 1 and ½ cups stevia
- 2 eggs, whisked
- ½ tsp. nutmeg, ground
- 1 tbsp. avocado oil
- 1/3 cup almond milk

DIRECTIONS
1. In a blender, combine the rhubarb with the stevia and the rest of the ingredients, pulse well, divide into cups and serve cold.

NUTRITION
Calories 200
Fat 5.2g
Carbs 7.6g
Protein 2.5g

572. Cranberries and Pears Pie

PREP TIME: 10 mins
COOK TIME: 40 mins
SERVINGS: 4 people

INGREDIENTS
- 2 cup cranberries
- 3 cups pears, cubed
- A drizzle of olive oil
- 1 cup stevia
- 1/3 cup almond flour
- 1 cup rolled oats
- ¼ avocado oil

DIRECTIONS
1. In a bowl, mix the cranberries with the pears and the other ingredients except the olive oil and the oats, and stir well.
2. Grease a cake pan with the a drizzle of olive oil, pour the pears mix inside, sprinkle the oats all over and bake at 350°F for 40 minutes.
3. Cool the mix down, and serve.

NUTRITION
Calories 172
Fat 3.4g
Carbs 11.5g
Protein 4.5g

573. Lemon Cream

PREP TIME
60 mins

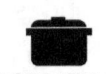
COOK TIME
10 mins

SERVINGS
6 people

INGREDIENTS

- 2 eggs, whisked
- 1 and ¼ cup stevia
- 10 tbsp. avocado oil
- 1 cup heavy cream
- Juice of 2 lemons
- Zest of 2 lemons, grated

DIRECTIONS

1. In a pan, combine the cream with the lemon juice and the other ingredients, whisk well, cook for 10 minutes, divide into cups and keep in the fridge for 1 hour before serving.

NUTRITION

Calories 200
Fat 8.5g
Carbs 8.6g
Protein 4.5g

574. Peach Sorbet

PREP TIME
2 hours

COOK TIME
10 mins

SERVINGS
4 people

INGREDIENTS

- 2 cups apple juice
- 1 cup stevia
- 2 tbsp. lemon zest, grated
- 2 lb. peaches, pitted and quartered

DIRECTIONS

1. Heat up a pan over medium heat, add the apple juice and the rest of the ingredients, simmer for 10 minutes, transfer to a blender, pulse, divide into cups and keep in the freezer for 2 hours before serving.

NUTRITION

Calories 182
Fat 5.4g
Carbs 12g
Protein 5.4g

575. Almond Rice Dessert

PREP TIME 10 mins
COOK TIME 20 mins
SERVINGS 4 people

INGREDIENTS

- 1 cup white rice
- 2 cups almond milk
- 1 cup almonds, chopped
- ½ cup stevia
- 1 tbsp. cinnamon powder
- ½ cup pomegranate seeds

DIRECTIONS

1. In a pot, mix the rice with the milk and stevia, bring to a simmer and cook for 20 minutes, stirring often.
2. Add the rest of the ingredients, stir, divide into bowls and serve.

NUTRITION

Calories 234
Fat 9.5g
Carbs 12.4g
Protein 6.5g

---

576. Blueberries Stew

PREP TIME 10 mins
COOK TIME 10 mins
SERVINGS 4 people

INGREDIENTS

- 2 cups blueberries
- 3 tbsp. stevia
- 1 and ½ cups pure apple juice
- 1 tsp. vanilla extract

DIRECTIONS

1. In a pan, combine the blueberries with stevia and the other ingredients, bring to a simmer and cook over medium-low heat for 10 minutes.
2. Divide into cups and serve cold.

NUTRITION

Calories 192
Fat 5.4g
Carbs 9.4g
Protein 4.5g

577. Mandarin Cream

PREP TIME
20 mins

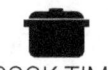
COOK TIME
0 mins

SERVINGS
8 people

INGREDIENTS

- 2 mandarins, peeled and cut into segments
- Juice of 2 mandarins
- 2 tbsp. stevia
- 4 eggs, whisked
- ¾ cup stevia
- ¾ cup almonds, ground

DIRECTIONS

1. In a blender, combine the mandarins with the mandarin's juice and the other ingredients, whisk well, divide into cups and keep in the fridge for 20 minutes before serving

NUTRITION

Calories 106
Fat 3.4g
Carbs 2.4g
Protein 4g

578. Creamy Mint Strawberry Mix

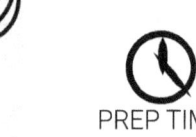
PREP TIME
10 mins

COOK TIME
30 mins

SERVINGS
6 people

INGREDIENTS

- Cooking spray
- ¼ cup stevia
- 1 and ½ cup almond flour
- 1 tsp. baking powder
- 1 cup almond milk
- 1 egg, whisked
- 2 cups strawberries, sliced
- 1 tbsp. mint, chopped
- 1 tsp. lime zest, grated
- ½ cup whipping cream

DIRECTIONS

1. In a bowl, combine the almond with the strawberries, mint and the other ingredients except the cooking spray and whisk well.
2. Grease 6 ramekins with the cooking spray, pour the strawberry mix inside, introduce in the oven and bake at 350°F for 30 minutes.
3. Cool down and serve.

NUTRITION

Calories 200
Fat 6.3g
Carbs 6.5g
Protein 8g

579. Vanilla Cake

PREP TIME: 10 mins
COOK TIME: 25 mins
SERVINGS: 10 people

INGREDIENTS

- 3 cups almond flour
- 3 tsp. baking powder
- 1 cup olive oil
- 1 and ½ cup almond milk
- 1 and 2/3 cup stevia
- 2 cups water
- 1 tbsp. lime juice
- 2 tsp. vanilla extract
- Cooking spray

DIRECTIONS

1. In a bowl, mix the almond flour with the baking powder, the oil and the rest of the ingredients except the cooking spray and whisk well.
2. Pour the mix into a cake pan greased with the cooking spray, introduce in the oven and bake at 370°F for 25 minutes.
3. Leave the cake to cool down, cut and serve!

NUTRITION

Calories 200
Fat 7.6g
Carbs 5.5g
Protein 4.5g

---

580. Pumpkin Cream

PREP TIME: 5 mins
COOK TIME: 5 mins
SERVINGS: 2 people

INGREDIENTS

- 2 cups canned pumpkin flesh
- 2 tbsp. stevia
- 1 tsp. vanilla extract
- 2 tbsp. water
- A pinch of pumpkin spice

DIRECTIONS

1. In a pan, combine the pumpkin flesh with the other ingredients, simmer for 5 minutes, divide into cups and serve cold.

NUTRITION

Calories 192
Fat 3.4g
Carbs 7.6g
Protein 3.5g

581. Chia and Berries Smoothie Bowl

PREP TIME
5 mins

COOK TIME
0 mins

SERVINGS
2 people

INGREDIENTS

- 1 and ½ cup almond milk
- 1 cup blackberries
- ¼ cup strawberries, chopped
- 1 and ½ tbsp. chia seeds
- 1 tsp. cinnamon powder

DIRECTIONS

1. In a blender, combine the blackberries with the strawberries and the rest of the ingredients, pulse well, divide into small bowls and serve cold.

NUTRITION

Calories 182
Fat 3.4g
Carbs 8.4g
Protein 3g

582. Minty Coconut Cream

PREP TIME
4 mins

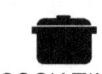
COOK TIME
0 mins

SERVINGS
2 people

INGREDIENTS

- 1 banana, peeled
- 2 cups coconut flesh, shredded
- 3 tbsp. mint, chopped
- 1 and ½ cups coconut water
- 2 tbsp. stevia
- ½ avocado, pitted and peeled

DIRECTIONS

1. In a blender, combine the coconut with the banana and the rest of the ingredients, pulse well, divide into cups and serve cold.

NUTRITION

Calories 193
Fat 5.4g
Carbs 7.6g
Protein 3g

583. Watermelon Cream

PREP TIME: 15 mins
COOK TIME: 0 mins
SERVINGS: 2 people

INGREDIENTS
- 1-lb. watermelon, peeled and chopped
- 1 tsp. vanilla extract
- 1 cup heavy cream
- 1 tsp. lime juice
- 2 tbsp. stevia

DIRECTIONS
1. In a blender, combine the watermelon with the cream and the rest of the ingredients, pulse well, divide into cups and keep in the fridge for 15 minutes before serving.

NUTRITION
Calories 122
Fat 5.7
Carbs 5.3
Protein 0.4

584. Grapes Stew

PREP TIME: 10 mins
COOK TIME: 10 mins
SERVINGS: 4 people

INGREDIENTS
- 2/3 cup stevia
- 1 tbsp. olive oil
- 1/3 cup coconut water
- 1 tsp. vanilla extract
- 1 tsp. lemon zest, grated
- 2 cup red grapes, halved

DIRECTIONS
1. Heat up a pan with the water over medium heat, add the oil, stevia and the rest of the ingredients, toss, simmer for 10 minutes, divide into cups and serve.

NUTRITION
Calories 122
Fat 3.7
Carbs 2.3
Protein 0.4

585. Cocoa Sweet Cherry Cream

PREP TIME
2 hours

COOK TIME
0 mins

SERVINGS
4 people

INGREDIENTS

- ½ cup cocoa powder
- ¾ cup red cherry jam
- ¼ cup stevia
- 2 cups water
- 1-lb. cherries, pitted and halved

DIRECTIONS

1. In a blender, mix the cherries with the water and the rest of the ingredients, pulse well, divide into cups and keep in the fridge for 2 hours before serving.

NUTRITION

Calories 162
Fat 3.4g
Carbs 5g
Protein 1g

586. Apple Couscous Pudding

PREP TIME
10 mins

COOK TIME
25 mins

SERVINGS
4 people

INGREDIENTS

- ½ cup couscous
- 1 and ½ cups milk
- ¼ cup apple, cored and chopped
- 3 tbsp. stevia
- ½ tsp. rose water
- 1 tbsp. orange zest, grated

DIRECTIONS

1. Heat up a pan with the milk over medium heat, add the couscous and the rest of the ingredients, whisk, simmer for 25 minutes, divide into bowls and serve.

NUTRITION

Calories 150
Fat 4.5g
Carbs 7.5g
Protein 4g

587. Ricotta Ramekins

PREP TIME
10 mins

COOK TIME
60 mins

SERVINGS
4 people

NUTRITION

Calories 180
Fat 5.3g
Carbs 11.5g
Protein 4g

INGREDIENTS

- 6 eggs, whisked
- 1 and ½ lb. ricotta cheese, soft
- ½ lb. stevia
- 1 tsp. vanilla extract
- ½ tsp. baking powder
- Cooking spray

DIRECTIONS

1. In a bowl, mix the eggs with the ricotta and the other ingredients except the cooking spray and whisk well.
2. Grease 4 ramekins with the cooking spray, pour the ricotta cream in each and bake at 360°F for 1 hour.
3. Serve cold.

588. Papaya Cream

PREP TIME
10 mins

COOK TIME
0 mins

SERVINGS
2 people

NUTRITION

Calories 182
Fiber 2.3g
Carbs 3.5g
Protein 2g

INGREDIENTS

- 1 cup papaya, peeled and chopped
- 1 cup heavy cream
- 1 tbsp. stevia
- ½ tsp. vanilla extract

DIRECTIONS

1. In a blender, combine the cream with the papaya and the other ingredients, pulse well, divide into cups and serve cold.

589. Almonds and Oats Pudding

PREP TIME
10 mins

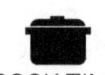
COOK TIME
15 mins

SERVINGS
4 people

NUTRITION

Calories 174
Fat 12.1g
Carbs 3.9g
Protein 4.8g

INGREDIENTS

- 1 tbsp. lemon juice
- Zest of 1 lime
- 1 and ½ cups almond milk
- 1 tsp. almond extract
- ½ cup oats
- 2 tbsp. stevia
- ½ cup silver almonds, chopped

DIRECTIONS

1. In a pan, combine the almond milk with the lime zest and the other ingredients, whisk, bring to a simmer and cook over medium heat for 15 minutes.
2. Divide the mix into bowls and serve cold.

590. Strawberry Sorbet

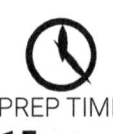
PREP TIME
15 mins

COOK TIME
10 mins

SERVINGS
6 people

NUTRITION

Calories 30,
Fat 0.4 g,
Carbs 14.9 g,
Protein 0.9 g

INGREDIENTS

- 1 cup strawberries, chopped
- 1 tbsp. of liquid honey
- 2 tbsp. water
- 1 tbsp. lemon juice

DIRECTIONS

1. Preheat the water and liquid honey until you get homogenous liquid.
2. Blend the strawberries until smooth and combine them with honey liquid and lemon juice.
3. Transfer the strawberry mixture in the ice cream maker and churn it for 20 minutes or until the sorbet is thick.
4. Scoop the cooked sorbet in the ice cream cups.

591. Vanilla Apple Pie

PREP TIME: 15 mins
COOK TIME: 50 mins
SERVINGS: 8 people

INGREDIENTS
- 3 apples, sliced
- ½ tsp. ground cinnamon
- 1 tsp. vanilla extract
- 1 tbsp. Erythritol
- 7 oz yeast roll dough
- 1 egg, beaten

DIRECTIONS
1. Roll up the dough and cut it on 2 parts.
2. Line the springform pan with baking paper.
3. Place the first dough part in the springform pan.
4. Then arrange the apples over the dough and sprinkle it with Erythritol, vanilla extract, and ground cinnamon.
5. Then cover the apples with remaining dough and secure the edges of the pie with the help of the fork.
6. Make the small cuts in the surface of the pie.
7. Brush the pie with beaten egg and bake it for 50 minutes at 375°F.
8. Cool the cooked pie well and then remove from the springform pan.
9. Cut it on the servings.

NUTRITION
Calories 140, Fat 3.4 g, Carbs 23.9 g, Protein 2.9 g

592. Cinnamon Pears

PREP TIME: 2 hours
COOK TIME: 0 mins
SERVINGS: 6 people

INGREDIENTS
- 2 pears
- 1 tsp. ground cinnamon
- 1 tbsp. Erythritol
- 1 tsp. liquid stevia
- 4 tsp. butter

DIRECTIONS
1. Cut the pears on the halves.
2. Then scoop the seeds from the pears with the help of the scooper.
3. In the shallow bowl mix up together Erythritol and ground cinnamon.
4. Sprinkle every pear half with cinnamon mixture and drizzle with liquid stevia.
5. Then add butter and wrap in the foil.
6. Bake the pears for 25 minutes at 365°F.
7. Then remove the pears from the foil and transfer in the serving plates.

NUTRITION
Calories 96, Fat 4.4 g, Carbs 3.9 g, Protein 0.9 g

593. Ginger Ice Cream

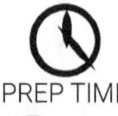
PREP TIME
15 mins

COOK TIME
10 mins

SERVINGS
6 people

INGREDIENTS

- 1 mango, peeled
- 1 cup Greek yogurt
- 1 tbsp. Erythritol
- ¼ cup milk
- 1 tsp. vanilla extract
- ¼ tsp. ground ginger

DIRECTIONS

1. Blend the mango until you get puree and combine it with Erythritol, milk, vanilla extract, and ground ginger.
2. Then mix up together Greek yogurt and mango puree mixture. Transfer it in the plastic vessel.
3. Freeze the ice cream for 35 minutes.

NUTRITION

Calories 90,
Fat 1.4 g,
Carbs 21.9 g,
Protein 4.9 g

594. Cherry Compote

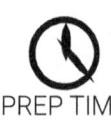
PREP TIME
2 hours

COOK TIME
0 mins

SERVINGS
6 people

INGREDIENTS

- 2 peaches, pitted, halved
- 1 cup cherries, pitted
- ½ cup grape juice
- ½ cup strawberries
- 1 tbsp. liquid honey
- 1 tsp. vanilla extract
- 1 tsp. ground cinnamon

DIRECTIONS

1. Pour grape juice in the saucepan.
2. Add vanilla extract and ground cinnamon. Bring the liquid to boil.
3. After this, put peaches, cherries, and strawberries in the hot grape juice and bring to boil.
4. Remove the mixture from heat, add liquid honey, and close the lid.
5. Let the compote rest for 20 minutes.
6. Carefully mix up the compote and transfer in the serving plate.

NUTRITION

Calories 80,
Fat 0.4 g,
Carbs 19.9 g,
Protein 0.9 g

595. Creamy Strawberries

PREP TIME: 15 mins
COOK TIME: 10 mins
SERVINGS: 6 people

INGREDIENTS

- 6 tbsp. almond butter
- 1 tbsp. Erythritol
- 1 cup milk
- 1 tsp. vanilla extract
- 1 cup strawberries, sliced

DIRECTIONS

1. Pour milk in the saucepan.
2. Add Erythritol, vanilla extract, and almond butter.
3. With the help of the hand mixer mix up the liquid until smooth and bring it to boil.
4. Then remove the mixture from the heat and let it cool.
5. The cooled mixture will be thick.
6. Put the strawberries in the serving glasses and top with the thick almond butter dip.

NUTRITION

Calories 192,
Fat 14.4 g,
Carbs 10.9 g,
Protein 1.9 g

596. Chocolate Cups

PREP TIME: 2 hours
COOK TIME: 0 mins
SERVINGS: 6 people

INGREDIENTS

- ½ cup avocado oil
- 1 cup, chocolate, melted
- 1 tsp. matcha powder
- 3 tbsp. stevia

DIRECTIONS

1. In a bowl, mix the chocolate with the oil and the rest of the ingredients, whisk really well, divide into cups and keep in the freezer for 2 hours before serving.

NUTRITION

Calories 174
Fat 9.1g
Carbs 3.9g
Protein 2.8g

597. Honey Walnut Bars

PREP TIME
20 mins

COOK TIME
30 mins

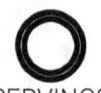
SERVINGS
8 people

NUTRITION
Calories 243,
Fat 4.4 g,
Carbs 15.9 g,
Protein 1.9 g

INGREDIENTS
- 5 oz puff pastry
- ½ cup of water
- 3 tbsp. of liquid honey
- 1 tsp. Erythritol
- 1/3 cup butter, softened
- ½ cup walnuts, chopped
- 1 tsp. olive oil

DIRECTIONS
1. Roll up the puff pastry and cut it on 6 sheets.
2. Then brush the tray with olive oil and arrange the first puff pastry sheet inside.
3. Grease it with butter gently and sprinkle with walnuts.
4. Repeat the same steps with 4 puff pastry sheets.
5. Then sprinkle the last layer with walnuts and Erythritol and cove with the sixth puff pastry sheet.
6. Cut the baklava on the servings.
7. Bake the baklava for 30 minutes.
8. Meanwhile, bring to boil liquid honey and water.
9. When the baklava is cooked, remove it from the oven.
10. Pour hot honey liquid over baklava and let it cool till the room temperature.

598. Yogurt Parfait

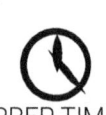
PREP TIME
5 mins

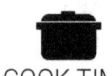
COOK TIME
0 mins

SERVINGS
1 people

NUTRITION
Calories 44,
Fat 0.4 g,
Carbs 6.9 g,
Protein 1.9 g

INGREDIENTS
- 1 oz blueberries
- 2 tbsp. Plain yogurt
- ½ tsp. vanilla extract

DIRECTIONS
1. Mix up together Plain yogurt and vanilla extract.
2. Then put ½ oz of blueberries in the glass.
3. Cover the berries with ½ part of Plain Yogurt.
4. Then add the layer of berries.
5. Top parfait with remaining Plain yogurt.

599. Raspberry Tart

PREP TIME: 15 mins
COOK TIME: 10 mins
SERVINGS: 6 people

NUTRITION
Calories 311,
Fat 11.4 g,
Carbs 14.9 g,
Protein 1.9 g

INGREDIENTS
- 3 tbsp. butter, softened
- 1 cup wheat flour, whole wheat
- 1 tsp. baking powder
- 1 egg, beaten
- 4 tbsp. pistachio paste
- 2 tbsp. raspberry jam

DIRECTIONS
1. Knead the dough: combine together softened butter, flour, baking powder, and egg. You should get the non-sticky and very soft dough.
2. Put the dough in the springform pan and flatten it with the help of the fingertips until you get pie crust.
3. Bake it for 10 minutes at 365°F.
4. After this, spread the pie crust with raspberry jam and then with pistachio paste.
5. Bake the tart at 365°F for another 10 minutes.
6. Cool the cooked tart and cut on the servings.

600. Quinoa Energy Bars

PREP TIME: 20 mins
COOK TIME: 15 mins
SERVINGS: 8 people

NUTRITION
Calories 240,
Fat 6.4 g,
Carbs 29.9 g,
Protein 1.9 g

INGREDIENTS
- ½ cup puffed quinoa
- ¼ cup oats
- 2 oz dark chocolate
- 2 tbsp. almond butter
- ¾ cup maple syrup
- 1 tbsp. butter
- 1 tbsp. coconut flakes

DIRECTIONS
1. Place dark chocolate, butter, maple syrup, and almond butter in the saucepan.
2. Melt the mixture and add oats, puffed quinoa, and coconut flakes.
3. Mix up well and remove it from the heat.
4. After this, line the baking tray with baking paper and transfer the quinoa mixture in it.
5. Flatten it well with the help of the spatula and cut on the bars (8 pieces).
6. Bake the quinoa bars for 10 minutes at 365°F.
7. After this, remove the tray with quinoa bars from the oven and cool well.

601. Cinnamon Stuffed Peaches

PREP TIME
10 mins

COOK TIME
15 mins

SERVINGS
4 people

NUTRITION
Calories 213,
Fat 1.4 g,
Carbs 23.9 g,
Protein 1.9 g

INGREDIENTS
- 4 peaches, pitted, halved
- 2 tbsp. ricotta cheese
- 2 tbsp. of liquid honey
- ¾ cup of water
- ½ tsp. vanilla extract
- ¾ tsp. ground cinnamon
- 1 tbsp. almonds, sliced
- ¾ tsp. saffron

DIRECTIONS
1. Pour water in the saucepan and bring to boil.
2. Add vanilla extract, saffron, ground cinnamon, and liquid honey.
3. Cook the liquid until the honey is melted.
4. Then remove it from the heat.
5. Put the halved peaches in the hot honey liquid.
6. Meanwhile, make the filling: mix up together ricotta cheese, vanilla extract, and sliced almonds.
7. Remove the peaches from honey liquid and arrange in the plate. Fill 4 peach halves with ricotta filling and cover them with remaining peach halves.
8. Sprinkle the cooked dessert with liquid honey mixture gently.

602. Blueberry Muffins

PREP TIME
15 mins

COOK TIME
25 mins

SERVINGS
4 people

NUTRITION
Calories 241,
Fat 12.4 g,
Carbs 24.9 g,
Protein 1.9 g

INGREDIENTS
- 1 cup whole wheat flour
- 1 tsp. baking powder
- ¼ cup blueberries
- 1 tsp. vanilla extract
- 1 tbsp. butter, softened
- ¾ cup sour cream
- 1 tbsp. Erythritol
- Cooking spray

DIRECTIONS
1. In the mixing bowl combine together wheat flour and baking powder.
2. Then add sour cream, vanilla extract, butter, and Erythritol.
3. Stir the mixture well until smooth. You should get a thick batter. Add more sour cream if needed.
4. After this, add blueberries and carefully stir the batter.
5. Spray the muffin molds with the cooking spray.
6. Fill ½ part of every muffin mold with batter.
7. Preheat the oven to 365F.
8. Place the muffins in the prepared oven and cook them for 25 minutes.
9. The cooked muffins will have a golden color surface.

603. Lime Grapes and Apples

PREP TIME 10 mins
COOK TIME 25 mins
SERVINGS 2 people

NUTRITION
Calories 142,
Fat 4.4 g,
Carbs 40.9 g,
Protein 1.9 g

INGREDIENTS

- ½ cup red grapes
- 2 apples
- 1 tsp. lime juice
- 1 tsp. Erythritol
- 3 tbsp. water

DIRECTIONS

1. Line the baking tray with baking paper.
2. Then cut the apples on the halves and remove the seeds with the help of the scooper.
3. Cut the apple halves on 2 parts more.
4. Arrange all fruits in the tray in one layer, drizzle with water, and bake for 20 minutes at 375F.
5. Flip the fruits on another side after 10 minutes of cooking.
6. Then remove them from the oven and sprinkle with lime juice and Erythritol.
7. Return the fruits back in the oven and bake for 5 minutes more.
8. Serve the cooked dessert hot or warm.

604. Almond Citrus Muffins

PREP TIME 10 mins
COOK TIME 30 mins
SERVINGS 6 people

NUTRITION
Calories 204,
Fat 7.4 g,
Carbs 57.9 g,
Protein 1.9 g

INGREDIENTS

- 2 eggs, beaten
- 1 ½ cup whole wheat flour
- ½ cup almond meal
- 1 tsp. vanilla extract
- 1 tbsp. butter, softened
- 1 tsp. orange zest, grated
- 1 tbsp. orange juice
- ¾ cup Erythritol
- 1 oz orange pulp
- 1 tsp. baking powder
- ½ tsp. lime zest, grated
- Cooking spray

DIRECTIONS

1. Make the muffin batter: combine together almond meal, eggs, whole wheat flour, vanilla extract, butter, orange zest, orange juice, and orange pulp.
2. Add lime zest and baking powder.
3. Then add Erythritol.
4. With the help of the hand mixer mix up the ingredients.
5. When the mixture is soft and smooth, it is done.
6. Spray the muffin molds with cooking spray from inside and preheat the oven to 365F.
7. Fill ½ part of every muffin mold with muffin batter and transfer them in the oven.
8. Cook the muffins for 30 minutes.
9. Then check if the muffins are cooked by piercing them with a toothpick (if it is dry, the muffins are cooked; if it is not dry, bake the muffins for 5-7 minutes more.)

605. Butter Cookies

PREP TIME
15 mins

COOK TIME
15 mins

SERVINGS
6 people

NUTRITION

Calories 103,
Fat 6.4 g,
Carbs 11.9 g,
Protein 1.9 g

INGREDIENTS

- 1/3 cup wheat flour
- ¼ cup coconut flour
- 2 egg whites
- 3 tbsp. butter, softened
- ½ tsp. vanilla extract
- 1 tbsp. Erythritol

DIRECTIONS

1. In the mixing bowl combine together Erythritol, wheat flour, and coconut flour.
2. Whisk the eggs whites in the separated bowl till you get soft peaks.
3. After this, combine together the wheat mixture and egg whites.
4. Add vanilla extract and softened butter.
5. Carefully mix up the cookies mixture with the help of the fork/spoon.
6. After this, line the baking tray with baking paper.
7. Make six balls from the coconut mixture, press them little with the help of the palm and arrange in the tray. Make enough space for every cookie in the tray.
8. Bake the cookies for 15 minutes at 375°F.
9. When the cookies are lightly golden but not brown, they are cooked.
10. Chill them well and store in the glass jar.

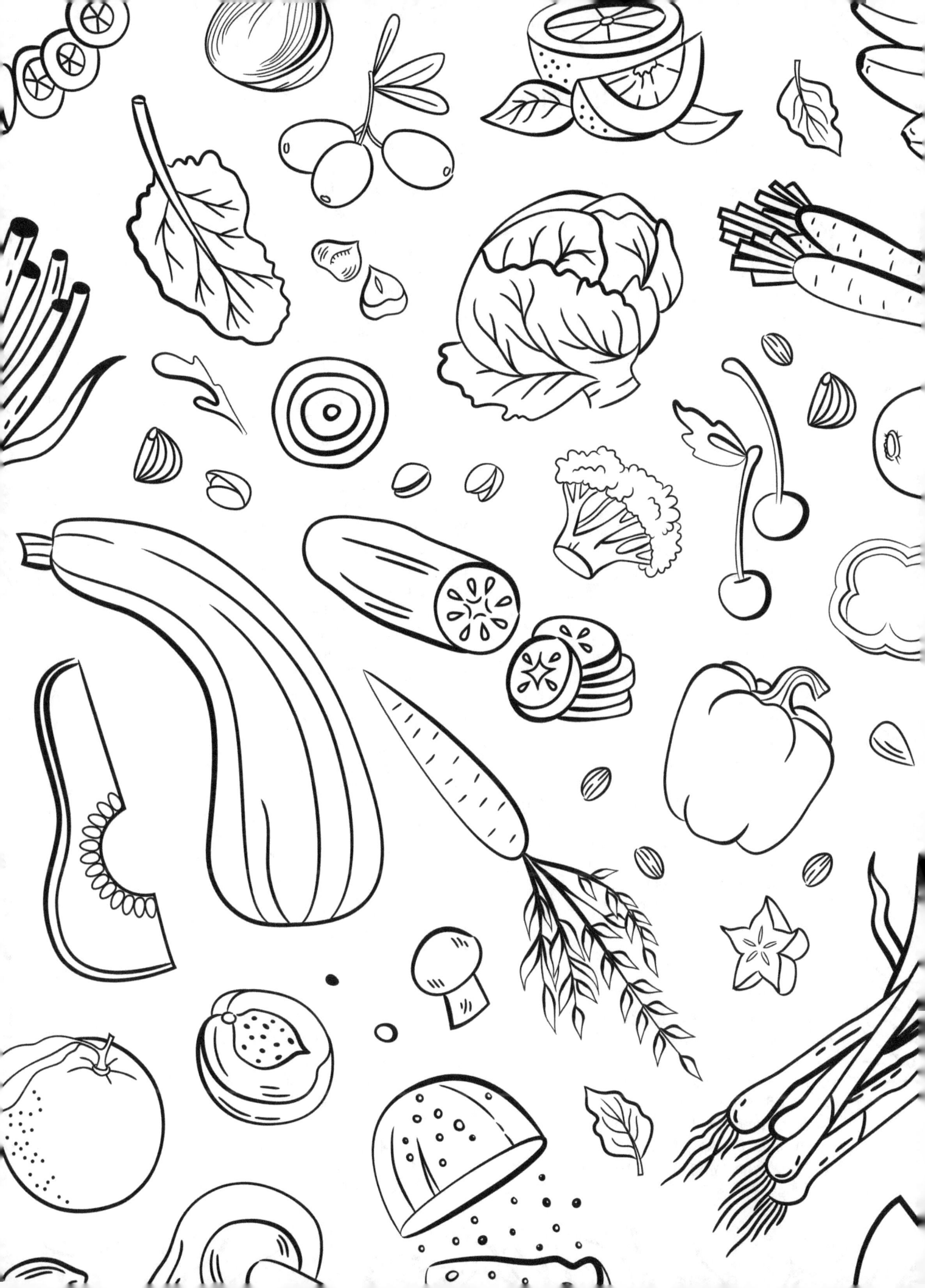

RECIPES TABLE OF CONTENTS

BREAKFAST 30
1. Banana and Quinoa Casserole 30
2. Ham Muffins 31
3. Cheesy Yogurt 31
4. Avocado Spread 32
5. Artichokes and Cheese Omelet 32
6. Walnut Poached Eggs 33
7. Almond Cream Cheese Bake 33
8. Chili Egg Cups 34
9. Dill Eggs Mix 34
10. Hummus and Tomato Sandwich 35
11. Buttery Pancakes 35
12. Cream Olive Muffins 36
13. Herbed Fried Eggs 36
14. Chili Scramble 37
15. Couscous and Chickpeas Bowls 37
16. Banana Oats 38
17. Slow-cooked Peppers Frittata 38
18. Veggie Bowls 39
19. Avocado and Apple Smoothie 39
20. Avocado Toast 40
21. Mini Frittatas 40
22. Berry Oats 41
23. Sun-dried Tomatoes Oatmeal 41
24. Quinoa Muffins 42
25. Quinoa and Eggs Pan 42
26. Stuffed Tomatoes 43
27. Scrambled Eggs 43
28. Watermelon "Pizza" 44
29. Baked Omelet Mix 44
30. Anti-Inflammatory Blueberry Smoothie 45
31. Cherry - Pomegranate Smoothie Bow - Gluten-Free & Vegetarian 45
32. Breakfast Banana Green Smoothie 46
33. Strawberry Oatmeal Breakfast Smoothie 46
34. Kale and Banana Smoothie 47
35. Summer Stone Fruit Smoothie 47
36. Pumpkin Pie Fall Smoothie 48
37. Green Tart Smoothie 48
38. Coconut Milk Smoothie 49
39. Creamy Strawberry Smoothie 49

ANTIPASTI, TAPAS, MEZE AND STARTER .. 50
40. Cheddar Potato Crisps 50
41. Stuffed Sweet Potato 51
42. Rosemary Bulgur Appetizer 51
43. Cauliflower Fritters 52
44. Mediterranean Chickpea Snack 52
45. Avocado Chickpea Pizza 53
46. Pita Wedges with Almond Bean Dip 53
47. Ginger Antipasti 54
48. Mediterranean Chickpea Spread 54
49. Rosemary Beets 55
50. Scallions Dip 55
51. Dill Tapas 56
52. Sour Cream Dip 56
53. Arugula Antipasti 57
54. Goat Cheese Dip 57
55. Mozzarella Dip 58
56. Spicy Salsa 58
57. Cheese Spread 59
58. Prosciutto Beans 59
59. Carrot Chips 60
60. Antipasti Salad 60
61. Black Olives Spread 61
62. Bell Pepper Antipasti 61
63. Hummus Rings 62
64. Fish Strips 62
65. Vegetable Balls 63
66. Italian Style Eggplant Chips 63
67. Lentil Dip 64
68. Cheese Baby Potatoes 64
69. Tuna Paste 65
70. Zucchini Chips 65
71. Crunchy Chickpeas 66
72. Stuffed Dates 66
73. Almond Gazpacho 67
74. Turkey Chowder 67

PASTA AND COUSCOUS 68
75. Herb-Topped Focaccia 68
76. Caramelized Onion Flatbread with Arugula ... 69
77. Quick Shrimp Fettuccine 69
78. Simple Pesto Pasta 70
79. Flat Meat Pies 70
80. Meaty Baked Penne 71
81. Mediterranean Pasta with Tomato Sauce and Vegetables 71
82. Very Vegan Patras Pasta 72
83. Cheesy Spaghetti with Pine Nuts 72
84. Creamy Garlic-Parmesan Chicken Pasta 73
85. Artichoke Chicken Pasta 73
86. Spinach Beef Pasta 74
87. Asparagus Parmesan Pasta 74
88. Mussels Linguine Delight 75
89. Arugula Pasta Soup 75
90. Pasta with garlic and Hoat Pepper 76
91. Stuffed Pasta Shells 76
92. Homemade Pasta Bolognese 77
93. Asparagus Pasta 77
94. Penne Bolognese Pasta 78
95. Quick Pasta Bolognese 78

96. Pilaf with Cream Cheese 79
97. Herbed Pasta 79
98. Pasta with Veggies 80
99. Pasta with Chicken & Veggies 80
100. Pasta with Shrimp & Spinach 81
101. Carbonara Pasta With Champignons 81
102. Spaghetti Carbonara With Red Onion 82
103. Cuttlefish Pasta With Carbonara Sauce 82
104. Spaghetti Carbonara 83
105. Chanterelle Pasta 83
106. Pasta "Verochka" 84
107. Pasta e Patate 84
108. Pasta with Fresh Tomatoes 85
109. Spaghetti Carbonara With Chicken 85
110. Carbonara With Fettuccine 86
111. Fast Spaghetti Carbonara 86
112. Pasta with Greens 87
113. Harvest Pasta 87
114. Pollo Mediterranean 88
115. Pasta Fagioli Soup 88
116. Pasta al Mediterraneo 89
117. Tomato Basil Penne Pasta 89
118. Whole Wheat Pasta Toss 90
119. Quick Mediterranean Pasta 90
120. Mediterranean Fish and Pasta Stew 91
121. Parsley Pesto Paste 91
122. Potato in Tomato Paste 92
123. Hummus 92
124. Hollandaise Sauce 93
125. Creamy Tahini Dip 93
126. Basil Lime Dip 94
127. Cilantro Dip 94
128. Tahini Sauce 95
129. Arugula Salsa 95

RICE AND GRAINS 96
130. Fragrant Basmati Rice 96
131. Cranberry Rice 97
132. Italian Style Wild Rice 97
133. Brown Rice Saute 98
134. Pesto Rice 98
135. Rice Salad 99
136. Rice Meatballs 99
137. Mediterranean Paella 100
138. Fast Chicken Rice 100
139. Rice Jambalaya 101
140. Jasmine Rice with Scallions 101
141. Cremini Mushrooms Pilaf 102
142. Vegetable Rice 102
143. Tomato Rice 103
144. Rice with Grilled Tomatoes 103
145. Rice and Meat Salad 104
146. Rice Bowl 104
147. Zucchini Rice 105
148. Rice Soup 105
149. Rice with Prunes 106
150. Rice and Fish Cakes 106
151. Salsa Rice 107
152. Seafood Rice 107
153. Vegetarian Pilaf 108
154. Rice Rolls 108
155. Rice Stew with Squid 109
156. Creamy Millet 109
157. Oatmeal Cakes 110
158. Yogurt Buckwheat 110
159. Halloumi Buckwheat Bowl 111
160. Aromatic Green Millet 111
161. Quinoa with Pumpkin 112
162. Almond Quinoa 112
163. Spring Rolls with Quinoa 113
164. Mushroom Quinoa Skillet 113
165. Strawberry Quinoa Bowl 114
166. Quinoa Meatballs 114
167. Stir-Fried Farro 115
168. Quick Farro Skillet 115
169. Bulgur Bowl 116
170. Boiled Bulgur with Kale 116
171. Chicken and Rice Soup 117
172. Tomato Bulgur 117
173. Bulgur Mix 118
174. Aromatic Baked Brown Rice 118
175. Aromatic Barley Pilaf 119
176. Basmati Rice Pilaf Mix 119
177. Brown Rice Salad with Asparagus, Goat Cheese, and Lemon 120
178. Carrot-Almond-Bulgur Salad 120
179. Chickpea-Spinach Bulgur 121
180. Classic Baked Brown Rice 121
181. Classic Italian Seafood Risotto 122
182. Classic Stovetop White Rice 122

SOUPS AND STEWS 123
183. Moroccan Lentil Soup 123
184. Roasted Red Pepper and Tomato Soup 124
185. Greek Spring Soup 124
186. Fast Seafood Gumbo 125
187. Minestrone Soup 125
188. Lemon Chicken Soup 126
189. Tuscan Vegetable Pasta Soup 126
190. Dairy Free Zucchini Soup 127
191. Farro Stew with Kale & Cannellini Beans 127
192. Italian Meatball Soup 128
193. Tuscan White Bean Soup with Sausage and Kale 128
194. Vegetable Soup 129
195. Sweet Yogurt Bulgur Bowl 129
196. Spring Farro Plate 130

#	Recipe	Page
197.	Sorghum Taboule	130
198.	Roasted Sorghum	131
199.	Sorghum Stew	131
200.	Sorghum Salad	132
201.	Sorghum Bake	132
202.	Lamb and Chickpeas Stew	133
203.	Chorizo and Lentils Stew	133
204.	Lamb and Potato Stew	134
205.	Meatball and Pasta Soup	134
206.	Peas Soup	135
207.	Minty Lamb Stew	135
208.	Spinach and Orzo Soup	136
209.	Minty Lentil and Spinach Soup	136
210.	Chicken and Apricots Stew	137
211.	Fish and Veggie Stew	137
212.	Tomato Soup	138
213.	Chickpeas Soup	138
214.	Fish Soup	139
215.	Chili Watermelon Soup	139
216.	Shrimp Soup	140
217.	Halibut and Veggies Stew	140
218.	Cucumber Soup	141
219.	Chickpeas, Tomato and Kale Stew	141
220.	Veggie Stew	142
221.	Beef and Eggplant Soup	142

SALAD AND SIDE DISHES 143

#	Recipe	Page
222.	Melon Salad	143
223.	Orange Celery Salad	144
224.	Roasted Broccoli Salad	144
225.	Tomato Salad	145
226.	Feta Beet Salad	145
227.	Cauliflower & Tomato Salad	146
228.	Tuna Salad	146
229.	Corn and Shrimp Salad	147
230.	Tahini Spinach	147
231.	Asparagus Couscous	148
232.	Easy Spaghetti Squash	148
233.	Garbanzo Bean Salad	149
234.	Spiced Chickpeas Bowls	149
235.	Tomato and Lentils Salad	150
236.	Egg and Arugula Salad	150
237.	Roasted Veggies	151
238.	Roasted Eggplant Salad	151
239.	Penne with Tahini Sauce	152
240.	Parmesan Barley Risotto	152
241.	Zucchini Pasta	153
242.	Quinoa and Eggs Salad	153
243.	Feta & Spinach Pita Bake	154
244.	Pistachio Arugula Salad	154
245.	Easy Salad Wraps	155
246.	Margherita Slices	155
247.	Vegetable Panini	156
248.	Baked Tomato	156
249.	Mediterranean Humus Filled Roasted Veggies	157
250.	Cucumber and Nuts Salad	157
251.	Courgette, Fennel, and Orange Salad	158
252.	Potato Salad	158
253.	Tomato, Cucumber, and Feta Salad	159
254.	Goat Cheese Stuffed Tomatoes	159
255.	Classic Tabbouleh	160
256.	Mediterranean Greens	160
257.	Classic Greek Salad	161
258.	North African Zucchini Salad	161
259.	Tunisian Style Carrot Salad	162
260.	Caesar Salad	162
261	Avocado Salad	163
262.	Spanish Salad	163
263.	Parsley Couscous Salad	164
264.	Cress and Tangerine Salad	164
265.	Prosciutto and Figs Salad	165
266.	Garden Vegetables and Chickpeas Salad	165
267.	Peppered Watercress Salad	166

VEGETARIAN DISHES 167

#	Recipe	Page
268.	Rustic Vegetable and Brown Rice Bowl	167
269.	Roasted Brussels sprouts And Pecans	168
270.	Eggs with Zucchini Noodles	168
271.	Roasted Root Veggies	169
272.	Roasted Vegetables and Zucchini Pasta	169
273.	Sautéed Collard Greens	170
274.	Savoy Cabbage with Coconut Cream Sauce	170
275.	Slow Cooked Buttery Mushrooms	171
276.	Steamed Squash Chowder	171
277.	Steamed Zucchini-Paprika	172
278.	Stir Fried Brussels sprouts and Carrots	172
279.	Stir Fried Eggplant	173
280.	Summer Vegetables	173
281.	Stir Fried Bok Choy	174
282.	Summer Veggies in Instant Pot	174
283.	Sumptuous Tomato Soup	175
284.	Superfast Cajun Asparagus	175
285.	Sweet and Nutritious Pumpkin Soup	176
286.	Sweet Potato Puree	176
287.	Sweet Potato Soup	177
288.	Sweet Potatoes Oven Fried	177
289.	Tasty Avocado Sauce over Zoodles	178
290.	Tomato Basil Cauliflower Rice	178
291.	Vegan Sesame Tofu and Eggplants	179
292.	Vegetarian Coconut Curry	179
293.	Veggie Lo Mein	180
294.	Veggie Jamaican Stew	180
295.	Vegetable Soup Moroccan Style	181
296.	Veggie Ramen Miso Soup	181
297.	Yummy Cauliflower Fritters	182
298.	Zucchini Garlic Fries	182

299. Zucchini Pasta with Mango-Kiwi Sauce 183
300. Quinoa with Almonds and Cranberries 183
301. Mediterranean Baked Chickpeas 184
302. Falafel Bites 184
303. Quick Vegetable Kebabs 185
304. Tortellini in Red Pepper Sauce 185
305. Freekeh, Chickpea, and Herb Salad 186
306. Kate's Warm Mediterranean Farro Bowl 186
307. Creamy Chickpea Sauce with Whole-Wheat Fusilli 187
308. Linguine and Brussels sprouts 187
309. Peppers and Lentils Salad 188
310. Cashews and Red Cabbage Salad 188
311. Apples and Pomegranate Salad 189
312. Cranberry Bulgur Mix 189
313. Chickpeas, Corn and Black Beans Salad 190
314. Olives and Lentils Salad 190
315. Lime Spinach and Chickpeas Salad 191
316. Beans and Cucumber Salad 191
317. Minty Olives and Tomatoes Salad 192
318. Tomato And Avocado Salad 192
319. Corn and Tomato Salad 193
320. Orange and Cucumber Salad 193
321. Parsley and Corn Salad 194
322. Radish and Corn Salad 194
323. Arugula and Corn Salad 195
324. Balsamic Bulgur Salad 195

SNACKS 196
325. Healthy Coconut Blueberry Balls 196
326. Crunchy Roasted Chickpeas 197
327. Tasty Zucchini Chips 197
328. Roasted Green Beans 198
329. Savory Pistachio Balls 198
330. Roasted Almonds 199
331. Banana Strawberry Popsicles 199
332. Chocolate Matcha Balls 200
333. Chia Almond Butter Pudding 200
334. Refreshing Strawberry Popsicles 201
335. Dark Chocolate Mousse 201
336. Warm & Soft Baked Pears 202
337. Healthy & Quick Energy Bites 202
338. Creamy Yogurt Banana Bowls 203
339. Chicken Wings Platter 203
340. Carrot Spread 204
341. Chocolate Mousse 204
342. Veggie Fritters 205
343. White Bean Dip 205
344. Eggplant Dip 206
345. Bulgur Lamb Meatballs 206
346. Cucumber Bites 207
347. Stuffed Avocado 207
348. Hummus with Ground Lamb 208

349. Wrapped Plums 208
350. Cucumber Sandwich Bites 209
351. Cucumber Rolls 209
352. Olives and Cheese Stuffed Tomatoes 210
353. Tomato Salsa 210
354. Chili Mango and Watermelon Salsa 211
355. Creamy Spinach and Shallots Dip 211
356. Feta Artichoke Dip 212
357. Avocado Dip 212
358. Goat Cheese and Chives Spread 213
359. Stuffed Chicken 213
360. Cinnamon Baby Back Ribs Platter 214
361. Buttery Carrot Sticks 214
362. Cajun Walnuts And Olives Bowls 215
363. Mango Salsa 215
364. Hot Asparagus Sticks 216
365. Pork Bites 216
366. Meatballs Platter 217
367. Yogurt Dip 217
368. Tomato Bruschetta 218
369. Artichoke Flatbread 218
370. Red Pepper Tapenade 219
371. Coriander Falafel 219
372. Red Pepper Hummus 220

PIZZA 221
373. White Pizza with Prosciutto and Arugula 221
374. Za'atar Pizza 222
375. Broccoli Cheese Burst Pizza 222
376. Mozzarella Bean Pizza 223
377. Olive Oil Pizza Dough 223
378. Crispy Pizza Dough 224
379. Thin Crispy Pizza Dough 224
380. Yeast Pizza Dough 225
381. Fresh Sour Cream Pizza Dough 225
382. Fast, Yeast-Free Pizza Dough 226
383. Thin Pizza Dough With Honey 226
384. Pasta (Pizza Dough) 227
385. Pizza Dough Without Yeast In Milk 227
386. Puff Pastry Pizza 228
387. Ideal Pizza Dough (On A Large Baking Sheet) ... 228
388. Vegetable Oil Pizza Dough 229
389. Pizza Dough On Yogurt 229
390. American Pizza Dough Recipe 230
391. Eggplant Pizza 230
392. Mediterranean Whole Wheat Pizza 231
393. Chicken Pizza 231
394. Spinach & Feta Pita Bake 232
395. Beef Pizza 232
396. Shrimp Pizza 233
397. Veggie Pizza 233
398. Watermelon Feta & Balsamic Pizza 234
399. Fruit Pizza 234

#	Recipe	Page
400.	Sprouts Pizza	235
401.	Cheese Pinwheels	235
402.	Ground Meat Pizza	236
403.	Quinoa Flour Pizza	236
404.	Greek Style Bread with Black Olives	237
405.	Turkey Flatbread	237
406.	Pepper Flatbread Bites	238
407.	Artichoke Pizza	238
408.	3-Cheese Pizza	239
409.	Chickpea Pizza	239

POULTRY AND MEAT 240

#	Recipe	Page
410.	Arugula Fig Chicken	240
411.	Parmesan Chicken Gratin	241
412.	Chicken Saute	241
413.	Grilled Marinated Chicken	242
414.	Chicken Fillets with Artichoke Hearts	242
415.	Chicken Loaf	243
416.	Chicken Meatballs with Carrot	243
417.	Chicken Burgers	244
418.	Duck Patties	244
419.	Creamy Chicken Pate	245
420.	Curry Chicken Drumsticks	245
421.	Chicken Enchiladas	246
422.	Chicken Fajitas	246
423.	Chicken Stroganoff	247
424.	European Posole	247
425.	Mango Chicken Salad	248
426.	Chicken Zucchini Boats	248
427.	Urban Chicken Alfredo	249
428.	Tender Chicken Quesadilla	249
429.	Light Caesar	250
430.	Chicken Parm	250
431.	Chicken Bolognese	251
432.	Jerk Chicken	251
433.	Crack Chicken	252
434.	Pomegranate Chicken Thighs	252
435.	Butter Chicken	253
436.	Santa le Skillet Chicken	253
437.	Tender Lamb Chops	254
438.	Smoky Pork & Cabbage	254
439.	Seasoned Pork Chops	255
440.	Beef Stroganoff	255
441.	Lemon Beef	256
442.	Herb Pork Roast	256
443.	Greek Beef Roast	257
444.	Tomato Pork Chops	257
445.	Greek Pork Chops	258
446.	Pork Cacciatore	258
447.	Pork with Tomato & Olives	259
448.	Pork Roast	259
449.	Easy Beef Kofta	260
450.	Lemon Pepper Pork Tenderloin	260
451.	Jalapeno Lamb Patties	261
452.	Basil Parmesan Pork Roast	261
453.	Sun-dried Tomato Chuck Roast	262
454.	Lemon Lamb Leg	262
455.	Lamb Stew	263
456.	Flavorful Beef Stew	263
457.	Herb Ground Beef	264
458.	Olive Feta Beef	264
459.	Italian Beef Casserole	265
460.	Roasted Sirloin Steak	265
461.	Easy Pork Kabobs	266
462.	Meatballs	266
463.	Baked Patties	267
464.	Keto Beef Patties	267
465.	Tender & Juicy Lamb Roast	268
466.	Basil Cheese Pork Roast	268
467.	Feta Lamb Patties	269
468.	BBQ Pulled Chicken	269
469.	Flavorful Lemon Chicken Tacos	270
470.	Crisp Chicken Carnitas	270
471.	Cilantro Lime Chicken Salad	271
472.	Shredded Turkey Breast	271
473.	Delicious Chicken Tenders	272
474.	Grilled Pesto Chicken	272
475.	Easy & Tasty Salsa Chicken	273
476.	Tender Turkey Breast	273
477.	Chicken Bacon Salad	274
478.	Green Salsa Chicken	274
479.	Chicken Chili	275
480.	Tasty Chicken Kabobs	275
481.	Cheesy Salsa Chicken	276
482.	Ranch Chicken Salad	276
483.	Harissa Chicken	277
484.	Almond Cranberry Chicken Salad	277
485.	Simple Baked Chicken Breasts	278

FISH AND SEAFOOD 279

#	Recipe	Page
486.	Baked Cod Fillets with Ghee Sauce	279
487.	Avocado Peach Salsa on Grilled Swordfish	280
488.	Breaded and Spiced Halibut	280
489.	Berries and Grilled Calamari	281
490.	Coconut Salsa on Chipotle Fish Tacos	281
491.	Baked Cod Crusted with Herbs	282
492.	Cajun Garlic Shrimp Noodle Bowl	282
493.	Crazy Saganaki Shrimp	283
494.	Creamy Bacon-Fish Chowder	283
495.	Crisped Coco-Shrimp with Mango Dip	284
496.	Cucumber-Basil Salsa on Halibut Pouches	284
497.	Curry Salmon with Mustard	285
498.	Dijon Mustard and Lime Marinated Shrimp	285
499.	Dill Relish on White Sea Bass	286
500.	Garlic Roasted Shrimp with Zucchini Pasta	286
501.	Easy Seafood French Stew	287

502. Fresh and No-Cook Oysters 287
503. Easy Broiled Lobster Tails 288
504. Ginger Scallion Sauce over Seared Ahi 288
505. Healthy Poached Trout 289
506. Leftover Salmon Salad Power Bowls 289
507. Lemon-Garlic Baked Halibut 290
508. Minty-Cucumber Yogurt Topped Grilled Fish..... 290
509. One-Pot Seafood Chowder 291
510. Orange Rosemary Seared Salmon 291
511. Orange Herbed Sauced White Bass 292
512. Pan Fried Tuna with Herbs and Nut 292
513. Paprika Salmon and Green Beans 293
514. Pecan Crusted Trout 293
515. Pesto and Lemon Halibut 294
516. Red Peppers & Pineapple Topped Mahi-Mahi... 294
517. Roasted Halibut with Banana Relish 295
518. Roasted Pollock Fillet with Bacon and Leeks 295
519. Scallops in Wine 'n Olive Oil 296
520. Seafood Stew Cioppino 296
521. Simple Cod Piccata 297
522. Smoked Trout Tartine 297
523. Steamed Mussels Thai Style 298
524. Tasty Tuna Scaloppine 298
525. Thyme and Lemon on Baked Salmon 299
526. Warm Caper Tapenade on Cod 299
527. Yummy Salmon Panzanella 300
528. Fish and Orzo 300
529. Baked Sea Bass 301
530. Fish and Tomato Sauce 301
531. Halibut and Quinoa Mix 302
532. Lemon and Dates Barramundi 302
533. Fish Cakes 303
534. Catfish Fillets and Rice 303
535. Halibut Pan 304
536. Baked Shrimp Mix 304
537. Shrimp and Lemon Sauce 305
538. Shrimp and Beans Salad 305
539. Pecan Salmon Fillets 306
540. Salmon and Broccoli 306
541. Salmon and Peach Pan 307
542. Tarragon Cod Fillets 307
543. Salmon and Radish Mix 308
544. Smoked Salmon and Watercress Salad... 308
545. Salmon and Corn Salad 309
546. Cod and Mushrooms Mix 309
547. Sesame Shrimp Mix 310
548. Creamy Curry Salmon 310
549. Mahi Mahi and Pomegranate Sauce 311
550. Smoked Salmon and Veggies Mix 311
551. Salmon and Mango Mix 312
552. Salmon and Creamy Endives 312
553. Trout and Tzatziki Sauce 313
554. Parsley Trout and Capers 313
555. Baked Trout and Fennel 314
556. Lemon Rainbow Trout 314
557. Trout and Peppers Mix 315

FRUITS, SWEETS AND DESSERTS 316

558. Banana Shake Bowls 316
559. Cold Lemon Squares 317
560. Blackberry and Apples Cobbler 317
561. Black Tea Cake 318
562. Green Tea and Vanilla Cream 318
563. Figs Pie 319
564. Cherry Cream 319
565. Strawberries Cream 320
566. Apples and Plum Cake 320
567. Cinnamon Chickpeas Cookies 321
568. Cocoa Brownies 321
569. Cardamom Almond Cream 322
570. Banana Cinnamon Cupcakes 322
571. Rhubarb and Apples Cream 323
572. Cranberries and Pears Pie 323
573. Lemon Cream 324
574. Peach Sorbet 324
575. Almond Rice Dessert 325
576. Blueberries Stew 325
577. Mandarin Cream 326
578. Creamy Mint Strawberry Mix 326
579. Vanilla Cake 327
580. Pumpkin Cream 327
581. Chia and Berries Smoothie Bowl 328
582. Minty Coconut Cream 328
583. Watermelon Cream 329
584. Grapes Stew 329
585. Cocoa Sweet Cherry Cream 330
586. Apple Couscous Pudding 330
587. Ricotta Ramekins 331
588. Papaya Cream 331
589. Almonds and Oats Pudding 332
590. Strawberry Sorbet 332
591. Vanilla Apple Pie 333
592. Cinnamon Pears 333
593. Ginger Ice Cream 334
594. Cherry Compote 334
595. Creamy Strawberries 335
596. Chocolate Cups 335
597. Honey Walnut Bars 336
598. Yogurt Parfait 336
599. Raspberry Tart 337
600. Quinoa Energy Bars 337
601. Cinnamon Stuffed Peaches 338
602. Blueberry Muffins 338
603. Lime Grapes and Apples 339
604. Almond Citrus Muffins 339
605. Butter Cookies 340

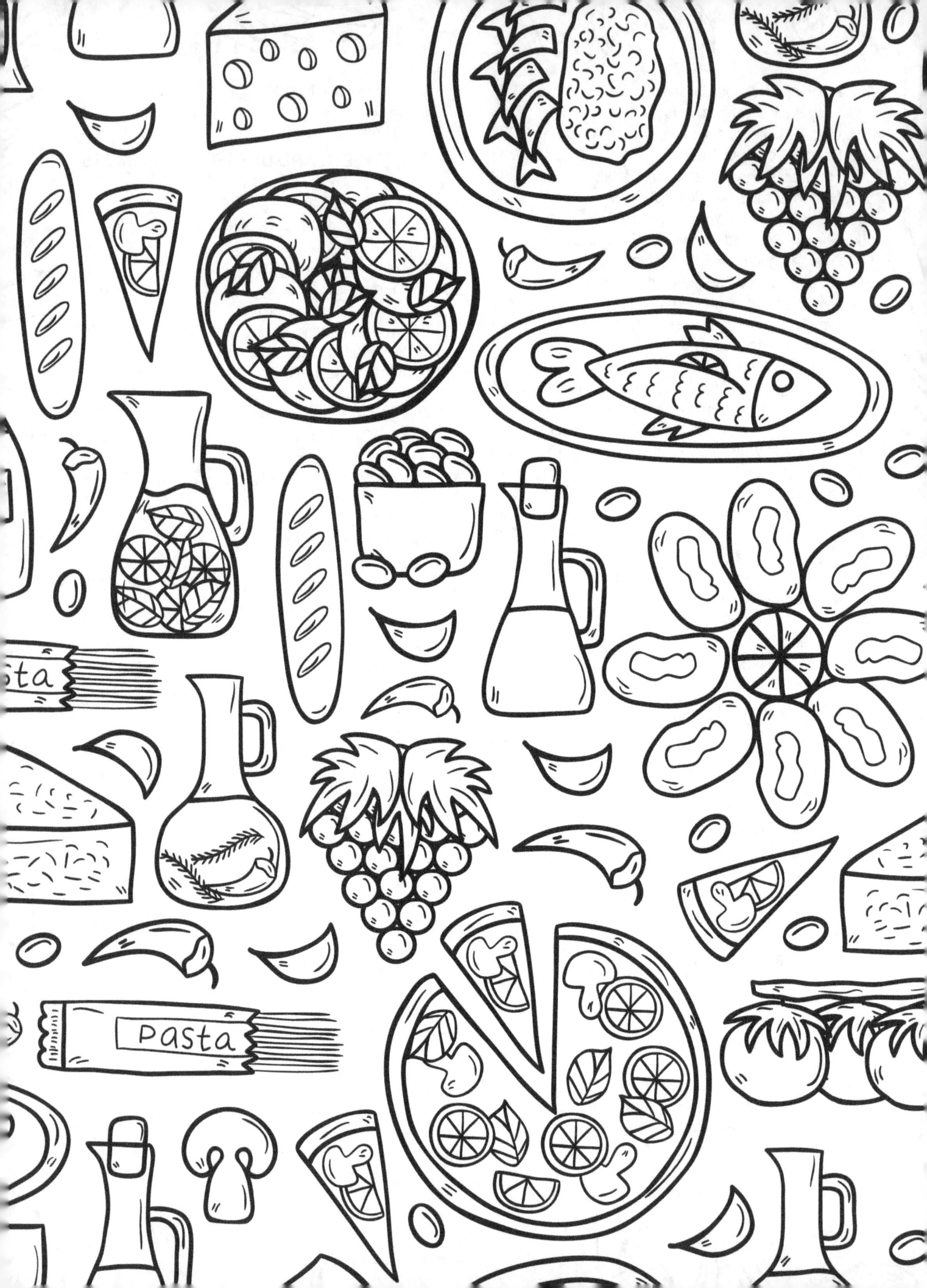

www.ingramcontent.com/pod-product-compliance
Lightning Source LLC
Chambersburg PA
CBHW081343070526
44578CB00005B/702